Wildlife Medicine and Health Management

NIPA GENX ELECTRONIC RESOURCES & SOLUTIONS P. LTD.
New Delhi-110 034

About the Authors

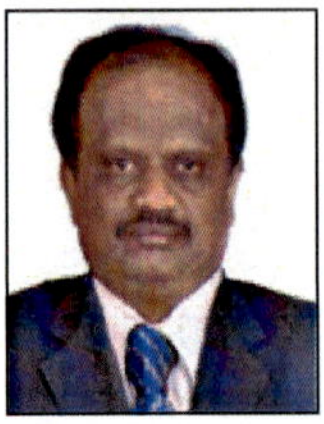

Dr. M.G. Jayathangaraj, published more than 140 research papers in reputed journals related to the field of both wildlife and domestic animal medicine. Guidance was offered for completion of 27 M.V.Sc. degree programmes and 3 Ph.D. research programmes in the field of wildlife science and has received the "Professional Excellence Award" for the outstanding contribution in Wildlife Veterinary Science Education" during the International Congress on Advances in Zoo and Wild Animals Health and Management" at Jammu, India on 26th April, 2007. Completed the Post graduate diploma in wildlife management (9 months duration) at Wildlife Institute of India, Dehradun and was recognised as a "Top Trainee" in this course. Received the Dr. R. Swaminatha Iyer Memorial Prize by Indian Veterinary Journal in the year 1995 for the best clinical article published in the year 1995 and the Professional Excellence Award from AIZ & WV (Association of Indian Zoo & Wildlife Veterinarians) in the year 2008. More than 100 nos. of special assessments and committee works were carried out successfully and as nominee of Central Zoo Authority of India, inspected many zoos, zoological parks etc. As Chairman of Advisory Committee, guided 7 nos. of students for the Post Graduate Diploma in Wild Animal Disease Management. As an Organizing Secretary, conducted an International Conference on "Wildlife Conservation, health and disease management - A Post Millennium Approach" at Madras Veterinary College, Chennai from 03.02.2010 to 05.02.2010. Served as Principal investigator in a project entitled "Development of an Indian Cooperative Wildlife Health Programme and Technical Assistance in Wildlife Institute of India's health project", funded by Wildlife Institute of India in collaboration with US Fish & Wildlife Services from Sept.1995 to Sept. 2001 and in a project entitled "Retrospective survey of diseases in free ranging a captive wild animals", funded by Wildlife Institute of India, from April 2000 to Nov. 2000 and in a project entitled "Strengthening of Madras Veterinary College as Nodal Centre of Wildlife Health and Disease Diagnosis", funded by Central Zoo Authority of India from July, 2002 to March, 2007 and in a project entitled "Health cover to captive wild animals (Prolifically breeding wild animals) maintained at Arignar Anna Zoological Park", funded by Arignar Anna Zoological Park from 17th October, 2007 to 17th October, 2010. He is one of the Recipients of The Murray Fowler International Conference Scholarship in the year 2015. Participated in the Joint Conference of the American Association of Zoo Veterinarians, the Wildlife Disease Association and the American Association of Wildlife Veterinarians in East Lansing, USA from 12-8-95 to 17-8-95. Currently serving as Professor and Head, Dept. of Veterinary Clinical Complex, CoVSc.& AH, Jalukie, CAU.

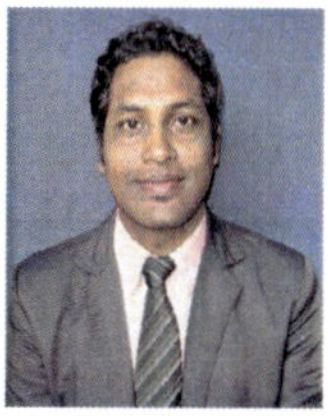

Dr. Gunjan Das, graduated from College of Veterinary Sciences and A.H, Khanapara, Guwahati in 1999 and later on obtained M.V.Sc degree in Veterinary Medicine in 2002 from West Bengal University of Animal & Fishery Sciences, Kolkata and awarded Ph.D in 2007 from prestigious Indian Veterinary Research Institute. He worked as RA (ICMR) in CDC Atlanta project before joining Ph.D programme for a brief period. During his Internship period he has undergone 1 month training at Assam Zoo and got hands on exposure to zoo and wild animal health management and also visited several wildlife sanctuaries and national parks of Assam and other states. He Served as Assistant Professor in the Dept. of Veterinary Preventive Medicine, Faculty of Veterinary Sciences, Sher-e-Kashmir University of Agricultural Sciences & Technology of Kashmir, Shuhama, Srinagar for nearly 2 years (2004-2006) and then joined Central Agricultural University as Assistant Professor in the Department of Veterinary Clinical Medicine, College of Veterinary Sciences & Animal Husbandry, Central Agricultural University, Selesih, Aizawl, Mizoram (2006-2009). On 2009 October he was selected as Associate professor in the same establishment. Have Experience of over 18 years in the field of Veterinary medicine (Teaching, Research and Extension), have guided 5 M.V.Sc Students as Major Advisor (Veterinary Clinical Medicine) and acted as Co-guide for sixteen M.V.Sc. Students. He has also guided two Ph.D. students as Co-guide. He has handled 3 DBT-funded project as PI and associated with 3 DBT-funded and one ICAR-funded projects as Co-PI. Published more than 80 research papers in national and international peer reviewed journal. Published an article on Conservation of wildlife resources of India in Livestock International. Attended advance Short Training course (21 days) on "Newer concepts and techniques in molecular and patho-anatomical diagnosis of farm animals, poultry, wildlife and laboratory animal diseases" Organized by Division of Pathology, IVRI, Izatnagar, U.P., from 01-10-2010 to 21-10-2010. Got Best Poster presentation award Under the Theme "Environment and Wildlife Health" and Session-3 at XVII Annual Conference of Indian Association of Veterinary Public Health Specialists (IAVPHS) on "One Health Concept: Opportunities and Perspectives in Present Scenario" held at GADVASU, Ludhiana, Punjab, India, during 28th to 29th May'2021. Taught courses on Zoo/Wild Animal breeding, management, nutrition and health care VMD-512 (1+1=2) and recently teaching Zoo and Wild Animal Medicine Unit III (4+1) and also prepared Practical manual for the same. Presently working as Professor & Head, Department of Veterinary, College of Veterinary Sciences & Animal Husbandry, Central Agricultural University, Jalukie, Peren, Nagaland.

Wildlife Medicine and Health Management

M.G. Jayathangaraj
Professor and Head
Department of Veterinary Clinical Complex
College of Veterinary Sciences & Animal Husbandry
Central Agricultural University
Jalukie, Peren, Nagaland

Gunjan Das
Professor & Head
Department of Veterinary Medicine
College of Veterinary Sciences & Animal Husbandry
Central Agricultural University
Jalukie, Peren, Nagaland

NIPA GENX ELECTRONIC RESOURCES & SOLUTIONS P. LTD.
New Delhi-110 034

NIPA GENX ELECTRONIC
RESOURCES & SOLUTIONS P. LTD.

101, 103, Vikas Surya Plaza, CU Block
L.S.C.Market, Pitam Pura, New Delhi-110 034
Ph : +91 11 27341616, 27341717, 27341718
E-mail: newindiapublishingagency@gmail.com
www: www.nipabooks.com

For customer assistance, please contact
Phone: + 91-11-27 34 17 17
Fax: + 91-11-27 34 16 16
E-Mail: feedbacks@nipabooks.com

ISBN: 978-93-94490-53-6

Composed and Designed by NIPA.

केन्द्रीय कृषि विश्वविद्यालय
लम्फेलपात, इम्फाल–795004, मणिपुर (भारत)

CENTRAL AGRICULTURAL UNIVERSITY
Lamphelat, Imphal-795004, Manipur (India)
Tel. : (0385) 2415933 (O)
Fax : (0385) 241041
Email : vcofficecau@yahoo.in

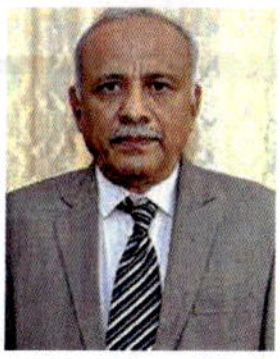

Dr. Anupam Mishra
Vice-Chancellor

No. SVC/CAU/182/2022/
Imphal, the 11th February, 2022

Foreword

It is a pleasure to give foreword of the book entitled "Wildlife Medicine and Health Management" written with a motive of creating awareness on the conservation of various wild fauna of this country. No doubt that globally much attention is being paid towards the protection of wild animals that are encountered by the common people in captivity as well as in free ranging regions.

It is a fact that India is one of the 17 mega diversities existing in this world and is a home to accommodate about 7.6% of all mammals, 12.6% of birds, 6.2% of reptiles and 6.0% of flowering plant species. The country also accommodates some of the most biodiverse regions on the planet and it comprises of four of 35 biodiversity hotspots of the world like the Western Ghats, the Eastern Himalayas, Indo-Burma and Nicobar Islands. Hence, it becomes a need to pay additional attention towards conservation esp. the management of health and diseases in wild fauna of this country.

One of the admirable features in this book under release is that primarily it will satisfy the requirements of student-community at large in various veterinary colleges of this nation, with regard to the MSV-Regulations 2016. In this perspective, this book is a highly welcome one in the current scenery. Minimizing the probable struggles in getting the right kinds of the technical information pertaining to the health and disease management of various species of wild animals that include mammals, reptiles, aves etc., this book has duly catered to the aspirations of the veterinary students towards the technical information with regard to the health and the disease management related features, expected for the welfare of wild animals.

Various features of wild animals like the general taxonomical classification, maintenance of zoo hygiene, public health aspects and preventive measures with control of multiple diseases in wild animals have been dealt in this book. Another interesting feature is that it includes significance of biological features of important wild animals as well as different restraint procedures comprising physical and chemical immobilization of various species of wild animals.

Since elephants are being considered as one of the star species of wild fauna of this nation, emphasis has also been laid on the specific features of elephants, diseases and health management features in these pachyderms.

No doubt that all these measures will be of highly useful towards a better scientific management of various species of wild animals that are encountered in multiple zoos, zoological parks, zoological gardens etc., in addition to the various protected wildlife regions of this country like wildlife sanctuaries, national parks, biospheres, tiger reserves, elephant reserves etc. The procedures related to collection of samples, significance of vetero-legal issues and handling procedures in wild animals etc. have also been incorporated.

Let me sincerely appreciate the authors towards preparation of this book for catering to the wildlifers, scientists and esp. the veterinary students, pursuing their under-graduate degree in veterinary sciences and animal husbandry.

Anupam Mishra

Prof. Arun Kumar Sangwan
Dean
CoVSc. & AH., CAU, Jalukie, Nagaland

Foreword

As healthcare and disease management of wildlife is an essential feature and due attention needs to be paid to this important aspect in order to have scientific management in captive animal places as well as in the free ranging wildlife regions. In this perspective, the book entitled "Wildlife Medicine and Health Management" has been prepared.

The veterinary students pursuing the undergraduate degree in various veterinary colleges will get immensely benefited by this book aimed at catering to the syllabus pertaining to the wildlife health and disease management as per the MSVE-2016. Before treating or performing post-mortem of the wild animals that includes various species of wild mammals, reptiles and birds, it is prerequisite to know in details about the species of wild animal. The biology of the significant species of wild animals also has been dealt in order to assist the understanding of the life-style of different wild animals, in addition to the sampling procedures to be adapted by the veterinarians.

Various illustrations whenever required have been duly furnished by the authors with regard to the enhancement of knowledge about the health and disease management. Special features in reptiles are also dealt. Hence, though the primary purpose of this book is to cater to the syllabus laid by Veterinary Council of India, wildlife veterinarians can obtain technical information in various features of wildlife health and diseases.

The excellent contribution done, in the form of this book is highly appreciable. I am confident the book will be useful to the veterinary students as well as the veterinarians who are dealing with wildlife health and disease management in captive as well as in free ranging wildlife regions of this country.

-Sd-
Prof. Arun Kumar Sangwan

Preface

The book with a title of "Wildlife Medicine and Health Management" has been prepared primarily with an idea of satisfying the criteria of the wildlife related syllabus for the veterinary students undertaking their degree programme in various veterinary institutions of this country. However, this book has additional information with regard to the catering of wildlife veterinarians serving in various zoos or wildlife regions of this country as well as in other countries.

Different photographs pertaining to the health and disease management in wild fauna have been duly presented in places where they are required and the requirements pertaining to carrying out the therapeutic approaches in wild animals are also concurrently presented. Understanding about the various species of wild animals is the basis for exercising the wildlife medicine at any zoo or zoological park or zoological garden.

In this manner, this book has incorporations with regard to the identification of various parasitic fauna in captive wild animals. Various features pertaining to the captive breeding of wild animals, housing and feeding are being dealt in this book, carefully. To name the few special information, the technical features with regard to the management of health and diseases in elephants, reptilian features and clinical examination procedures to be adapted with regard to the aviary species have also been incorporated in this book.

Gadgets with regard to the physical as well as the chemical restraint of wild animals that are frequently encountered by the veterinarians in the field condition are also detailed elaborately, in addition to the dose rates of various drugs useful for the chemical control of wild animals. Different sampling procedures including the ones in crocodiles and elephants are presented in a good manner, so that the readers esp. the veterinary students doing their undergraduate degree in veterinary sciences and animal husbandry can understand about this subject in a clarified manner.

We hope that is book might be an eye opener with regard to the obtaining of good information about the wildlife health and disease management.

M.G. Jayathangaraj
Gunjan Das

Contents

1

Taxonomical Classification of Wild Fauna

It is crystal clear that India is one of the 12 mega biodiversity countries in the world. The country has been divided into 10 biogeographic regions. In our country, the diverse physical features and climatic situations have formed ecological habitats like forests, grasslands, wetlands, coastal and marine ecosystems and desert ecosystems, which harbor and sustain immense biodiversity. Many institutions including NGOs help the government towards the framing of different policies and designing of various strategies, thus favoring solutions that address wildlife conservation issues in today's changing circumstances, like wildlife conflict related problems which are highly emerging in these current periods at various parts of the world including our country.

In understanding about various species of wild fauna, the different grouping of wild fauna are given below for a quick-understanding and the conservation measures during the therapeutic or surgical or obstetrical management, the attempts often depend on the effective understanding about the various groups of wild fauna and their biologic features in a systematic manner.

Edentata

This group comprises armadillos, sloths, Anteaters like Giant anteater.

Proboscidea

- Asiatic elephant (*Elephas maximus*) and African elephants are grouped under this category.
- There are four sub-species in the Asiatic elephants (Indian, Ceylon, Sumatran and Malaysian)

Lagomorpha

This group comprises small to moderate sized animals like rabbit, hare and pikas.

Insectivora

This group comprises hedgehogs, true shrews, elephant shrews, true moles etc.

Primates

- This group comprises old world monkeys, new world monkeys, apes (Only ape in India is Hyalobates hoolock) etc.
- MACAQUES (Bonnet macaque, Rhesus macaque, Lion tailed macaque, Assamese macaque, Pig tailed macaque, Stump tailed macaque etc.)
- LANGURS (Common langur,Nilgiri langur,Golden langur,Leaf monkey or capped langur)
- APES (Lesser apes comprise Hoolock gibbon in India and Greater apes comprise Orang-utan, Chimpanzee and Gorilla)
- LORISES (Slender loris and Slow loris are the examples under this group)

Chiroptera

Microchiroptera

- Small insectivorous bats like Desmodus and Rhindophus are grouped in this category. These mammals hang in tree branches or crevices with their head down.

Macrochiroptera

- This order contains large sized bats like fruit bats or fruit eating bats which are commonly called as the flying foxes.

Rodentia

The animals under this group are squirrels, gerbils, rats, porcupines, bandicoots, beavers etc.

Hyracoidea

This order contains small rabbit like mammals i.e. hyraxes that but have reduced tail in addition to the presence of short ears.

Tubelidentata

This order comprises Aardvark which is the only representative of this order

Pholidota

This order comprises nocturnal animals eg. Scaly anteaters or Pangolins (Indian and Chinese Pangolins).

Carnivora

Felids (lion, tiger, cheetah, leopard, snow leopard, clouded leopard, jungle cat, golden cat, desert cat etc.), Canids(jackals, foxes, wolves and wild dogs),

Ursids(slothy bear, Himalayan black bear, Himalayan brown bear etc.), Mustelids(Otter, weasels, badgers,martens etc), Red Panda, Giant Panda, Hyaena, Mongoose, Civets etc. come under the carnivora order.

Perissiodactylids (Old toed)

Asiatic wild ass, Tibetian wild ass, Great one horned rhinoceros, tapirs and wild horses fall under this group.

Artiodactylids (Even toed)

This group comprises bovids (gaur, wild buffaloe, Himalayan tahr, Nilgiri tahr, antelopes like black buck, nilgai, four horned antelope and gazelle or chinkara etc.), suids (Indian wild boar) and cervids (Deer like spotted deer, swamp deer, hog deer, musk deer, mouse deer, barking deer, Barasingha etc.)

Dermopetra

Flying or gliding lemur which is also called as the Colugo comes under this order

Monotremata

The monotremes comprise echidnas and the platypus.

Marsupialia

These orders of wild mammals are large in numbers and kangaroos, honey possum, wombats, Tasmanian devil etc. fall under this group.

Cetacea

The animals of this order belong to marine mammals group. The cetaceans comprise whales, porpoises and dolphins.

Pinnipedia

The animals of this order also belong to marine mammals group. The pinnipes comprise seals, sea lions and walruses.

Sirenia

The animals of this order also belong to marine mammals group. This order comprises dugongs and manatees.

2

Biology of Important Wild Animal Species

Biology of deer

- Deer are true ruminants.
- The unique anatomical characteristic feature of cervids is antlers. Only two species of deer, the musk deer and Chinese water deer lack antlers. The reindeer is the only species in which the female has the antler.
- There is no gall bladder except in musk deer
- There are rudimentary large digits on each foot
- Scent glands: Deer utilize scent glands for territorial and hierarchical interaction. Most species have preorbital glands along with inter-digital glands
- Mammary gland – four nipples are present

Biology of felids and canids

Except lions, the tigers like other felids are highly solitary and however, during the breeding period, the males will approach the female for mating activity. Tigers are highly territorial in nature. Like other felids, retractile claws are present in felid which is an anatomically peculiar feature. They are crepuscular in nature and however, they are quite active in the morning hours.

Longevity of tiger is 12-19 years. Sexual maturity for males is 4 years and in case of females, it is 3 years. In general, the age of maturity for tigers is 3 to 5 years of age. Females are polyoestrus in nature all the year. Duration of heat is 3-10 days and average is 7.1 day. Duration and frequency of copulation is 0.5 to 3 minutes, with an average of 2 minutes. Frequency of copulation is 3-23 daily, for 3 to 21 days. Gestation period is about 98 to 110 days and majorityare born between October to November, in general. Litter size is about 1 to 6 with an average of 2 to 3.Weaning age is about 3 to 5 month

The weight of lion ranges from 180 to 225 Kg. Males are larger in size. Their feed consists of prey as large as elephants esp. the elephant calves, hyenas, hippos, rhinos, etc to something as small as lizard and mice. Lions feed mainly on hoofed wild animals like Gaur, Nilgai, spotted deer, Sambar, Wild pigs etc. Females are the prime hunters in the group but the males are the ones that eat the prey first despite the females usually catching it. It can take up to four hours to finish feeding.

Lions live in groups always. When males join a pride, they usually kill other cubs. Males defend their territory. Lions can be extremely aggressive. They are diurnal in nature but sometimes; engage in hunting in night hours also. Longevity of lions is about 15-30 years. A lion is in prime when it is about 5 years old. Females are polyoestrus in nature. Duration of heat is 4-16 days. Duration and frequency of copulation is 21 seconds and in general, number of copulations per day may be about 60 to 70 times. Period of gestation is about 116 days.

In the Gir forests of Junagadh district covering 1280 square kms of rugged area, the roars of lions are frequently heard throughout the night period and in the Gir may lions mate between October and November and the young one is produced at intervals of at least 18 months to 2 years. Litter size is about 1 to 6, with an average of 2 to 3. Females rearing young ones generally don't exhibit oestrus for several months and conceptions usually do not recur until the cubs become 19-23 months old. Weaning age is about 3 months or longer, in general.

Panthers are also called as leopards (*Panthera pardus)* and is the smallest of the four "big cats,". Each spot on a leopard is unique—similar to the fingerprints of humans. These spots are also called as Rosettes. Average body weight is about 50 Kg in case of females and in case of males, it is about 68 Kg. However, most of the times, they weigh about 52 Kg.Panthers eat mainly small and medium sized mammals. When unable to eat as single meal, it hauls up into a tree for storage in order to make feeding activity later (hoarding character).

Panthers feed in general on cervids like deer, non-human primates like bonnet macaques, rhesus macaques, rodents, aviary species like peafowls, porcupines etc. In period of hunger, the panthers may tend to eat anything like fowl, reptiles etc. including the carrion. These are arboreal in nature. They are adaptable to varied conditions in forest, unlike tiger or lions. These animals are cunning in nature and may become man-eaters at times and are notable for lifting of sheep, goat, dog and children sometimes, from the nearby villages. Longevity of panther is 12-17 years

Female produces the first litter when it is about 2.5 to 4 years of age. Females are polyoestrus in nature all the year and peak births occur in April in India. Duration of heat is 3-14 days and average is 6-9 days. Gestation period is about 87 to 94 days. Litter size is about 1 to 5, with an average of 2. They will stay with their mother for 18 to 24 months. Weaning age is about 4 months

Biology of fruit bats

- The suborder-*Microchiroptera*(Smaller insectivorous bats) has more than15 families but the suborder-*Megachiroptera*has one family, that comprises of Flying-foxes ie) Fruit bats, tubenosed bats and blossom bats.

Difference between mega bats and micro bats

- Megachiropterans : Rely on vision to orient in the dark of night, and thus have large, prominent eyes but ears are small.
- Hibernation is a common feature of Microchiropterans until insects become more abundant (unlike megabats).
- Megabats have claws on the second digits supporting their wings (with one exception); this is never the case in microbats.
- Microbats often have dentition or cheek teeth whose morphology can easily be related to dilambdodontteeth; (lambda shaped) but the megabats have simplified cheek teeth that are difficult to interpret.
- No echolocation feature is encountered in megabats like Fruit bats (unlike microbats) but have large eyes & small ears.Echolocation is a feature of microchiropteransie) microbats; locate and catch prey such as insects in midair and have large, complex pinnae-external ears, including an enlarged tragus or antitragus and small eyes.
- The patagium is the wing membrane; it is stretched between the arm and finger bones, and down the side of the body to the hind limbs and tail, in fruit bats.
- Upon their return, mothers and their respective infants can identify each other by their vocalizations and scent, and thus can successfully reunite. Scent marks and pheromones are also important in bats, as they are in other mammals.
- **Life span**: 30 years in the wild.

Body weight

- Smallest bat: The microchiropteran-Craseonycteristhonglongyai (2-3 grams)
- Largest bats may weigh about 1.5 Kg.
- All species of flying foxes feed mainly or only on nectar, blossoms, pollen, and fruit (A few species may on occasion take insects, located visually by the flying fox).
- The range of distance covered by Fruit bats: 3 to 166 Kms.
- Flying-foxes are placental mammals.

- The gestation period is approximately 7months.Females generally give birth to 1-2 pups per litter, but in some species in the genus Lasiurus, litter may reach 3 or 4 pups (e.g. Lasiurus borealis, L.seminolus, and L.cinereus). At birth, newborn bats(pups) weigh between 10 and 30% of their mother's weight, putting a large energetic strain on pregnant females and pups are born with fur and open eyes. From birth until 5-6 weeks old, the baby does not have the ability to control its own body temperature and hence, cling to its mother (Altricialin nature).
- A large number of bats breed seasonally (The function of seasonal breeding is to coordinate reproduction with the availability of resources to support newborn young.Many species have also evolved complex reproductive physiology including delayed ovulation, sperm storage, delayed fertilization, delayed implantation, and embryonic diapause).
- All species that are not seasonal breeders (occur in the tropics, where resources may not be as variable as in temperate regions).
- Temperate species often breed before they enter hibernation (only microbats hibernate) while many tropical species breed in a cycle that is linked to wet-dry seasonality.
- Many bats live in groups or colonies.
- Guano (excreta of bats) contains N,K,PO_4, which helps plant, root and flower health and growth.
- **Orchard-damage by Fruit bats:** Though they assist pollination to a greater extent, they damage fruits earning enemiy among agricultural communities.

The Fruit bats are placed in Vermin category as per WILDLIFE PROTECTION ACT, 1972 and as LC (Least Concern) category in IUCN red data list.

Biology of asiatic elephants

Elephants are gregarious in nature and have a matriarchy type of living led by the eldest female in the group.

Free ranging wild elephants consume about 270-320 Kg feed materials in a day and will be spending almost 18 hours a day in foraging and is migratory in nature generally.

Drinks about 200-250 litres of water per day; about 50-60 litres of water at a time can be consumed by these animals and a trunk can retain 7-8 liters or even as much as 10 liters of water.

Habitat in general

Mixed deciduous and evergreen forests scrub & grass lands. Movements are in generally near the water resources in forest regions.

Other significant data on asiatic elephants

- Range of body weight in adults in kg: 3700-4500
- Number of chromosomes is 56
- Age of maturity for female elephants is about as early as six years of age
- Age of maturity for male elephants is about nine or ten years of age
- Oestrus cycle is about 18-27 days and oestrus lasts for about 3-4 days
- Gestation period is 20-22 months.
- Weight of the new born elephant calf in Kg : 90-110
- Time taken to be up on its legs after the birth by the new born elephant calf is generally 5-10 minutes
- Calves are milk dependent for the first two years and may often suckle up to the age of four to five years
- The calf should gain the body weight of about 0.5 to 1.4 Kg per day, averaging 0.9 Kg weight as th weight gain on daily basis, during the first year of life
- Period for weaning is 2 years
- Walking speed is 4 km /hour.
- Running speed is 25 /km/hour for a short distance (or) 30-40 km/hr. (even with hobbles they can hop very fast but cannot jump or gallop or run like cattle)
- Able to swim and loves wallowing
- Continuous growth of tusk may be seen, even subsequent to the trimming or cutting of tusks due to management related causes
- Eye sight is very poor
- Smell and hearing capacity are the significant ones
- Longevity is generally 65-75 years
- Lives in herd with matriarchy as the social system.

Biology of wildpigs

- **Wild boars and domesticated pigs are the same species** (They can interbreed and produce viable offspring). Physically, domesticated pigs are fatter and have a shorter snout than their cousins. However, feral pigs that descended from escaped domesticated pigs develop long snouts and sleek bodies like wild boars.

- Wild pigs form the important **prey base** for wild carnivores in forests and are also considered as **pests** by farming community due to the damage to their crops, in the agricultural fields, esp. during the harvesting periods.
- **Wild boars are found throughout Asia (including throughout India) and Europe**, particularly in primary and secondary forests and along the edges of agricultural areas (Generally, the Asian wild boars are smaller than their Eurasian cousins. They average around 100 kilograms and some weigh only weigh around 50 kilograms; by contrast, Siberian boars can reach up to 300 kilograms in body weight).
- Wild boars usually live in groups of between 6 and 20 individuals, although large herds of around 100 have been seen.
- **Habitat of wild pigs**
  - Wild Pigs can live almost anywhere.
  - Habitat generalists.
  - Highly adaptable.
  - Can live in many different habitats.
  - Can tolerate a wide range of climates.
  - Can live as far away as a day's walk from water.
- Wild pigs have two sets of tusks and the more fearsome set, on the upper jaw, is used primarily to push through the thorn-bush (The upper tusks are sometimes called whetters) and the sharper, small tusks are on the lower jaw and are used in defense against attackers and in fights against other wild pigs. The tusks grow as long as a wild pig lives. Both the boars and the sows have tusks.
- Wild pigs are good swimmers and they often snort when they swim.
- Foraging nature:Wild pigs are opportunistic omnivores and generally feed on vegetation but will eat small mammals, new-borns of larger mammals, and eggs and young of ground-nesting birds and reptiles. TheWild boars forage primarily at night. During the day they spend most of their time hiding in dense thickets. The presence of wild boars can be ascertained in the forest regions by the following features:

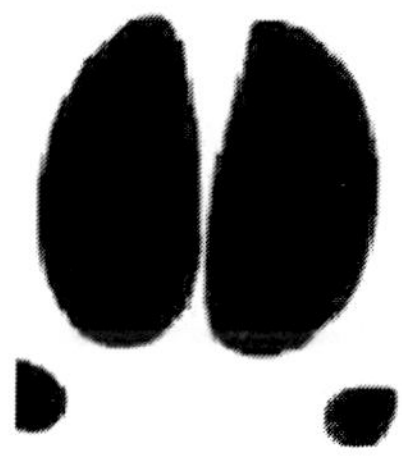

- **Foot prints (four toe prints of wild pigs)** of wild pigs shall be found out on ground esp. on wet areas.
- **Rooting signs** in the land (overturning of grassland to grub for worms & insects and dug out areas in vegetations-tubers, carrots, groundnut etc.)
- **Trees with signs of peeling of bark** at bottom of tree above earth (this is due to get rid off the external parasites and itching), coupled with **signs of dried mud sticking at the bottom of the trees**
- Presence of **wallow (marshy areas)** near the suspected signs of wild pig-existence.
- A characteristic **arch shape is left by the wild boar in the fence** above ground where they have breached stock fencing.
- **Hair of wild boar** is found snagged on barbed wire (the long guard hairs can be seen, with a clump of thicker underhair).
- Presence of **faecal pellets**
- Presence of **nests** (with dried leaves, broken stems, plants etc.)
- **History of sighting** of wild pigs in the concerned regions which often are located near the periphery of forest regions.

Breeding in wild swines

Highly prolific in breeding. Gestation period is 114 days & the sows reach sexual maturity at age one and can farrow twice a year and litter size is 4 to 10 piglets, at one time. According to the Guinness Book of Records, the world's largest pig litter contained 37 piglets and the breeding season lasts for about month. Females are only fertile for four days and males follow female until the female allows mating which takes about 8 minutes. Males release a large amount of sperm & then the male follows the female around to make sure the female doesn't mate with another wild pig. After mating, females remain with their drift for about 4 months and then retire to give birth alone in a cave, a den of another animal, an abandoned building or leaf-lined holes in the ground. Mother wild pigs are always hungry as they divide time between eating and taking take care of their

Crop damage due to wild boar attacks has increased considerably in the last few years, especially in Dharmapuri, Tirunelveli, Virudhunagar and Perambalur districts of Tamil Nadu state and in many agricultural regions in India that are adjoining the protected wildlife areas and in the year 2012-13, about 290 cases of crop damage were reported and is almost on rise in recent years, in most of the regions.

BIOLOGY OF BEARS (SYN: URSIDS)

Bears belong to ursidae family

There are four species of bears found in India, Bears family of India includes Sloth bear, Asiatic Black bears (Syn: Moon bear), Himalayan brown bear and Sun bear. In India The Black bear and the Brown bear are found in the Himalayan ranges whereas the Sloth bear is found all over the peninsular India. The Brown bear is known to live in the higher reaches of the Himalayas whereas the Black Bear inhabits the forests of lower Himalayan range.

In general, there are eight species in the world and they comprise the. Asiatic black bears, brown bears (which include grizzly bears), giant pandas, North American black bears, polar bears, sloth bears, spectacled bears (Syn: Andean bears), and sun bears. The Sun bear (***Helarctos malayanus***) is a species in the family Ursidae occurring in the tropical forests of Southeast Asia. Sun bear is the smallest bear, standing nearly 70 centimetres (28 inches) at the shoulder and weighing 25-65 kilograms. On average, bears can live up to 25 years in the wild and 50 in captivity.

The Himalayan brown bear is one of the largest carnivores in the highlands of Himalayas. It occupies the higher reaches of the Himalayas in remote, mountainous areas of Pakistan and India, in small and isolated populations, and is extremely rare in many of its ranges. The Himalayan brown bear, also known as the Himalayan red bear, isabelline bear (or) Dzu-Teh, is a subspecies of the brown bear and is known esp. the from northern Afghanistan, northern Pakistan, northern India, west China and Nepal. In India, brown bears are present in 23 protected areas in the northern states of Jammu and Kashmir, Himachal Pradesh, and Uttaranchal, but only in two of these the bears are regarded as fairly common. There are likely less than 1,000 bears, and possibly half that in India and they weigh from 55 to 95 kg. They are capable of galloping faster than a person can run.

Sloth bears (*Melursus ursinus*) live in a variety of dry and moist forests and in some tall grassland, where boulders, scattered shrubs and trees provide shelter. It is a nocturnal animal. Their range includes India, Sri Lanka and southern Nepal. The *sloth bear* is a bear species native to the Indian subcontinent. It feeds on fruits also in addition to the ants and termites. They rarely feed on carrion. Hence, it is often grouped as an omnivore, like the case with non-human primates.

Sltoh bears have also been called "labiated bears" because of their long lower lip and palate used for sucking insects. Their long lower lips can be stretched over the outer edge of their noses, and lack upper incisors, thus allowing the bears to suck up large numbers of insects. Sloth bears have a long, shaggy fur, a mane around the face, and long, sickle-shaped claws. Their fur is completely black mostly and in some, it is rusty.

Sloth bear, (*Melursus ursinus*), also called **honey bear,** Hindi **bhalu,** forest-dwelling member of the family Ursidae that inhabits tropical or subtropical regions of India. Sloth bears mainly live in tropical areas including the Sri Lanka. Named for its slow-moving habits, the sloth bear has poor senses of sight and hearing but has a good sense of smell. Various adaptations actually equip this animal for raiding insect colonies. With long, curved front claws (extending from large paws), it digs toward and rips open a nest of bees or termites. Inserting its long snout into the nest and closing its nostrils (thereby preventing entry of insects into its respiratory passages), the sloth bear opens its protrusible lips and sucks in the insects through the gap caused by the lack of central upper incisors. Supplements to this diet include fruit, honey, grains, and small vertebrates. Sloth bears are myrmecophagous, meaning that they specialize in eating termites and ants.

Sloth bears have a light "U" (or) "Y" shaped patch on their chest.

It is listed as Vulnerable on the IUCN Red List, mainly because of habitat loss and degradation. Historically, humans have drastically reduced these bears' habitat and diminished their population by hunting them for food and products such as their bacula, skin, bile, teeth and even the claws

Sloth bear is a small bear species characterized by having a long lower lip and palate for sucking insects.

Bears, however, lack the physiological characteristics (lower heart rate, body temperature, breathing rate, and blood pressure) exhibited by animals that truly hibernate, as the case with American and Asiatic black bears.

Gestation periods vary, the fertilized egg remaining dormant in the uterus (delayed implantation), which ensures the birth of young while the female is in the winter den and guarantees that the cubs will emerge from the den in the spring, when food is abundant. Ursids breed once per year at most, and many bears breed only every two to four years.

Biology of wild dog (*Cuon alpinus)*

Wild dog *(***Syn: Dhole)** is an **opportunistic feeder** and eats fruit, insects, lizards and hunt medium sized mammals like spotted deer, rodents etc. and they may hunt from small rodent to large deer size, including hares, wild boar, various ruminants, antelopes, gaur and even monkeys.

Though they are not fast runners, they are capable of pursuing the prey species for long distances until the prey species get exhausted. They communicate by making whistling like sounds and often they hunt in packs.

In silence, they follow the prey species and attack in groups (communal hunting) with more aggressions. Usually hunt by day though sometimes hunt by night. When hunting as a pack it can subdue prey over 10 times its own body weight, and can even fend off a tiger! Longevity of wild dog is about 15 years in captivity. The main breeding season for wild dogs in India is between November and December. Gestation period is about 60-62 days. Litter size is about 2-5.

Biology of jackals

Jackals are omnivores and scavenge from kills made by larger animals, and will also eat insects, plant materials (Jackals raid on melon patches as well as sugarcane fields and may even go for the fallen fruits of ber trees etc.) and carrion. They are nocturnal in nature. Jackals are secretive in habits, in general. They are however, in hot days; they come out even in day time. Jackals inhabit crevices in rocks and dens made by other animals and are in order to keep the jackals cool while they sleep. These animals are territorial in nature.

Jackals have no hesitation in defending their marked territory. The main breeding season for jackals in India is between November and December. The golden jackal's courtship rituals are remarkably long, lasting for 26–28 days. Gestation period is about 57-70 days.Many female golden jackals usually give birth in burrows. Litter size is about 2-7 pups. Pups are born blind and the pups get their sight in about 8-11 days. Longevity of jackals is about 10-12 years.

Biology of Hyaena

Primarily hyaenas are scavengers. These animals are particularly bone-eaters. Copulation lasts an average of 10 minutes. Gestation period is about 98 days in striped hyaena and 110 days in case of spotted hyaena and 90 days in case of Brown hyaena. Litter size is about 2-4 cubs. Spotted hyena cubs are born with their eyes open.

Biology of Giraffe

Giraffe is an African even-toed ungulate mammal and is the tallest living terrestrial animal and the largest ruminant (Camelids are pseudo-ruminants ie. omasum is absent in them). Both male and female giraffes have two distinct, hair-covered horns called ossicones.

Cervical vertebrae are seven in nos. like most of the mammals. Male giraffes use their horns to sometimes fight with other males. Both male and female giraffe have 'horns' already at birth. A giraffe's neck is too short to reach the ground. Blood pressure related valves are significant in giraffe and the heart weighs approx. 11 kg and is the biggest of any land mammal. It is used to pump

60 litres of blood around its body every minute at a blood pressure twice that of an average human.

Pregnancy periods in wild animals

Chimpanzee	227 days
Gorilla	257 days
Orangutan	260 days
Baboon	187 days
Bonnet macaque	168 days
Rhesus macaque	164 days
Pattas monkey	167 days
Elephant	660 days
Gaur	270 days
Llama	330 days
Sloth bear	210 days
Leopard	94 days
Lion	108 days
Tiger	105 days
Spotted deer	227 days
Black buck	167 days
Sambar deer	246 days
Barasingha	245 days
Jackal	60 days
Bengal Fox	52 days
Wolf	64 days
Striped hyaena	90 days
Camel / Giraffe	450 days
Rhinoceros	465 days
Hippopotamus	243 days

3

Principles of Zoo Hygiene Public Health Problems Arising from Zoos

Poor hygiene leads to occurrence of diseases and disorders among various captive wild animal species in zoos.

Important associated factors in zoo hygiene

- Usage of suitable disinfectant (natural or synthetic)
- Proper disposal of carcass.
- Speedy disposal of feed wastes.
- Supply of hygienic water.
- Animal keepers and handlers - hygiene.
- Bush clearance (vector control).
- Disposal of polythene bags.
- White washing of water containers and walls and feeding tanks in a periodical manner.
- Adaptation of suitable fly control measures (fly catcher lights) esp. in fed–receiving spots or stores room.
- Speedy clearance of sheds/ cages after the occurrence of diarrheic stools/ after the conducting of operation.
- Strengthening of rodent or pest proof barriers (Vermin control) or cages or fences esp. in aviaries or bird-exhibit places to avoid diseases.
- Usage of aseptic infrastructures like sterilized needles, syringes, sample-collecting containers etc.
- Laboratory should be a clean one without giving chances for any types of infections.

Sanitation measures related to the Anthrax -carcass disposal

- **Glutaraldehyde** shall be chosen for the disinfections processes after the disposal of the carcass, subsequent to the post- mortem (however, it is carcinogenic in nature).
- Anthrax affected carcass or suspected carcass should not be opened and the burial should be carried out atleast with 2 metre-depth, with a sample spread-over of quicklime ($CaCO_3$). It may be better to bury the carcass, together with the bedding and soil contaminated with discharge. If spore formation occurs (within few hours of exposure to air), strong-disinfectants may be used like Lysol (this should be in contact with spores for atleast 2days) or strong solution of formalin (or) 5 to 10% of NaOH. Incinerator shall be good for disposal of the animal carcass affected by anthrax disease.

Sanitation related to "Wastes"

Waste-materials of Zoos have been listed below

- Animal faeces from multiple spp of wild animals
- Animal carcasses
- Used animal bedding
- Straw and other materials from animal enclosures
- Food waste, including fruits, vegetables and bones
- Veterinary and medical waste
- Waste materials from cage/door/exhibit/office repairs and maintenance
- Waste from visitors to your zoo

Metods for waste-disposal

- Some types of waste require a specific method of disposal. One of the most effective and efficient ways to eliminate all waste from your zoo or safari park is through incineration.
- Municipalities
- Biowaste-disposal agencies (MoU)

Burial of carcases

Burial is good in terms of ecologicalwell being of the environment.

Demerit: Scavenging wild animals/diggers like wild pigs / jackals / foxes / hyaena-the scavenger animal etc. may dig and/eat; hence, contamination of disease causing agents.

Incinerator-usage

Removing waste offsite is costly and often requires specialist support. Zoo waste incineration reduces those waste disposal costs and speeds up processes but initial cost may be more and one has to take care of the public-protests also, if any.

Burning by using an incinerator (with rotary kiln) will be a better practice of disposal of carcass, since it avoids the digging & subsequent feeding/wasting of the infected carcasses by scavengers like hyena, jackals etc. and also helps to prevent the contamination of the environment: crows/rodents etc. may also get subsequently affected.

There is a need of large incinerators to support disposal of the biggest of animals of the zoological park.

Types of incinerators

Regular incinerators and Specialist-incinerators

Recycling of energy by special-incinerators

(The benefits of incineration extend beyond the safe, secure disposal of your zoological waste i.e.One can now a days- also generate energy from the zoo wastes, with specialist-incinerators that are fitted with the latest, state-of-the-art technology) and large incinerators (to accommodate even large sized wild animals like the elephants/giraffe/gaur/rhinos/hippos etc).

Each **incinerator can harness the energy generated** (from burning waste) to heat water for cleaning purposes or to blow hot air to aid with drying and heating enclosures or work areas i.e. such incinerators are the ideal solutions to recycle energy, dispose of waste in an environmentally way, and prevent outbreaks of disease.

Sanitation related to parturition

- Documentations are available on the high incidence of enteric infections in cages with has not been cleaned well after the cubbing/ farrowing/ calving/ whelping etc.
- Unhygienic status maintained within the wild animal cages especially the ones with the new born wild animals lead to infection in the young ones.

Gadgets for cleaning

- Cotton and clothes
- Broom: soft bristled broom and hard broom

- Mops: dry and wet
- Brushes: soft and hard
- Vacuum-cleaner
- Water-hose with sufficient length
- Buckets/ Jugs

Sanitation with regard to Zoo- laboratory

Laboratory should be a clean one without giving chances for any types of infections.

- Gadgets: Sterility (sterile needles, syringes, sample-containers)
- Disposing of clinical wastes
- Gloves
- Cover-alls

UV LIGHT-STERILIZATION

Types of UV lamps

UV-A lamps (UVA: UVA radiation is less hazardous than UVB radiation but is also significantly (approximately 1000 times) less effective than either UVB or UVC radiation at inactivating viruses. The UVA is also implicated in skin aging and risk of skin cancer).

UV-B lamps (UVB): UVB radiation is less effective than UVC against the viruses and is also more hazardous to humans than UVC radiation because UVB radiation can penetrate deeper into the skin and eye. UVB is known to cause **DNA damage** and is a risk factor in developing **skin cancer and cataracts**.

UV-C lamps (UVC): UVB radiation is highly effective against the viruses and is less hazardous in general and can be used for disinfection purposes but safety risks are present depending on followings:

- UVC wavelength, dose, and duration of radiation exposure (the risk may increase, if the unit is not installed properly or used by untrained individuals.

Actual risks of UV-C lamps

- Direct exposure of skin and eyes to UVC radiation from some UVC lamps may cause painful eye injury and burn-like skin reactions (Never look directly at a UVC lamp source, even briefly).

- Some UVC lamps generate ozone. Ozone inhalation can be irritating to the airway.
- UVC can degrade certain materials, such as plastic, polymers, and dyed textile.
- Some UVC lamps contain mercury. Because mercury is toxic even in small amounts, extreme caution is needed in cleaning a lamp that has broken and in disposing of the lamp.

The Ultraviolet-C lamps (UVC) are now a days being used for disinfection of surfaces in the home, lab (or) similar spaces

The UVC radiation is effective at inactivating a particular virus.

But,there are also limitations to how effective UVC radiation can be at inactivating viruses, generally.

- **Direct exposure:** UVC radiation can only inactivate a virus if the virus is directly exposed to the radiation. Therefore, the inactivation of viruses on surfaces may not be effective due to blocking of the UV radiation by soil, such as dust (or) other contaminants such as bodily fluids.
- **Dose and duration:** Many of the UVC lamps sold for home use are of low dose, so it may take longer exposure to a given surface area to potentially provide effective inactivation of a bacteria or virus.
- **UVC radiation is commonly used inside air ducts to disinfect the air**: This is the safest way to employ UVC radiation because direct UVC exposure to human skin or eyes may cause injuries, and installation of UVC within an air duct is less likely to cause exposure to skin and eyes. There have been reports of skin and eye burns resulting from improper installation of UVC lamps in rooms that humans can occupy.

Sanitation with regard to vessels

- White washing of water containers and walls and feeding tanks in a periodical manner.
- Any stainless steel surfaces (feeding vessels if any) may be cleaned and disinfected with **trisodium phosphate**.
- During adaptation of the sanitation measures in the animal room, it is to be noted that since the **alkalis are non-toxic**, when adequately diluted they leave no residual odor and are even used in the treatment of floor in food factories and hence can be safely used for floors.
- Particularly these materials will be of useful in places where layers of fatty materials may accumulate.

Sanitation with regard to floor

- Documentations are available on the high incidence of enteric infections in cages with has not been cleaned well after the cubbing/ farrowing/ calving/ whelping etc.
- Unhygienic status maintained within the wild animal cages especially the ones with the new born wild animals lead to infection in the young ones.

Sanitation with regard to vectors and other unwanted animals/ invertebrates esp. vectors

- **Stray dogs, cats, rodents, snails and insects** transmit various diseases both in active and passive manners. Hence, a strict control is to be made on the breeding and elimination of them within the zoo premises, to the possible extent.
- **Moats** wet (or) dry need to be cleaned in a periodical manner and the prompt cleaning measures need to be undertaken with adequate drying of wet moat.
- **Algae** development may be monitored on the **wet moats** in particular. Enteric infections may occur when the confined wild animals develop the habit of drinking water.
- **Bush** needs to be cleared with regard to minimizing of incidences with trypanosomes.
- Use **insect/fly-catchers (electronic equipments)** / **avoid water-stagnation** near animal cages (or) enclosures
- **Avoid the establishment of the manure pits nearby** (reduce sodium in diet, so less sodium excreted/less thirst for birds/less moisture or water in droppings/less attraction of flies).

Sanitation with regard to clinical and non-clinical wastes including surgery related events (scissiors/broken pieces of thermometers / needles / BP blades etc

- These procedures need to be maintained in a perfect condition in appropriate polythene bags **without any spillage** in the environment.
- **FB syndrome** may occur if the wild animal in the cage / enclosure swallows any when left in cage (or) enclosures.
- More **frequencies of cleaning** are required in animal-cages / enclosures of the sick animals.

Sanitation within captive wild animal-room:

- Despite proper cleaning and one or two times of washing of floor, there are more chances for the accumulation of feces and feces which often get mixed with urine and they get embedded in the crevices of floor or wall. Hence there may be a possibility of a heavy "build-up-of-Potentially Pathogenic Bacteria".
- Often, due to the conditions like suitable climate that comprises the apt temperature, humidity and rain fall changes, there is increase in the spread and survival of these bacterial organisms especially, when cleaning works are not done in a proper manner.
- Application of effective disinfectants like the glutaraldehyde will be of highly useful in destroying the bacterial, viral, fungal and parasitic pathogens.

Sanitation withregard to water:

- Periodical examination of water-hygiene is to be taken care of well, in a zoological park atmosphere.
- **Rusted pipe**s need to be removed and good ones are to be replaced
- Presence of algae, bacterial load esp. any contamination with *E. coli*, Salmonella sp., toxic materials etc. have to be ruled out, always.

Waste-water disinfection in zoos

- Add five drops of 2% tincture of iodine to each quart i.e.946 ml (or) liter of water that you are disinfecting. If the water is cloudy or colored, add 10 drops of iodine. Stir and let the water stand for at least 30 minutes before use (Iodine is most effective against most of bacteria and not against viruses (or) protozoa and generally, short term usage shall be carried out in order to avoid the iodine-toxicity).
- Per day drinking water with more than 0.02 mg of iodine should not be allowed, in general for humans.
- Lower end range of the recommended upper limit is 0.5 mg/day in humans.
- **Bromine** is also being used as water (even the drinking water)-disinfectant and is active against most bacteria, some viruses and some protozoa including *Entamoebahistolytica, Cryptosporidum* spp. etc.
- **Chlorination** (chloramine and chlorine shall be used for water-disinfections, even for the drinking water) is the process of adding chlorine to drinking water to kill parasites, bacteria, and viruses. Different processes can be used to achieve safe levels of chlorine in drinking water. Using or drinking

water with small amounts of chlorine does not cause harmful health effects and provides protection against waterborne disease outbreaks.

- **Chlorine** levels up to 4 mg/L of liter (or) 4 parts per million (ppm) are considered safe in the drinking water for man (The small amount of chlorine added to water will not affect mammals and birds in general and can be used regularly for watering and bathing animals.

Chlorine and chloramine are toxic to fish, other aquatic animals, reptiles, and amphibians.

Ban on carrying of Polythene bags and canned eatable items:

Throw into wild - animal enclosure (indiscriminate feeders!)

Eg) gunny bags in llama / coco-cola cans, brush etc. in hippo/croc stomach.

White washing

White washing of water containers and walls and feeding tanks should be carried out in a periodical manner.

Zookeepers - hygiene

The zoo keepers need to be advised the necessity to adjust their cleaning strategies (some times) according to the status of the animal (eg: recently given-birth animal: scent marks or removal of body fluids).

Personal hygiene / cleanliness are to be emphasized and examined periodically.

Their health status also needs to be investigated periodically (scabies /TB/ Pulmonary infections etc.), including their visual and auditory reflexes etc., with a medical team.

They have to practice the approved methods of cleanings only (high pressure water-hose flow may disseminate larvae/eggs in the floor to the walls) and cleaning related protocols shall be provided to the animal keepers.

Public health problems

Visitors should be free from highly recognizable respiratory system-disorders and it is better to have properly placed mask that covrs the nostrils also.

Zoonotic diseases & Visitors of Zoos

Public are prone for acquiring of diseases from zoo animals (Zoonotic diseases)Zoonoses are diseases that can be passed from animals to humans. Wild animals may carry more pathogens but there may not be identifiable clinical symptoms in them, most of the times ie) Wild animals may carry a range of pathogenic organisms, without showing any signs of disease.

Most zoonoses are uncommon and can usually be treated when detected. While there are dozens of zoonotic diseases, there are a few that are particularly dangerous to humans.

EXAMPLES OF ZOONOTIC DISEASES (SPREADING AT ZOOS)

Zoonoses include

Toxin-producing *E.coli, Campylobacteriosis,* Cryptosporidiosis, Orf.

Scabies, Fungal infections (eg.Blastomycosis), Toxocariasis, CD, Rabies

Avian influenza, Psittacosis, Salmonellosis, New Castle disease, *Staphylococcus* spp., *Yersinia* spp., Pasteurella spp., Shigella spp., Congo Red fever.

Toxoplasmosis, Q fever, Amoebiasis, Giardiasis

Tuberculosis, Anthrax, Leptospirosis, Brucellosis, Listeriosis, Hydatidosis

Strongyloidosis, KFD, Herpes and Pox viruses, Viral hepatitis, Measles, Ebola virus, Malaria, *Hymenolepsis nana*.

Nipah virus, Lyssa virus, etc.

Aquatic oriented: *Cl.botulinum, Enterobacter* spp., *Vibrio* spp., Leptospira l serovars, *Mycobacterium* spp.

Mode of transmission of diseases from ZOO-Animals to the visitors (Public)

Diseases can be spread through direct contact with animals and then placing contaminated fingers (or) other items in the mouth. Diseases can also be spread through animal bites and scratches / contact with their carcasses / through indirect contact with their faeces, urine, saliva, blood, aerosols, birth products (or) enclosures contaminated with these materials.

Diseases can also be spread through contaminated dust (or) aerosol.

Precautions to be taken by general public during visiting of the zoos

Hand washing is the key; the infectious diseases may be spread from either animals (or) the environment to people by contaminated hands. Hence, the proper-hand washing is a must for the visitors for the prevention of the zoonotic diseases at the zoos esp. in the petting zoos (zoos with some domesticated animals and docile wild animals and public esp. the children are allowed to touch, hold and even to feed such animals and such petting zoos are more profitable in many countries).

Always wash hands with soap (for <1 to 2 minutes) and running water before eating (or) drinking (or) before smoking.

Followings are the "don'ts" for the visitors at the zoos

- Touching of the mouth with hands (or) licking of the fingers.
- Eating of food that is intended for the captive wild animals.
- Leaving their open-wounds uncovered.
- Wipe hands on clothing, if avoidable.
- Avoid contact with soil or faeces of WA-areas.

Always wash hands and other exposed body parts with soap and running water, particularly aftertouching animals, their enclosures or food containers. Any part of the animal or its surrounds can be contaminated with faeces or urine

- being licked, bitten (or) spat on by animals.
- having contact with soil or faeces.

Precautions to be undertaken esp. for children

Zoo / School / Wildlife Centre - Staff (perhaps with the assistance of some parents) should closely supervise children who are petting animals by using the precautions outlined above

Hand-washing of children should be ensured, immediately after the visits (or) petting the wild animals / animals.

Ensure that the hand-washed children do not become re-contaminated by playing with children who have not washed their hands.

Precautions to be taken at zoos by officials to reduce spread of zoonotic diseases among general public

Veterinarians (or) the zoo-operators should take precautions to reduce the risk of ill health to visitors of the zoo especially the petting zoo by adapting following measures.

- **Providing only healthy animals** for public display or contact by establishing a close association with a vet to ensure animals are clinically healthy, appropriately vaccinated, and maintaining a comprehensive parasite control program for all species.
- **Promoting thorough hand washing** with soap and running water after contact with animals (o.r) their enclosures
- **Positioning hand washing facilities**, so that visitors are encouraged to wash their hands with soap and running water on exiting animal enclosures and before entering designated eating areas.
- Separating animal contact areas from visitor eating areas.

- Keeping animals out of visitor eating areas.
- Providing adequate well-secured waste bins (so no scavengers/raiding wild animals like rodents).
- Maintaining a first aid kit
- Keeping birthing animals out of public areas
- Placing wild-caught animals out of public areas.
- If providing milk (or) milk products for tasting, only doing so after they have been pasteurised (or) heat treated
- Banning known aggressive animals from coming into direct contact with visitors
- Maintaining animals in an environment conducive to maintaining their health and well-being
- Reducing stress of WA and overcrowding of animals to reduce the possibility of disease
- Regularly removing and appropriately disposing of faeces and other wastes, including birth products
- Periodical deworming and vaccinations of vulnerable and other wild animals
- Providing adequate barriers to prevent touching animals that are not available for touching (or) that should not be touched.

EXTENSION ACTIVITIES ON ZOONOTIC DISEASES AND THE PREVENTIVE MEASURES FOR THE PUBLIC VISITING THE ZOOS

Signages

Place obvious and prominent hand washing and directional signs in appropriate locations, such as the entrance (or) exits of the zoo, and in eating areas (or) in drinking areas to remind visitors to:

- To carry out good hygiene practices in the petting zoo environment.
- To eat (or) drink only in the designated areas & not in animal contact areas.
- To place signages or display boards about the significance of washing of hands for zoo-visitors ie) the general public.
- To use only the designated toilets and not in open places of zoos.
- Audio as well as the video-programmes on these.

Pamphlets: Preparation and distribution of illustrative pamphlets on these. Conducting of quiz for few minutes on hygiene and zoonosis among visitors esp. children to enrich their knowledge on zoonosis and preventive steps. Nominal-cost based selling of printed T-shirts / Printed Tea-cups etc. on these.

4

Prevention and Control of Significant Infectious Diseases of Animals

Disease	Hosts affected
Trypanosomosis	Boids, equids, canids,felids, equids, suids etc.
Glanders (*Pseudomonas malle*)	Equids like wild ass, zebra etc.
FMD	All artiodactylids
Hog cholera (Toga virus)	Suids
Haemorrhagic septicemia	Bovids in particular
Japanese B encephalitis (Flavivirus)	Suids, Equids and Homosapiens
Louping ill (Flavi virus)	Bovids, shrew, wild sheep, wood mouseand man
Dourine (*Trypanosoma equiperdum*)	Equids
African swine fever	Suids
African horse sickness	Equids and Dogs
Teschen disease (Enterovirus porcine 1)	Suids
East coast fever (Therileriasis)	Bovids
Rift Valley fever, Bunyavirus	Wild sheep and Wild goat
Peste des petits ruminants (Paramyxo viruses)	Ruminants

Disinfectants as preventive and control measures

Diseases	Specific disinfectant to be used
FMD	• 4% solution of sodium bi carbonate (washing soda) • Formaldehyde fumigation of materials like straw, grain etc. • Citric acid
Anthrax	2-5% HCl acid to disinfectant the hides and hides contaminated with Anthrax as in taxidermy
Rabies	Formaldehyde or Cresol may be of used
Tuberculosis	70% Isopropyl alcohol in 5mtes time or 3% phenol in 2-3 hrs
Herpes virus	Gluteraldehyde /Chlorine/Ethanol
Fowl pox virus	Formaldehyde /Methyl bromide
New castle diseases	Formaldehyde /Chlorinated lime /Chloramine lime

Disease	Prevention and/or Treatment
Foot and Mouth Disease	• Antiseptic mouth wash and application of antiseptic solutions on foot lesions. • Proper immunization.
Anthrax	• Administration on antibiotics and annual vaccination. • Carcass should not be opened and is to be burnt or deeply buried. • Restrict animal movement.
Hemorrhagic Septicemia	• Use fluroquinolone compounds like enrofloxacin for treatment. • Vaccination • Isolate the affected ones
Black Quarter	• Anitibiotics • Vaccination • Isolate the affected ones
Theileriosis	• Treat with Buparvaquone @ 20 mg/kg i/m • Control of tick population. • Vaccination of animals in enzootic areas. • Isolate the affected ones
Anaplasmosis	• Treat with tetracycline and supportive therapy with B-complex vitamins.
Babesiosis	• Treat with Diaminazene aceturate @ 4 mg/kg i/m or Imidocarb dipropionate @ 1 mg/kg i/m • B-complex injection. • Adoption of tick control measures.
Coccidiosis	• Administration of sulphonamides, etc • Strict sanitary measures
Trypanosomosis	• Use quinapyramine sulphate and chloride for both curative and prophylactic purpose. • Use diminazine aceturate for curative purpose • Control of fly population.
Cestodiasis	• Praziquantel may be used. • Strict sanitary measures.
Helminthiasis	• Use Albendazole (or) Pyrantel pamoate for deworming purpose. • Strict sanitary measures
Malaria	• Administration of quinine • Control of mosquitoes
Amoebiasis	• Metronidazole @ 30-60 mg/kg b.wt daily for 5-10 days (orally)
Leptospirosis	• Doxycycline, Ceftriaxone, etc. may be used
Tuberculosis	• Administration of Isoniazid and related drugs (rifampicin, ethambutol and pyrazinamide)

5

Organizations Related to Zoo and Wild Animals

NATIONAL AND INTERNATIONAL ORGANIZATIONS AND INSTITUTIONS INTERLINKED TO WILD & ZOO ANIMALS

Role and functioning

National organizations

Bombay Natural History Society (BNHS)

BNHS is one of the oldest scientific organizations in India, working for nature conservation since 1883. Our primary goal is to spread awareness about nature through science-based research, conservation advocacy, education, scientific publications, nature tours, and other programs. Natural history collections that tell of great scientific discoveries in the Indian subcontinent, dating back to the 19th century, occupy pride of place in the Hornbill House. There are over 18,500 mammals, 29,000 birds, 5,430 bird eggs, over 8,500 amphibians and reptiles, 50,000 insects and 5,000 other taxa, which are regularly referred to by wildlife researchers and amateur naturalists from India and abroad. It was established on 15th September, 1883.

It is the largest Non-government organization engaged in nature conservation research. The role and functions were mainly related to the fact that conservation must be based on scientific view. Dr.Salim Ali was the first Indian Honorary Secretary in this organization.

Wildlife Institute of India (WII)

Established in December, 1982, Wildlife Institute of India (WII) is an internationally acclaimed Institution, which offers training program, academic courses and advisory in wildlife research and management. The Institute is actively engaged in research across the breadth of the country on biodiversity related issues.This institution was established with an objective of becoming a significant centre for wildlife training, research, publication and extension in India.

The functions and roles are related to the followings

- Training of personnel for protected area management and wildlife research.
- Training of education and extension specialists for protected area management and wildlife research.
- Offering of orientation courses for those who are involved in land use management.
- Provision of advisory and consultant service to central and state governmental agencies, universities, colleges, institutions and other official and non-official agencies.
- Creation of databases by employing modern computerized analytical techniques.
- To conduct and co-ordinate applied wildlife research.

Indian Board for Wildlife (IBWL)

Indian Board for Wildlife (*IBWL*), a body created for conservation of Wild Life, was constituted in the year 1952 by the Central Government of India.

- Prevents cruelty against birds and beasts caught alive.
- Promotes public involvement in wildlife and its preservation in harmony with natural and human environment.
- 1st phase of IBWL was confined to protection of wildlife from poachers and unscrupulous hunters.
- 2nd phase was associated with development and creation of National Parks and Sanctuaries where threatened species are protected.
- 3rd phase was associated to the detailed study and improvement in the existing food and water reserves, offering of effective protection to threatened species and fast development of wildlife sanctuaries.

Botanical Survey of India (BSI)

BSI is the apex taxonomic research organization of the country which is under the Ministry of Environment, Forest & Climate Change.The BSI was established on 13th February, 1890 with the basic objective to explore the plant resources of the country and to identify the plant species with economic values.

Roles assigned to BSI for study

- Develop and maintain **Botanical** Gardens, Museums and Herbaria. Preparation of Pollen, Seed and Spore Atlas of Indian Plants. Qualitative analysis of nutritive value of ethno-food plants and other economically useful species.

- To carry out the Impact Assessment of areas, assigned.
- To carry out surveys on faunal resources of India.

Zoological Survey of India (ZSI)

ZSI was established on 1st July, 1916. ZSI provides information and vital data for the in-situ conservation of various species in different ecosystems, both within and outside the protected areas. The current mandate of ZSI is survey, collection documentation (including the traditional knowledge associated with animals) and ***ex-situ*** conservation of wild animal diversity of the country.

The main **objective** of the Centre is to conduct survey, exploration and research on the faunal diversity of estuaries, backwaters, lagoons and mangrove ecosystems of India and to develop a regional museum exhibiting the fauna of Estuaries and associated ecosystem. ZSI carries out surveys on the faunal resources of India and has published the Red Data Book on Indian animals.

Indian Institute of Sciences (IIS)

This is located at Bangalore and is involved in studies on ecology and wildlife of Western Ghats.

Wildlife Protection Society of India (WPSI)

- It is a NGO founded in 1958 at Dehradun. Promotes interest and knowledge among people in the field of preservation and conservation of all kinds of fauna and flora and management.
- Supports in enforcement of wildlife protection act.
- Promotes wildlife tourism.
- Co-operates with state Government of India as well as other societies and institutions for the interest of wildlife protection.
- Protects, propagates and conserves the wildlife.

Central Zoo Authority (CZA)

The **CZA** is a statutory body under the Ministry of Environment, Forest and Climate Change. This highly empowered statutory body was constituted in 1992, under the Wildlife (Protection) Act, 1972. Members: It is chaired by the Environment Minister and has 10 members and a member-secretary.

Mission

To provide better upkeep and veterinary care to the wild animal housed in zoos in India to ensure their conservation through best practices of management and bringing education & awareness among the people.

Vision

To complement and strengthen the national efforts in conservation of the biodiversity of the country, particularly the fauna through the *ex-situ* conservation linked with in-situ practices.

Objective

To enforce minimum standards and norms for upkeep and healthcare of animals in Indian zoos and to control mushrooming of unplanned and ill-conceived zoos.

Main functions of CZA are

- To specify the minimum standards for housing and veterinary care of the zoo animals.
- To provide technical and other assistance to zoos for their proper management.
- To identify endangered species of wild animals for the purpose of captive breeding.
- To recognize or derecognize zoos
- To evaluate the functioning of a zoo.
- To co-ordinate research in captive breeding and educational programmes
- To ensure maintenance of stud book of endangered species of wild animals bred in captivity.
- To restrict the power of a zoo regarding acquisition or transfer of any wild animal specified in schedule I and II.

National Board for Wildlife (NBWL)

It was started in 1952 as the highest advisory body of the Government of India regarding wildlife. The NBWL is the apex body for conservation of wildlife and its habitat, and the NBWL's role is of critical importance to ensure the long-term protection of India's biodiversity. The National Board for Wildlife (NBWL) is a "statutory board" constituted under the Wild Life (Protection) Act, 1972 (wildlife act).

The Prime Minister of the country is the ex officio chairperson of the NBWL. The Minister of Environment, Forests and Climate Change is the Vice-Chairperson of the Board. As per the WLPA, every time a new government is formed, a new NBWL has to be constituted with the Prime Minister as the chairperson.

NBWL helps to solve the policy matters. It is instrumental for legislation of wildlife protection act and guides central and state government on matters pertaining to wildlife through legislative and practical measures.

Wildlife Trust of India (WTI)

It is a leading Indian nature conservation organization committed to the service of nature. Established in November 1998, in response to the rapidly deteriorating condition of the country's wildlife, with only three staff members, WTI now has a team of over 100 full-time professionals and consultants, in addition to volunteers from all walks of life. The core team includes scientists, field biologists, conservation managers, veterinarians, lawyers, finance, business management and communication specialists, who operate diverse conservation projects across India.

The Wildlife Trust of India (WTI), a non-profit conservation organisation, committed to urgent action that works towards the protection of India's wildlife. It's mission is to conserve nature, especially endangered species and threatened habitats, in partnership with communities and governments.

In 20 years, WTI has grown to be one of India's premier wildlife NGOs. The principal concerns of WTI include crisis management and provision of quick, efficient aid to individuals, species or habitats that require it the most. In its 21 years of operations, WTI has saved more than 42,000 animal lives, trained and equipped 20,000 frontline forest staff and covered them under India's pioneering supplementary accident assurance scheme that also covers Covid-19, assisted the govt. in creating 7 Protected Areas, sensitised 25 lakhs children to conservation, protected almost 1200 sq km of natural habitat including mangroves and coral reefs, assisted enforcement agencies in almost 240 seizures.

- It is a non-profit conservation organization located in Delhi.
- It works on conservation related programmes in India through a team of professionals comprising of biologists, veterinarians, communication specialists, lawyers, etc.
- This organization has special programmes pertaining to sloth bear. Elephant, tiger, rhinoceros, etc.

Indian Board of Wildlife (IBWL)

It is first constituted in 1952 as the advisory body under the name Central Board for Wildlife which is later renamed as Indian Board for Wildlife. It is mainly responsible for Wildlife conservation with the assistance of the central and state governments. It works in close co-operation of WWF.

The functions of the IBWL, among others are

1. To devise ways and means for the preservation and control of wildlife through coordinated legislative and practical measures;
2. To sponsor the setting up of national parks, wildlife sanctuaries and zoological gardens;
3. To promote public interest in wildlife and the need for its preservation in harmony with natural and human environment;
4. To advise the Government on policy in respect of export of plants and animals.
5. To prevent cruelty to birds and beasts caught alive with or without injury.

National Biodiversity Authority of India (NBA)

NBA has its headquarters in Chennai,Tamil Nadu. NBA has not more than five members from amongst experts in matters relating to conservation of biological diversity, sustainable use of biological resources and equitable sharing of benefits arising out of the use of biological resources.

The Biological Diversity Act, 2002 is an Act enacted by the Parliament of India for the preservation of biological diversity in India, and provides mechanism for equitable sharing of benefits arising out of the use of traditional biological resources and knowledge.

Following are the important definitions in this

1. 'Chairperson' means the chairperson of the National Biodiversity Authority (NBA) or as to case may be of the State Biodiversity Board.
2. 'Member' means a member of the National Biodiversity Authority (NBA) or a State Biodiversity Board and includes the Chairperson.
3. Bio-survey and Bio-utilization means survey or collection of species, sub species, genus, components and extracts of biological resource for any purpose and includes characterization, inventorisation and bioassay.
4. "Value added products" means products containing potions or extracts of animals as well as the plants in unrecognizable and physically inseparable

World Wildlife Fund- India (WWF-India)

It was established in India **as a Charitable Trust on 27 November, 1969,**at the time of XII General Assembly of the IUCN, held at Delhi. It was founded as a branch of WWF-International formed in 1961 with its headquarters at Glands, Switzerland.

WWF-India set out with the aim of reducing the degradation of Earth's natural environment and building a future in which humans live in harmony with nature.

In 1987, the organization changed it's name from the World Wildlife Fund to World Wide Fund for Nature India.

Mission Statement of World Wide Fund for Nature India

- To stop the degradation of the planet's natural environment and build a future in which humans live in harmony with nature, by:
- Conserving the world's biological diversity
- Ensuring that the use of renewable natural resources is sustainable
- Promoting the reduction of pollution and wasteful consumption

Academic Institutions Related to Wildlife Research

Department of Wildlife Science, Tamil Nadu Veterinary and Animal Sciences University, Chennai and Centre for Wildlife Forensic and Health, M.P. Veterinary University, Jabalpur and Indian Veterinary Research Institute, Bareilly, UP state and Karnataka Veterinary, Animal and Fisheries Sciences University, Karnataka state and veterinary colleges in Kerala state.

These institutions are currently involving in teaching, research and extension activities pertaining to wildlife science.

International Union for Conservation of Nature and Natural Resources (IUCN)

The International Union for Conservation of Nature's Red List of Threatened Species has evolved to become the world's most comprehensive information source on the global extinction risk status of animal, fungus and plant species.The IUCN Red List has listed 132 species of plants and animals from India as "Critically Endangered".

As per IUCN, following ten species of wild fauna are quoted as the most famous endangered species of wild fauna at global level:

- Giant panda (*Ailuropodamela noleuca*)
- Tiger (*Panthera tigris*)
- Whooping crane (*Grusamericana*)
- Blue whale (*Balaenoptera musculus*)
- Asian elephant (*Elephas maximus*)
- Sea otter (*Enhydralutris*)
- Snow leopard (*Panthera uncia*)
- Gorilla (*Gorilla beringei* and *Gorilla gorilla*)

Now this is called as World Conservation Union. It is the world's largest and most important conservation network. It is a multi-lingual, multi-cultural organization.

Role and Functions

- It links both research and results to local, national, regional and global policy by convening dialogues between Governments, civil society and private sector.
- It supports and develops cutting-edge conservation science and implements this research in field projects around the world.
- It facilitates paths for peace between countries in areas of conflict and works with the corporate sector on energy and bio-diversity.
- Species Survival Commission (SSC) is one of the Commissions of IUCN which has aim of conservation of bio-diversity.

Convention on International Trade in Endangered Species (CITES)

This organization helps to prevent the over-exploitation of wild fauna and flora. Government of India signed this convention in July 1974 and became a party to it from 18th Oct, 1976.

Role and Functions

- People and states are linked for best protection of their own wild fauna and flora.
- Stresses on need of International collaboration.
- Stresses on need of undergoing the ever-growing value of wild fauna and flora from aesthetic, scientific, cultural, recreational and economic point of view.
- Emphasizes that the wild fauna and flora in their many beautiful varied forms are on irreplaceable part of the natural systems of the earth.

UNITED NATIONS DEVELOPMENT PROGRAMME (UNDP) AND FOOD AND AGRICULTURE ORGANIZATION (FAO)

UNDP

It is the global development network recommending for the modidication and connection of various countries to experience, knowledge and appropriate resources that are beneficial to public at large. India is in liaisonship with this UNDP since 1951 for poverty eradication and environmental management, Infact, the North East India Conservation Initiative (NEICI) is in collaboration with this UNDP only.

FAO

It has a long history of maintaining a sustainable form of agricultural development and biodiversity, Conservation of biodiversity is protectioin, scientific management of biodiversity and upliftment, so as to maintain the sustainable benefits for the present and future generation.These organizations are overall said to be associated with all features of conservation, in general.

Trade Records Analysis of Flora and Fauna in Commerce (TRAFFIC)

TRAFFIC rules need to be meticulously followed up during exchange or procurement of any species of wild fauna.

- It is a wildlife trade watch group of IUCN and WWF for nature.
- Started in 1975 with the aim of monitoring wildlife trade worldwide.
- It collects and analyses the data on wildlife trade.
- TRAFFIC – India was established on 1/01/1992 as a division of WWF – India and a part of global TRAFFIC network.

United Nations Educational, Scientific and Cultural Organization (UNESCO)

It launched various bio-diversity programmes like establishment of different biospheres. The UNESCO biosphere reserves are basically central to education, and research, in addition to the awareness-raising works in order to foster the innovative sustainable development practices and combat the loss of biodiversity.Such measures are found to be basically essential for the better protection of environment in various protected regions of this country.

World Wide Fund for Nature (WWF)

- It was set up in 1961 and giant panda is the official symbol of WWF.
- It was earlier called as world wildlife fund but in 1990 it was renamed as world wide fund for nature.

Role and Functions

It helps to raise funds for urgent conservation requirements and promoting conservation through the world wide education campaign and public consciousness. Grants are raised by donations from public, heritable foundations, regular members, etc.

International Commission on Zoological Nomenclature (ICZN), International Commission on Botanical Nomenclature (ICBN), Global Tiger Forum (GTF)

It is an International platform to discuss features pertaining to the protection of tiger population in the world.

Role and Functions

- Establishment of wildlife sanctuaries and national parks.
- Establishment of special squad to discover poaching etc.
- Focuses on welfare of the tiger-populations.

6

Acts and Rules Related to Zoo and Wild Animals

It pays emphasis on the conservation of ecosystem and support to the management of the country in protected area-network. To prevent wildlife depletion, several Acts have been made from time to time, by the State as well as the Central Government.

The important ones related to wildlife conservation and protections in India are

1. Madras Wildlife Act, 1873
2. All- India Elephant Preservation Act, 1879
3. The Indian Fisheries Act, 1897
4. The Wild Birds and Animals Protection Act, 1912
5. The Indian Forest Act, 1927
6. Bengal Rhinoceros Preservation Act, 1932
7. Bombay Wild animal and wild birds Protection Act, 1951
8. Assam Rhinoceros Preservation Act, 1954
9. The Cruelty against animals Act, 1960.
10. All-India Wildlife Protection Act, 1972, amended in 1983, 1986 and 1991.
11. The Forest (conservation) Act, 1982

Several non-government organizations in the country are engaged in specific areas of target species in-situ conservation measures through external or Natural assistance or through a combination of assistance from both.

Wildlife Protection Act, 1972

Reasons for the framing and implementation of the Wildlife Protection Act.

Wildlife is a part of 'forests' and this was a state subject until the Parliament passed this law in 1972. Now it is Concurrent List.

Reasons for a nationwide law in the domain of environment esp. the wildlife

- India is a treasure-trove of varied flora and fauna. Many species were seeing a rapid decline in numbers.
- For instance, it was mentioned by Edward Pritchard Gee (A naturalist), that at the turn of the 20th century, India was home to close to 40000 tigers. But, a census in 1972 showed this number drastically reduced to about 1827.
- A drastic decrease in the flora and fauna can cause ecological imbalance, which affects many aspects of climate and the ecosystem.
- The most recent Act passed during the British era in this regard was the Wild Birds and Animals Protection, 1935. This needed to be upgraded as the punishments awarded to poachers and traders of wildlife products were disproportionate to the huge financial benefits that accrue to them.
- There were only five national parks in India prior to the enactment of this Act.

This was amended in the year 1991 and 2002

According to this act, "Wildlife" is defined as any animal, bee, butterflies, crustaceae, fish and moths and aquatic or land vegetation. Thus it is to be understood that Wildlife is the term that embraces all life forms that are wild or care themselves.

There are many important sections of this act which are to be understood.

IMPORTANT SECTIONS OF THIS ACT

Section-18 - Declaration of Sanctuary

The State Government may by notification declare its intention to constitute any area or area comprised with any reserve forest or territorial waters as Sanctuary if it considers that such area is of adequate ecological faunal, floral, geomorphological, natural or zoological significance for the purpose of protecting, propagating or developing wildlife or its environment.

Section 27- Restriction of entry in Sanctuary

No person other than

i) A public servant on duty.

ii) A person who has been permitted by the Chief Warden or the authorized officer to reside within limits of the sanctuary.

iii) A person who has any right over immovable property within limits of the sanctuary.

iv) A person passing through the sanctuary along a public highway.

v) And the dependents of the person classified in class (a), (b), (c) shall enter and reside in the sanctuary, except under and in accordance with the conditions of a permit granted under section 28.

Section 28- Grant of permit

1. The Chief Wildlife Warden may on application grant to any person a permit to enter or reside in a sanctuary for all (or) any of the following purpose:
    - Investigation or study of Wildlife and purposes of ancillary or incidental threats.
    - Photography
    - Scientific research
    - Tourism
    - Transaction of any lawful business with any person residing in the sanctuary.
2. A permit to enter or reside in a sanctuary shall be issued subject to such conditions and on payment of such fee as may be prescribed.

Section 33- A- Immunization of Livestock

1. The Chief Wildlife Warden shall take such measures in such manner as may be prescribed, for immunization against communicable diseases of livestock kept in or within 5 kms of the sanctuary.
2. No person shall take or cause to be taken or grazed any livestock in a sanctuary without getting it immunized.

Schedule I to VI dealt by Wildlife Protection Act 1972 with amendments during 1986 and 1991. Important animals in each schedule are given below.

Part I- Mammals

Indian Chinkara, Indian Lion, Indian Wild Ass, Indian Wolf, Leopard, Leopard cat, Lion-tailed macaque, Loris, Gaur or Indian Bison, Cheetah, Indian ggazelle, Dugong, NilgiriTahr, NilgiriLangur, Musk deer, Sloth bear, Tiger, Wild Buffalo, Mouse Deer, Honey Badger, Hispid Hare, Chinese pangolin, Crab-eating Macaque, Desert Fox, Fishing Cat, Four-horned Antelope, Indian One-horned Rhinoceros, Rusty Spotted Cat, Serow, Swamp Deer etc.

Part II- Amphibians and Reptiles

Pythons, Water lizard, Gharial, Estuarine (or) Salt water crocodile, Golden Gecko, Green sea turtle, Leathery turtle, Logger head turtle, Howksbill turtle, Indian egg-eating snake.

Part III A- Fishes

Whale shark, Shark, Ray, Sea horse, Giant grouper.

Part III B- Birds

Hornbills, Mountain quail, Peafowl, Andaman teal, Nicobar megapods, Nicobar pigeon, Bengal florican, Black-necked crane etc.

Part IV- Insects

Butterflies and Moths.

Part IV A- Coelentrates

Fire coral, Sea fan, Roof building coral.

Part IV B- Mollusca

Part IV C- Echinodermata

Sea cucumber (all Holothurians)

Schedule II

Part I- Bonnet macaque, Common langur, Wild dog, Chameleon, Spiny tailed lizard or Sanda.

Part II- Beetles.

Schedule III

Chital, Barking deer or Muntjac, Gorals, Hog deer, Wild pig, Nilgai, Sponges.

Schedule IV

Indian Hedgehogs, Indian porcupine, Mongooses, Polecats.

Schedule V

Common crow, Fruit bats, Mice, Rats, Five striped palm squirrel, Black napped hare, Common Indian hare, Desert hare, Himalayan mouse hare.

Schedule VI

Birds like Coots, Cranes, Cormorants, Flamingos, Ibises.

Ladies slipper orchids, Red Vanda, Blue Vanda.

Indian Biological Diversity Act, 2002

This is act to provide for constitution of biological diversity, sustainable use of its components and fair and equitable sharing of the benefits arising out of the use of biological resources, knowledge and for matters connected there with or incidental threats.

7

Basics on the Management of Captive Elephants

Important facts about elephants

Elephants are the simple stomached animals and colon is associated with digestion, predominantly. Elephants are the herd animals (gregarious in nature) and belong to the matriarchal groups (Leader of herd is usually a cow elephant)

Geological distribution in Asia has led to the classification of seven numbers of sub-species of elephants and the names are given below

- *Elephas maximus indicus* (India)
- *Elephas maximus bengalensis* (North India)
- *Elephas maximus dakhamensis* (South India)
- *Eleph maximus ceylonicus* (Sri Lanka)
- *Elephas maximus burminicus* (Burma / Myammar)
- Elephas maximus hirsutus (Malaysia / Thailand)
- *Elephas maximus sumatranus* (Sumatra)

Physiological and Anatomical Peculiarities in Elephants

- Asian elephants can be tamed early in life and taming is difficult with regard to the African elephants.
- Teeth get completely worn at 6^{0th} year & some times, the wearing of last pair of teeth may be seen at 5^{0th} year itself.
- Elephants can tolerate cold than the heat and elephants are highly vulnerable to heat stroke like conditions.
- Skin has a poor circulation of blood in general.
- Caecal digestion is a prominent feature (hind-gut fermenter) due to large caecum.
- Ears are large and are associated with maintenance of thermo-regulation.

- Since pleural space is absent in adult elephants, it is better to avoid the elephant to assume sternal recumbency esp. for more than 7 minutes.

ANTOMICAL FEATURES OF ELEPHANTS

Dental Formula

$$I\frac{1-1}{0-0}\quad C\frac{0-0}{0-0}\quad PM\frac{3-3}{3-3}\quad M\frac{3-3}{3-3}$$

Molar Number	Lamella	Appears	Loss
1	4	4 Months	2-2.5 years
2	8	6 Months	6 years
3	12	3 years	9 years
4	12	6 years	25 years
5	16	20 years	50-60 years
6	24	40 years	60+ years

Vertebral formula

C7 T19-20 L4 S4 Cy30

- **SKIN is** very thick and hence the name "PACHYDERM" but one can even see the mild signs of mosquito bites on the skin. Skin is thicker over the hind limbs and hind quarters but is thinner over the forelimbs.
- **HAIR** ismost significant in case of younger elephants than in adult or older elephants.
- **SWEAT GLANDS** are fewer on the skin may be observed – just above the toe nails.
- **SKULL** has a large area of air–filled sinus cavity and has doom shape and this anatomical peculiarity leads to less burdon despite the existing body weight in these naturally huge sized mega herbivores.
- **TUSK** is an extension or outgrowth of upper incisors and is embedded in the sulcus.
- Tushes are tusk like structures present in female elephants
- **TRUNK** is formed by extension / fusion of upper lip and the nose and there are no bones or cartilage in the trunk.

- **TONGUE** has restricted movement (Non-prehensile) and can't be protruded out, as in case of crocodilians.
- **TEETH** are in two pairs at a time and in general, elephants have six complete sets of grinding teeth and these teeth are referred by few authors as simply molars.
- **NASOLACRIMAL DUCT** is absent in case of elephants.
- **EAR VEINS** are prominent and is used for IV injections
- **MAMMARY GLANDS (in pair)** arepectoral in position, as the case with non-human primates.
- **KNEE CAP** is placed in the lower position and hence, this helps the bending of knees by the elephants to bend their knees like humans.
- **ANAL FLAP** is one of the unique features in elephants.
- **LIMBS** hasfibro-elastic pad at extremities.
- **HEART** has a bifid apex and anterior vena cavae are double.
- **BRAIN has** highly convoluted cerebrum and cerebellum.
- **LUNGS** have no pleural space (pleural cavity) in ease of elephants unlike in calf stage.
- **GALL BLADDER** is absent.
- **KIDNEYS** are multilobed (5-7 lobes).

Like equines, elephants are hind-gut fermenters (Caecal digestion).

The special position of vulva makes the erected penis, to a cobra shaped hood, to facilitate penetration. Glans penis is absent. Testicles are intra-abdominal.Duringmusthstage, testes enlarge in size very much Functional Hypertrophy).

Clitoris can reach the length of about forty cm. Vulva is located between the hind legs of female and is not located under the tail as seen in other mammals.Vagina is long and vertical.

The vagina is separated from the vulva by a urogenital canal that is about 40-100 cm long and the urethra enters the urogenital canal of the female just posterior to the juncture between the vagina and the canal.

- **PENIS** has cobra shaped hood, to facilitate penetration & glans penis is absent
- **TESTICLES** are intra-abdominal and have testicondy condition.

- **VAGINA AND VULVAL OPENING** are located between the hind legs of female and is not located under the tail as seen in other mammals. Vagina is long and vertical.
- **ESTIMATION OF BODY WEIGHT**

W = 12.8 (Cg + ng) – 4281 (or) 4152 + 14.76 cg + 8.84 ng (W: Weight in Kg & Cg: Chest girth in Cms & Ng: neck girth in cms)

ESTIMATION OF HEIGHT

H-21.04 + 1.77 CF (H: Height in cm & CF: Circumference of front foot in cms)

MUSTH AND ITS MANAGEMENT

Musth – a peculiar physiological phenomenon

This is the temporarily occurring physiological condition in case of male elephants. Moda (or) Juvenile musth is observed in the age group of 15-20 years. Duration of musth lasts for 1-3 months and sometimes for 5 months. Occurrence of musth in female elephants is often insignificant. Unlike in Asiatic elephants, musth occurs in both sexes of African elephants.

Key changes during musth

- Swelling of temporal gland region.
- Black coloured fluid oozing from the temporal gland regions flowing down the cheek region. Drainage from the temporal gland is insignificant in case of Asiatic female elephants and cow elephant may reveal drainage when in estrus or when excited.
- Smell of droppings from the fowls may be felt at a distance.
- Dribbling of urine.
- Disobedience.
- Aggressive behaviour.
- Exhibition of goring any moving or non-moving objects that catches its attention.
- Enlargement of the perineal region which is an obvious feature observed.
- Duration of musth ranges from 3 weeks to 3 months.
- However, variations may be observed with elephants.

Medical Management of Musth in Elephants

First, properly restrain the animal by using insulated chain.

Clinical approach to postponement of Musth and the related aggression

Postponement of musth temporarily	Administer Flutamide 2500 mg /elephant, orally
Postponement of musth for longer time for more than many months	Administer Flutamide 7500 mg / elephant, orally
Control of musth in pre-musth state	Administer Flutamide 5000 mg per animal, orally

Chemical Immobilization of Elephants

S.No.	Drug	Dose-rate	Antidote
1.	Xylazine	0.08 – 0.14 mg / kg body weight I/M (use atropine sulphate @ rate of 0.04 – 0.05 mg / kg body weight S/C)	Yohimbine (Needs double the dose rate of Xylazine, in general)
2.	Etrophine	0.0022 – 0.0044 mg / kg body weight (1 mg / 450 kg body weight I/M)	Diprenorphine HCL/Norcan

Note

During usage of etorphine, the duration of immobilization is 40-50 minutes and hyperthermia is to be managed effectively.

Signs of health in elephants

- Frequent movements of extremities.
- Free passage of dung and urine.
- Apparently normal feeding activities.
- Watering activities without much change, as reported by the care-takers of the elephants.
- Free movements of the body.
- Absence of abnormal posture or appearance or unusual behaviour.
- Proper obeying to the commands of mahouts or the care takers of the elephants
- Tip of the trunk is moist.
- Good appetite.
- Well-formed dung.
- Clear and bright eyes
- Small amount of clear discharge from the conjunctiva is normal.

- Skin is soft and resilient.
- Neither too fat nor too lean.
- Urine is copious in amount, faintly yellow, with a pleasant odour.
- Absence of straining during urination or defecation.
- Rosy pink color is seen on tongue, mouth and inside of the trunk.

Signs of diseases are also to be well known during the clinical examination of the elephant and are mentioned below

- Disobedience or less obedience to mahout's commands
- Anorexia
- Pyrexia
- Constipation or diarrhea depending on the condition
- Change in urine or feces (i.e. change in colour as well as in quantity and smell)
- Lameness
- Any unusual swelling or protrusion
- Frequent sitting and standing
- Restlessness
- Aggression
- Dullness
- Passing of lesser amounts of urine
- Apparent swellings or injuries may be seen on parts of body regions
- Totally reduced or partial movements of trunk or legs
- Absence of swaying of body regions
- Frequent trumpeting
- Placement of trunk frequently in oral region
- Pressing of fore head or tusk if it is a male animal against some hard object like wall or tree
- Limping or reluctant walking.
- Weight loss
- Partial closure of eyes
- Eyes with increased tear flow

- Eyes with thick discharge
- Sunken abdomen
- Prominent ribs
- Dry skin
- Loss of elasticity
- Obvious pain
- Discharge from the trunk
- Coughing
- Abdominal respiratory sounds
- Mucous membranes become pale, muddy, bright red or dry
- Unusualbehaviour
- Decreased movement
- Exercise intolerance

Signs of pain in elephants

- Frequent trumpeting or screaming
- Frequent changing of limbs
- Defective obedience
- Aggression
- Frequent turning to sides
- Vigorous shaking of head regions
- Standing without any movement for a long time
- Uncontrollable aggression related signs
- Violent behaviour, all time
- Spreading of ears with making of hissing like sounds
- More alert appearance of the eyes
- Unpredicted movement patterns
- Biting the tip of trunk for a long time.
- Beating of trunk on the ground as a mark of discontent or anger
- Pushing against some objects like pillar, wall etc.
- Frequent sitting and getting up
- Frequent lifting and kicking activities of limbs

Feeding

- Quantity of feed consumed in a day during 18 hours of feeding is about 280 Kg of feed.
- Time spent by free ranging elephants in feeding is about 18 hours.
- Nature of feed consumed in wild may be low in nutrients but high in fibers.

RATION (ON EMPIRICAL BASIS) FOR ELEPHANTS WEIGHING 3000 KGS/DAY

Roughages

150-200 kgs/day, in the form of bamboo leaves, grasses, ficus, twigs, palm leaves etc.

Concentrates

Horse gram	5 kgs
Ragi	7 kgs
Rice	3 kgs
Salt	100 gms
Mineral mixture	100 gms
Jaggery	50 gms

VACCINATION

Anthrax

Prophylactic vaccination is recommended in elephants, as follows:

Elephants of 2-5 years of age 1 ml (S/C route)

Elephants of 5-10 years 1.5 ml (S/C route)

Elephants of 10-15 years 2 ml (S/C route)

Elephants of 15-20 years 2.5 ml (S/C route)

Elephants of 20 years and older 3 ml (S/C route)

Note: In elephants, the caudal fold may be chosen for the subcutaneous administration of anthrax spore vaccine.

FMD

Animal may be vaccinated against FMD esp. In the endemic regions or during OBR.

Haemorrhagic septicaemia

Animal may be vaccinated against HS in endemic areas or during OBR.

Tetanus

Vaccination against tetanus may be carried out. One 1ml by I/M as the first dose at 3 months of age and booster at 4 months of age may be given. (Tetanus antitoxins may be given to elephants that are suspected to have chances of infection with *Clostridium tetani*). Prophylaxis is by administration of tetanus toxoid at rate of 6 – 10 ml by I/M route.

Rabies

Animal may be vaccinated against Rabies esp. in endemic regions.

HERPES VIRAL INFECTIONS

In Asian elephants, Endotheliotrophic Elephant Herpes Virus (EEHV) causes fatal haemorrhagic disease, attacking endothelial cells (blood vessels, heart and similar organs). This disease is 90 per cent fatal and preferentially targets juvenile captive zoo elephants. These are the emerging infections esp. in elephant calves and cardiac region is highly affected and swelling is noticed in cheek and thorax regions.

8

Disease Management in Wild Animals

Wildlife diseases have gained some good momentum in the recent years due to the complex-linkage with zoonosis, conflicts between wild fauna and homo sapiens in an ascending manner, environmental health care measures etc. Due to this, considerable pressure is there on zoo veterinarians or the field veterinarians working in free ranging areas of forests like national parks, wildlife sanctuaries etc.

Whenever dealing with wildlife health and diseases in various wild animals of this country, veterinarians often encounter technical-embarrassment due to the lack of adequate technical information related to the health and diseases in wild animals.

With regard to disease conditions affecting wild fauna, though many disease conditions have been documented in South India, it is also equally true that still there are large number of conditions that may warrant in-depth analysis towards establishing the confirmatory diagnosis in case of wild fauna of this part or most parts of this country, and this situation exists often, regardless of whether the wild animals are reared in captive (or) in free ranging regions that are being administered by forest department officials-the custodians of the forests, in this country. Important wildlife diseases are dealt in this paper.

Management of diseases in captivity is an art to be exercised by the Zoo Veterinarians and often it becomes a team work in which zoo personnel like Director of the zoo or zoological park or zoological garden, Range officers and animal keepers and biologists of the zoos have coordinating roles in the field of wildlife conservation and management.

Priority measures for the effective management of diseases in the captive wild animals

Veterinarians working in the zoological parks often get perplexed by the complex nature of the concerned species which are totally different from each other in terms of biology, physiology, anatomy, exhibition of symptoms, reactions to the therapeutic management measures. Though the treatment of many diseases or disorders in captive wild animals is often a complex one which is routinely carried out by the concerned zoo veterinarians, it becomes the duty of the other officials like the range–officers to understand some fundamental features like the common symptoms that are likely to be encountered in the concerned disease or disorder and middle level officers always need to think on how best the contributions are to be made towards the up keeping of the health status of the wild animal species under investigation as well as towards how best they can apprise the symptomatology encountered in different species of wild fauna.

The clinical problem might be dealt in the initial stages by the veterinarians serving in the zoo. However, the middle level officer may supervise whether the tablets or drugs are administered in time by the concerned animal keeper of the cage.

Direct supervision needs to be executed by the middle level officers on the spot in this regard. Such activities exercised will not only help increase the morale of the animal keepers in up keeping the health status of the captive wild animal species but also, will help in speedy recovery of the concerned wild animal species by the timely drug administration, subsequent to the technical suggestions offered by the concerned zoo veterinarian.

Role in management of vector and vector based diseases

First-hand knowledge on the various features of the causative agents that are associated with disease occurrence is an important factor in this regard. The eradication of vector and the related diseases is often used in disease management programmes that are directed against various types of causal agents prevalent in the zoos.

Extra efforts need to be carried out in the control measures against vectors like clearance of bushes around the enclosures of different wild animals belonging to various species and taxonomical groups with varying peculiarities in biology etc. Captive wild animals are highly vulnerable to vector based diseases like felids etc. and wild animal species like those belonging to felidae family are more generally more vulnerable to occurrence of diseases like trypanasomosis, as the case with camelids.

Habitat modification as a measure of management of diseases in captive wild animals

This can be done in a systematic manner. The most direct type of habitat modification is the usage of appropriate disinfectants in the captive wild animal places. Lyme may be used to destroy the helminthic eggs on the sites used for feeding. Glutaraldehyde may be used to disinfect premises in the event of microbial agent based disease-occurrence.

Habitat modification helps to reduce the number or availability of disease causing agents. The substrate has to be changed most of the times, since many parasitic stages may occur in a recurring manner, frequently posing problems to the healthy status of the wild animals confined in different types of enclosures. Hence, the period of change of substrate should be noted down in a register and this has to be monitored in a periodical manner.

Effective rodent management control measures as a measure of disease management

Many a times, persons tend to ask the reasons for need of rodent control programme in the zoos and one should understand that the rodents are associated with species related to ecology in the environment despite the fact that they also at times become finally a prey species to the concerned wild animal species.

It is to be remembered that diseases get transmitted from rodents to other wild animals. If urine from rodents fall on water resources of the concerned wild animal species, there is a likey chances of occurrence of leptospirosis in them which may cause jaundice or even abortion in the affected wild animal species that are in the immuno-compromised status.

Proper disposal of feed wastes as one of the disease management measures

It is an accepted fact that the feed wastages do occur in many zoos due to multifaceted factors. If they are not properly disposed off, then the scavenging animal in the surrounding areas may often tend to congregate at that place and hence, there may be a spread of wildlife disease causing agents in that area, ultimately affecting the weak animals. Hence, this feature needs to be specifically monitored in a periodical manner by the middle level officials of the zoos. However, the concerned animal keeper needs to be enlightened about the proper disposal of feed wastes in the zoo atmosphere and cleanliness of the disposal place need to be maintained in a perfect manner in a continuous manner.

Management of disease by proper carcass disposal

The practice of scattering of carcases in the premises needs to be avoided. To avoid the disease contamination, the carcass needs to be incinerated in the properly installed and maintained incinerator and the functioning of the incinerator needs to be monitored on a continuous basis. Lyme may be added to the pits if the small sized carcasses are buried due to management based reasons.

Disease management during quarantine or relocation

The strict control of avoiding the visitors to the quarantine section needs to be exercised. Only designated individuals should be permitted in the quarantine section which houses the usually a charming wild animal species. Foot paths should be provided at the entrance of the quarantine section and it's usage needs to be ensured by the visiting personnel of the zoo regularly. Similarly, whenever wild animals are being dislocated or relocated, this should be carried out in a systematic manner. Particularly the sick animals under transport to the veterinary hospital need an additional health care measures. The falling of discharge if any may be avoided and suitable disinfectants may be used in the concerned spots to minimize the contamination of the environment with disease causing agents.

Effective liaison with animal keepers as disease management measure

The middle level officers need to maintain the effective liaison with animal keepers who need a continuous monitoring during the upkeeping of the health care status of the captive wild animal species. Proper delivery of drugs in time needs to be supervised effectively.

Enlightening the role of animal keepers in disease management

Animal keepers need to be enlightened on their vital role in the disease management in the affected captive wild animal species. Followings are to be observed seriously and is to be reported to both range officer and in particular the zoo veterinarians who have to visit the enclosures on daily basis.

1. Feeding activity
2. Defecation and Urination activity
3. Resting activity
4. Time taken to go to the yard after the opening of the gate
5. External swellings / bleedings
6. Movement patterns
7. Excessive fly accumulation in any part of the body
8. Any abnormal activity like vomiting, diarrhoea
9. Signs of heat occurrence if it is a female animal.

9

Bacterial Diseases in Wild Animals

Wild life diseases are given more priority in the recent days due to the fact that conservation of any wild fauna can't be achieved fully, unless due efforts are equally given pertaining to the assessment of health status and the disease management, in the concerned wild animal species.

Bacterial diseases are in plenty in case of wild animals esp. the captive wild animals and they pose problems in the diagnosis as well as the treatment. Hence, one should have a thorough understanding of various bacterial disease conditions that affect commonly the wild animals belonging to multiple taxonomic classes or groups.

Significant Bacterial Diseases

- Tuberculosis
- Haemorrhagicsepticaemia
- Leptospirosis
- Anthrax
- Tetanus
- Enterotoxaemia
- Salmonellosis
- *Escherichia coli* infections
- Wound infections

Tuberculosis

- The disease is chronic in nature and is caused by Mycobacterium tuberculosis,
- Mycobacterium bovis and Mycobacterium avium.
- This disease caused by *Mycobacterium bovis* is very common in general.
- These organisms are acid-fast in nature.

Species affected

- Almost all species are affected in general. The disease is somewhat widely
- prevalent in a captive wild animal atmosphere.
- Commonly affected species are given below:
  - Mammals (Non-human primates, cervids, antelopes, felids, ursids, canids, elephants etc.).
  - Aves (Raptors, Psittacine birds, Passerine birds, Anseriform birds etc.).

Note

Documented frequently in cervids, antelopes, non-human primates under captivity and some times, tuberculosis is revealed in elephants esp. those reared under captivity and to a lesser extent in carnivores.

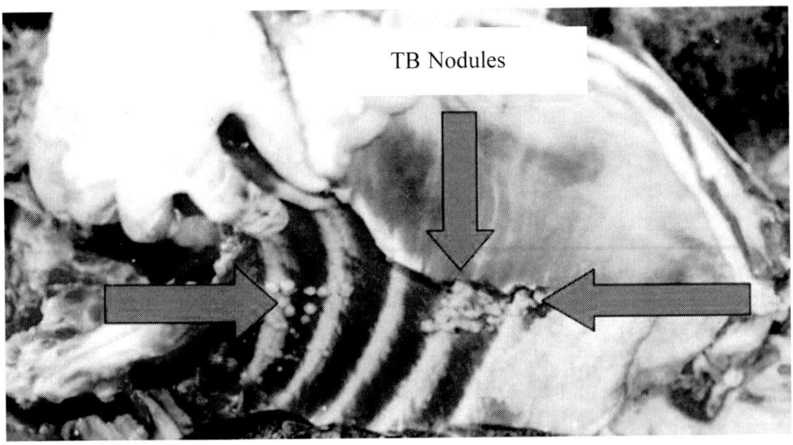

Fig. 1. (TB nodules on organs)

Mode of spread and significance

- Discharges from the body like vaginal discharge, exudates from the fistulous tracks, milk, sputum and excreta like feces and urine get contaminated with these microbes.
- The bacterial organisms are also shed in exhaled air also.
- This disease is zoonotic in nature.

Symptoms

- Emaciation despite moderate to good nutrition
- Anorexia

- Weakness
- Mild pyrexia
- Low pitched cough may be seen

Diagnosis and therapy

- By culture tests, ELISA tests, PCR tests etc. Tuberculin tests may have falsepositive results some times.
- In dead animals, the tubercles may be seen in various organs esp. the lungs. Smears from the lesions may be subjected to the staining for the diagnosticpurpose.
- The therapy consists of usage of combination of drugs like isoniazid, ethambutol, pyrizanamide and rifampin. Enrofloxacin may also be used in thecombination.

Treatment, Prevention and Control of TB in animals

Currently, treatment of bovine tuberculosis is not recommended due to its infectious nature. If an animal is found to be infected, it should be removed from the zoo. However, there are some preventative measures available. One way to ensure that cattle do not become infected is to eliminate any possible interaction with deer.

- Post mortem inspection (looking for tubercles in the lungs, lymph nodes, intestines, liver, spleen, pleura, and peritoneum), for detection of infected wild animals,
- Intensive surveillance including zoo-visits,
- Systematic individual testing of susceptible wild animal species in random manner.
- Removal of infected and in-contact animals,
- Effective movement controls,
- Individual animal identification
- Though vaccination is practiced in human medicine, it is not used as a prophylactic measure in case of wild animals under captivity and investigations with regard to the prophylaxis for tuberculosis in wild fauna are still going on through out the world.

Treatment of tuberculosis in elephants

This is not much advisable. However, following therapy regimen shall be adapted.

Treatment Phase	Drug	Frequency	Notes
Intensive	Isoniazid (INH) 2-5 mg/kg rectally plus Pyrazinamide 20 mg/kg rectally or Ethambutol (ETH) 15mg/ kg orally plus Rifampin (RIF) 10 mg/kg orally kg plus/or LEVO, 15 mg/ rectally	5 days per week	INH should be started as soon as possible and even before other drugs Combination of 3 drugs should continue for minimum of 8-10 weeks
Continuation	INH 5-7 mg/kg rectally plus RIF, 10mg/kg orally plus/ or LEVO, 15 mg/kg rectally	3 days per week	44 weeks

Public health problems

Post mortem inspection (looking for tubercles in the lungs, lymph nodes, and intestines) to be done. The most common form of TB in people is caused by *M. tuberculosis.* However, it is not possible to clinically differentiate infections caused by *M. tuberculosis* from those caused by *M. bovis*, which is estimated to account for up to 10% of human tuberculosis cases in some countries. Diagnosis may be further complicated by the tendency of *M. bovis* infections to be located in tissues other than the lungs (i.e. extrapulmonary infections) and the fact that *M. bovis* is naturally resistant to one of the antimicrobials that is commonly used to treat human tuberculosis, pyrazinamide.

Paratuberculosis

The disease is caused by *Mycobacterium paratuberculosis* and is a rod-shaped organism resembling the tuberculosis bacillus.

Species affected

- Mostly bovids, wild sheep, wild goat, antelopes, cervids etc. may get affected.
- It was even reported in equines and swines have been reported as the carriers.

Mode of spread and significance

- Ingestion of food and water contaminated by the feces of infected animals.
- Intra-uterine transmission occurs at a fifty percent incidence from the infected mother.
- This disease is the one causing specific-infectious enteritis, in the affected wild animals.

Symptoms

- Profuse diarrhea that is more often odorless, and there is no accompanying tetanus. There appears to be no correlation between the severity of the clinical syndrome and the severity of the lesions.
- Emaciation and intermandibular-oedema.

Diagnosis and therapy

- By culture, PCR tests and by staining with acid-fast preparations like Ziehl-Neelsen and Ponder-Kinyoun stains. Also, biopsies of lymph nodes, FAT, fecal culture, complement fixation tests, stained fecal smears also help the diagnosis.
- In dead animals, hypertrophied intestinal mucosa is seen and the primary site of infection is the lower gastro-intestinal tract mainly the posterior jejunum and ileum **(Most of the bacilli are seen in the macrophages and giant cells)**.
- There is no true therapy for Johnes disease but general therapy may be carried out, with broad spectrum antibiotics to ameliorate the clinical signs, esp. with fluidsand electrolytes.
- **Broadspectrum-antibiotics** are to be given to control the secondary bacterial infections.
- Fluids and vitamins may be given taking care of the animal's condition.

Prevention and control

- Reduce newborns' exposure to M. paratuberculosis at calving.
- Provide clean feed for youngstock (preferably to 24 months).
- Provide clean water for youngstock (preferably to 24 months).
- Keep youngstock separate from adults and their manure.

Pasteurellosis

The incidence of Pasteurellosis is a world wide. Pasteurellosis or haemorrhagic septicaemia has been documented in many wild animal species like gaur, hippopotamus, chital, barking deer, captive African lion cub, bear etc. Recently it was documented in elephants and tigress. The disease is caused by Pasteurella multocida organisms. Overcrowding, stress factors like long time- transport related event, inclement weather etc. may precipitate this disease. Pneumonia and septicaemia related signs are dominant. Acute deaths are commonly encountered in case of the pasteurellosis affected wild animals.

Avian cholera caused by *Pasteurella* spp. organisms is found commonly around the monsoon period in the captive semi-aquatic and aquatic aviary species and the haemorrhagic lesions over heart region and nectrotic foci on liver occur in aves like raptors, as furnished below.

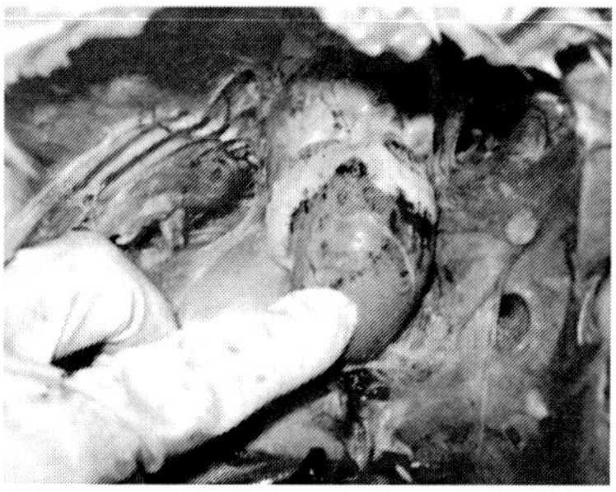

Fig. 2. (Haemorrhagic spots on heart)

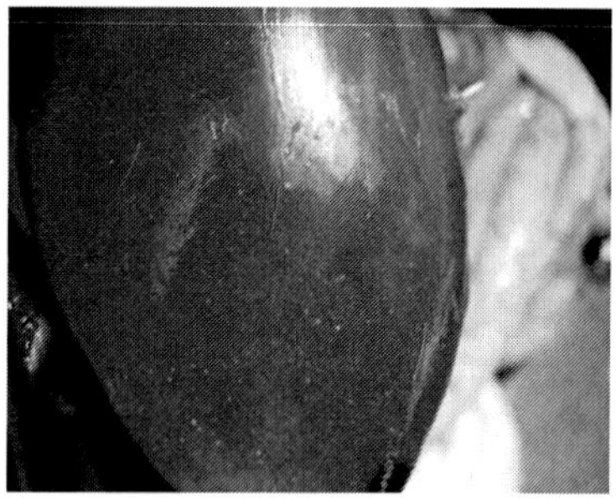

Fig. 3. (Necrotic foci on liver)

SIMILARLY, LIVER REVEALS WHITE SPOTS AS PRESENTED IN RAPTORS

Species affected

- This disease is documented in various species of animals including elephants, cervids, antelopes, ursids, felids, elephants etc.
- Even marsupials like kangaroo get affected by this infection.

Mode of spread and significance

- Organisms get passed through contaminated food materials by infected rodentsetc. Overcrowding and strenuous events like a prolonged transport etc. lead to the precipitation of this disease condition in case of wild animals. It is not uncommon to find the peracute occurrence of this disease condition.
- This is a highly infectious disease in general.

Symptoms

- In elephants, the symptoms may be similar to those of anthrax. The death occurs within 12 hours in case of acute cases.
- The clinical symptoms are often related to the pleuropneumonia, dyspnoea, gastroenteritis in addition to the pyrexia, anorexia and depression.

Diagnosis and therapy

- By PCR, examination of the heart blood-smear, biological test and culture from oral or nasal mucus and some times from feces help the diagnosis, in addition to the ELISA based tests etc.

- Post mortem reveals splenomegaly, petechial haemorrhage on lungs, epicardium, kidneys etc. Respiratory tract (upper regions)infections including tracheitis and red hepatization of the lungs are the common findings. Are common and if aves are affected, it may be having necrotic foci on liver along with the petechial hemorrhage on epicardium and lungs.
- Tetracyclines, sulphonamides and fluoroquinolone compounds may assist the treatment of this condition in a successful manner.

Leptospirosis

- This is a significant disease that is caused by multiple serovars of the leptospires. Affected animals whether it is wild in free ranging or captive status become highly dull and lethargic.
- This disease has been documented in multiple species of wild animals, in general.

Species affected

- Most of the wild animal species get affected like ruminants, ursids, proboscids, felids,canids, marsupials and monotremes, peccaries and suids, procyonids, rodents and lagomorphs, rodents, viverrids, insectivores, pinnipeds etc.
- Outbreaks have been documented in case of non-human primates esp. the baboons and macaques. Rodents including mongooses act as carriers for this disease.

Mode of spread and significance

- Spread is mainly by the contaminated urine sample by rodent-urine etc.
- This disease is of zoonotic significance and affected human may reveal symptoms like myalgia, head ache, fever, sore throat, joint and neck pain, abdominal cramps etc.

Diagnosis and therapy

- Serolgoical examinations, culture, MAT, PCR finding of the organisms in the tissues etc.
- Therapy consists of usage of compounds like streptomycin, penicillins, tetracyclines (10 mg/kg bwt, IV, IM & PO) esp. doxycycline (10 mg/kg bwt, PO or IV, daily for 24 days)

Anthrax

- Anthrax itself is a well-known disease with a great degree of public significance.

- In case of elephants, sub-cutaneous oedema may be found, along with bursting of few swellings on body.
- However, bloody discharge from natural orifices is a commonly found symptom in case of wild bovids, cervids, antelopes etc.
- This disease has been documented in felids, canids, perissodactylids, primates, wildsuids etc.
- Instant death is commonly encountered in anthrax affected elephants esp. in the free ranging pachyderms.

Brucellosis

Brucellosishas been documented in many wild animal species but in south India, the disease related documentations are not much in case of wild animals. A field veterinarian however should be aware of this condition leading to abortion in multiple species of wild animals.

- This has marked public health significance and the reports on the documentation of this dangerous disease among wild stock are many.
- This disease has been documented in case of chital, blackbuck etc. In general, it can be quoted that the hooved mammals, lagomorphs, rodents and canids get affected by this disease condition.
- Bacteria are shed in milk or via the aborted fetus, afterbirth or other reproductive tract discharges. In addition to the abortion,
- Abortion is a commonly found symptom in many animal species and is of zoonotic significance. Hence, dure precautions esp. during the attending of dystokia in immobilized animals in a zoo-environment.
- Treatment is not much satisfactory and vaccination is to be considered based on due research in the concerned species.

Tetanus

Documented frequently in non-human primates, cervids, antelopes and some times, tuberculosis is revealed in elephants esp. those reared under captivity and to a lesser extent in carnivores.Overall, tetanus hasbeen documented in animals like elephants and non-human primates, in general. Death of number of elephants due to affection by tetanus like conditions was documented over a period of many years, in Kerala state.

Trismus was partial (or) full in case of tetanus cases in the affected elephants. Salivation and inability to drink water in addition to the stiffness of gait and difficulty in movements with dilatation of pupils were the commonly encountered signs in case of affected elephants.

- Clostridial organisms cause this condition in which muscular rigidity is the prominent feature. This is commonly noticed in captive elephants that met with injuries or those undergone surgical interventions as during the management of deep wounds in foot pads of captive elephants, non-human primates, cervids etc.
- Clostridial organsisms live longer in moist regions and in soil ; these organisms may be found even in feces of equids, homosapiens, bovids etc. In case of affected elephants, this causes death in large number of elephants.
- In elephants affected with tetanus, after an incubation period of 15-20 days, neurotoxins are produced that damage the nervous system and cause typical muscular spasms. Through wounds by means of contamination from rubbing by trunk (or) though even the cut-ends of tusks, these anaerobic organisms spread fastly.

  Clinical symptoms comprise diarrhea, loss of appetite, listlessness and death, in addition to the stiffness of limbs.
- The therapy consists of administration of antitoxins and high levels of antibiotics, includinfg the muscle relaxants. Drugs like penicillin, (Amoxicillin trihydrate: Dose in elephants: 5.5 mg/kg bwt, IM) or fluoroquinolones like enrofloxacin (Dose in elephants: 5 mg/kg bwt, IM) shall be administered for treatment of tetanus.

Botulism

Botulismis one of the important bacterial diseases and documentations are not available about the occurrence of this condition in wild animals of South India. However, it is to be remembered that this disease caused by *Clostridium botulinum* has been documented in pheasantry unit at UP.

- This disease affects the birds belonging to Anseriformes and incidences were also found in the mink, also.
- There are seven separate forms of botulinum toxins (A to G) are noticed and among these, the botulinum toxin C is the most common among the wild animal species like wild ducks and geese, pheasants, chickens, mink, bovids (in bovids, Type D botulism is also commonly encountered) and equids. Type C botulism mainly occurs among the birds, in summer seasons.
- The ingestion and wound infections are the primary routes of this infection in case of wild animal species.
- Affected species may reveal the neurological symptoms that are often fatal.

Klebsiella infections

- Klebsiella and other vector borne gram negative bacteria (pseudomonas) are primary opportunistic pathogens, affecting the non-human primates.
- *Klebsiella* is present in stagnant water, dirty drinking receptacles and soil and as flora of alimentary tract.

Colibacillosis

- These infections are caused by *Escherichia coli* organisms affecting the wide variety of birds as well as the mammals esp. the neonatal animals and affected mammals often assume recumbency if reveals severe enteritis, as revealed below

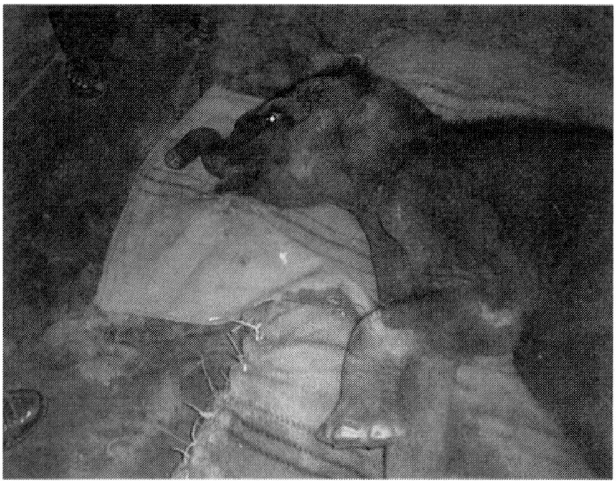

Fig. 4. (Elephant calf with severe diarrhoea)

- Incidences have been found throughout the world among the various wild animal species.
- Fecal-oral route is the mode of transmission of these organisms, in most of the conditions. The culture tests may assist the confirmation of thismicrobial infections.
- Enteritis occur in the affected wild animal species.

Bumblefoot

These conditions caused by bacterial infections have been documented in aviary species like pin tailed ducks and staphylococcal infection is generally attributed as the causal factor affecting the connective tissue of the foot and it often leads to the occurrence of podo-dermatitis or foot abscess in the aviary species, as the case with captive Galliformes, in general.

Campylobacteriosis

- This was earlier classified as a member of the family vibriacae but recently re-classified as a separate group.
- *Campylobacter jejuni* causes entero-colitis in a variety of mammals and birds including man. This is frequently reported in non-human primates.

Salmonellosis

- This is more common in most of the animal species esp. in case of non-human primates and reptiles.
- The affected animals may suffer from severe diarrhea and is of zoonotic significance.
- In wild animals like felids, *salmonella typhimurium* and other species cause this disease condition the
- Gastro-intestinal signs in addition to septicemia.
- Documentations are available on isolation of the most serious human pathogens of the groups namely-*Shigella dysenterriae type I* and *Salmonella typhi.*
- Symptoms comprise weakness, edema of face and neck and diarrhea with mucus and /or blood.

Other bacterial infections

- Most of the carnivores get affected by the infections with *Streptococcus* sp., *Staphylococcus* sp. and *Corynebacterium* sp. frequently.
- These organisms may be cultured from animals with neonatal polyarthritis, pneumonia, septicemia and abscesses.
- Similarly, *Corynebacterium pyogenes*is found with abscesses, arthritis, metritisand cystitis.
- Colic like disorders and corneal opacity like conditions may be encountered in animal like elephant.

10

Viral Disease in Wild Animals

Viral diseases in herbivores

- Viral diseases causing problems to the routine performance of the wild animals are caused substantially by many viral agents also.
- In both the captive and free ranging wildlife regions, the diseases caused by different viral agents are being documented throughout the world.
- However, the research findings are still to be improved in this regard due to variousreasons.

Foot and mouth disease (FMD)

- This disease occurs in case of wild ruminants and other artiodactylids, in general. Affected wild animal species may have lesions in the foot and mouth.
- This disease may lead to severe morbidity among the hooved stock.
- This disease has been documented in herbivores like gaurs, cervids, suids etc. and is common among wild fauna but needs documentation in most of the cases.
- Elephants, gaurs, deer, antelopes, wild pigs and camelids are often affected.

FMD lesion in gaur

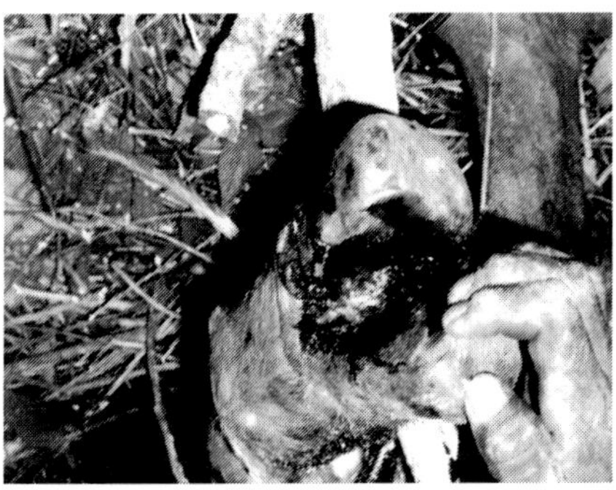

Fig. 5. Ulcer in inter-hoof area

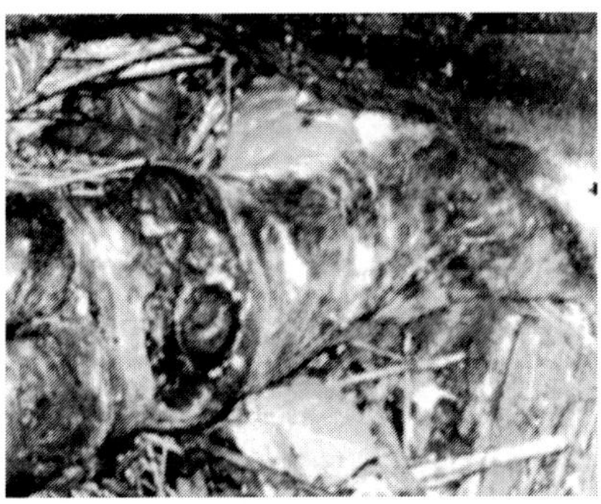

Fig. 6. Ulcer at skin near hoof

Rabies

Rabies may occur in many animal species including deer, antelope etc. This disease was documented in mongoose, deer like Sanghai deer and hog deer. An elephant calf was clinically suspected for rabies. Paralytic symptom was dominant in an elephant cow died due to rabies. Outbreak was quoted affecting jackals in Nilgiri and Dharmapuri areas of Tamil Nadu state.

Rabies has been documented in chital, rhino, elephants etc. Even oral infection has been documented in foxes and skunks by experimental means, following the ingestion of mouse carcasses infected by rabies virus.

It is noteworthy to mention that the exposure to rabies virus in peripheral nerves could potentially occur when a person with wounds on the hands does not wear any protective covering or gloves while skinning rabies suspected captive wild animal.

Signs & Lesions in Wild Animals affected by rabies esp.deer

- Ethology-charging in deer
- Reddish eyes
- Maniacal behaviour
- Signs of excitement for 3 days prior to death

Prophylaxis

In endemic regions, appropriate anti-rabies vaccines shall be administered in the concerned captive wild animal species.

Vaccination related details in general

- EPHEMERAL FEVER (insect borne virus): No vaccine
- PESTE-DES-PETITS disease (Goat plague): RP TC vaccine is being used.
- FMD (Aphthous fever): Raksha SC 3ml for captive wild bovids& calf.
- 1 ml for captive wild sheep and goat q 6 months.
- Hoechst FMD (O,A, C& ASIA-1) 10 ml for adult bovids; 5 ml for captive.

Sheep and goat and calves q 6 months

- WARTS (Contagious bovine virus: Papilloma virus).
- HERPES VIRUS: No vaccine.
- COW POX (Gel adsorbent vaccine).
- **BLUE TONGUE** (Avianised Live vaccine or tissue culture vaccine shall be used).

Blue tongue

Ruminant species like deer, antelopes etc. are commonly affected by this viral disease. Facial oedema, diarrhea, lameness etc. are the symptoms noticed in the affected wild animal species. Blue tongue like disease was documented in captive Indian wild ruminants.

- Intractable diarrhoea
- No specific therapy but fluid and electrolytes.
- Reduce newborns' exposure to paratuberculosis at calving
- Provide clean feed for youngstock (preferably to 24 months)
- Provide clean water for youngstock (preferably to 24 months)
- Keep youngstock separate from adults and their manure.
- Vaccination programme should be carried out.

VIRAL DISEASES IN CARNIVORES AND OMNIVORES

Feline panleukopenia of felids

Feline infectious enteritis (FIE) is a disease caused by infection with feline parvovirus (FPV), also known as feline panleukopenia virus. It is sometimes referred to as panleukopenia virus because one of the results of infection is the development of a low white blood cell count.The mortality rate is very high among the felids whether domestic or wild, in general and was the first viral disease identified among the domesticated cats.

In felids over three (or) four weeks of age and in adult felids, the virus causes a very severe gastroenteritis, following an incubation period of 5 to 9 days. Affected felids develop acute onset-haemorrhagic vomiting and diarrhoea and some felids may die rapidly. The virus causes severe damage to the lining of the intestine and some felids may die before even showing signs of gastroenteritis.

Acute in onset with haemorrhagic diarrhea; intestinal villi get damaged and the virus also travels via the blood to the bone marrow and lymph glands. Viral replication at these sites leads to a marked depletion of white blood cells.

Transplacental mode of infection in feline panleukopenia

Due to interference of virus in developing brain tissues of cubs, the cubs may then be born with a condition known as cerebellar hypoplasia (lack of development of the cerebellum- a part of the brain needed for fine coordination of movement). Cubs may initially seem fine, but as they start to move and walk it becomes obvious that they are highly uncoordinated.This may also happen in very young cubs of less than 4 weeks of age.

TREATMENT, PREVENTION AND CONTROL

Symptomatic treatment is to be carried out

- Interferons are chemicals made in the body that can exert an antiviral effect and shall be used.
- Recombinant feline interferon omega (or human interferon products) might be of some help in the treatment of severe cases (NOTE: Feline interferon has been shown to have successful usage in managing dogs with parvovirus infection).
- Highly effective vaccines are available and all felids including the cubs should be vaccinated.
- Modified live vaccines should not be used in pregnant felids (or) the felids that are immunosuppressed and, in such cases, inactivated (killed) vaccines are recommended.
- Control of the spread of FPV relies on both vaccination and good management practice, including disinfection (with appropriate disinfectants) and use of isolation procedures.
- When faced with an outbreak of FPV in a colony of felids, vaccinating all the felids will help and anti-FPV serum may be given to susceptible felids to help protect them by providing antibodies against the virus.

Feline leukemia virus-disease (FELV)

Feline leukaemia virus (FeLV) is an exogenous gamma-retrovirus (enveloped, single-stranded RNA) enzootic to domestic cat. The course of disease is somewhat variable pending the infectious strain of FeLV (FeLV-A, -B, or -C) and what endogenous retroviruses are present in the host's genome.

It is the recombination of these retroviruses within the host that influence pathogenicity (The surface glycoprotein and promoter region sequence of the infecting FeLV strain are the two most significant pathogenic determinants).

Feline lymphosarcoma

Four forms occur (based upon the location of the primary tumour), as follows.

- Multicentric- tumours originate from many lymphoid and non-lymphoid tissues
- Thymic- originate from the thymus; most often seen in neonates
- Alimentary- originate from gastrointestinal lymphoid tissues and/or mesenteric lymphnodes; most often seen in older individuals.
- Unclassified- all tumors originate in non- lymphoid tissue (skin, eyes, CNS).

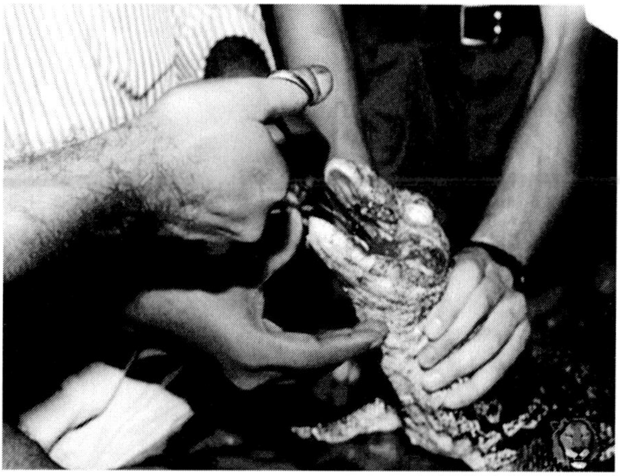

Fig. 7. Extraction of tumour like growth from oral region of reptile

Feline myeloproliferative diseases & anaemia (based on lineage targeted)

- Erythremic myelosis- erythroid progenitors occur.
- Granulocytic leukaemia- granulocytic myeloid progenitor, often neutrophil lineage.
- Erythroleukaemia- granulocytic myeloid and erythroid progenitors .
- Myelofibrosis- malignant proliferation of fibroblasts and cancerous bone; causes medullary osteosclerosis and myelofibrosis.

Neoplastic bonemarrow cells/Non-regenerative anaemia and/or immuno-suppression occur.

Immunopathologic disease associated with FeLV infection:

Prolonged high level of AG-AB complexes (trapped in glomerular capillaries damaging renal tissues) occurs. Antibody-dependent cytotoxicity against viral antigens expressed on lymphocyte surfaces may lead to lymphocyte depletion, increasing the animal's susceptibility to inflammatory and infectious diseases.

Fibrosarcoma: This may (or) may not be virus-associated, if FeLV associated; it is typically seen in younger individuals and is very proliferative with frequent metastases. This form, referred to as feline sarcoma virus, is replication defective and cannot be transmitted.

Transmission of feline leukemia virus

- The virus is shed in saliva, nasal secretions, urine, feces & milk of he infected felids.

- Felid-to-felid transfer of the virus may occur from a bite-wound, during mutual grooming, and (rarely) through the shared use of litter-places and feeding places/vessels.
- Transmission is also thro' transplacental / transmammary
- Virus survives only for a few hours outside the felid-body, under normal household conditions.

Followings are the clinical signs of feline leukemia viral disease

- Loss of appetite.
- Progressive weight loss.
- Poor coat condition.
- Enlarged lymph nodes.
- Persistent fever.
- Pale gums and other mucus membranes.
- Inflammation of the gums (gingivitis) and mouth (stomatitis)
- Infections of the skin, urinary bladder, and upper respiratory tract often occur.

Feline immunodeficiency viral disease (FIV)

Although FIV is similar to HIV (the human immunodeficiency virus), FIV causes a feline disease that is similar to AIDS (acquired immune deficiency syndrome) in humans. It is a highly species-specific virus that infects only felines.There is currently no evidence that FIV can infect (or) cause disease in humans.

Transmission: Mainly by bites.

Clinical symptoms of FIV

- Poor coat condition & persistent fever with a loss of appetite are common in infected felids.
- Gingivitis & stomatitis.
- Chronic (or) recurrent infections of the skin, eyes, urinary bladder, and upper respiratory tract are often present.
- Persistent diarrhoea like varieties of eye-conditions.
- Some felids may reveal seizures, behavior changes & other NS signs
- Generalized but usually temporary enlargement of the lymph nodes.

Corona viral infection

Documented by Wildlife Conservation Society in 2020 in one of the captive Malayan Tiger.

Measles (Rubeola), viral hepatitis, kyasanur forest disease (KFD) and others

- Measles is one of the most frequently reported viral diseases of non human primates and upon infection; the virus is shed and can re-infect man.
- This is a highly infectious exanthematous viral disease of children. This has been documented in marmosets, tamarins, owl monkeys etc. and is fatal to them.
- Several outbreaks of viral hepatitis have been documented in primate handlers and primate practitioners.
- The virus causing human infectious hepatitis (hepatitis A) can infect chimpanzees, patas, wooley monkey, gorilla, tamarins, cebus etc.
- KFD has been reported in non human primates in states like karnatka and kerala states and is of zoonotic importance. Periodical monitoring of free ranging as well as captive non-human primates is to be strengthened.
- The KFD was documented in non-human primates like common langurs and bonnet macaques of Karnataka state. Outbreak occurred among these non-human primates causing death in these species. This is a tick borne flavi viral disease and among ten species of ticks, it was the *Hemophysalis spinigera* that was found to be responsible for the occurrence of epizootics and epidemics in these areas.

Herpes virus and pox virus infections

- Herpes virus infections are documented in non-human primates, elephant calves etc. In man, herpes B virus can be fatal, causing an acute ascending myelitis.
- Rhesus macaques and cyanomolgus are considered as the primary natural hosts.
- Lesions in non-human primates are mostly confined to the mucosa of buccal cavity.
- Ulcers or vesicles do occur around the lips and external nares and the most common site is the tongue. Monkey bites and laboratory accidents lead to the most human infections.

- Pox virus infections often are classified into four types in non-human primates, elephants etc. All these four diseases are infectious to man but it is to be remembered that the monkey pox is the most frequent one.
- Pox virus infections often are infectious to man but it is to be remembered that the monkey pox is the most frequent one that may cause problems. Pox virus was documented in chimpanzees reared under captive conditions. Exotic ruminant under captive condition like mufflon revealed the evidences of this infection.
- Pox virus was documented in chimpanzee under captive condition reared at zoological gardens.

Management: Isolate the affected ones and treat the secondary bacterial infections which are common in general.

Respiratory infections

- These are common in case of felids. Feline viral rhinotracheitis is the most common of the diseases that affect the felid group.
- Transmission is through the saliva and respiratory secretions contaminating the feed resources.
- Incubation period of this viral infection is two to four days. In case of calci viral infections of felids, it is one to two days.
- Symptoms comprise the weight loss, signs of dehydration, anorexia, fever and salivation along with sneezing and reluctance to drink.

Canine Distemper

- This is a viral disease affecting the canids as well as the felids.
- The occurrence of canine distemper in case of felids as an outbreak has been documented among the free ranging lions in Africa.
- Affected ones reveal dullness, ataxia or deranged gait, anorexia, thick muco-purulent discharge etc. in general.

Prevention and control of viral diseases in carnivores

- Stray dog-entries are to be banned totally.
- Any violent animal inflicting injuries to human beings in the nearby fringe villages of the protected wildlife regions need to be captured and examined for evidences of rabies infection in them.
- Monitoring of such animals need to be intensified.

- Dogs reared in peripheral regions of the protected areas shall be duly vaccinated against rabies, canine distemper etc. in a periodical manner, in addition to the strengthening of health-care management –measures.
- Rabies infected domesticated dogs shall be euthanized subsequent the permission from the concerned authorities.
- Stray dogs always carry a disease related risks associated with Adeno virus, CD, Rabies, Tryps, Mange, Fungal infections etc.
- Stray dogs straying in WL areas of Tiger Reserves generally prey about more than 25. spp of wild fauna including wild pigs, cervids, antelopes, porcupines, rodents etc and hence, always, these dogs pose a health-risk problem for tigers.

National tiger conservation authority

SOP for stray dogs (COMMITTEE with government job holding veterinarian, veterinarian from other agency, NGO of that area, member of Animal Welfare Board are members), capture / breeding-control operatiion / release etc. are also dealt, in addition to the regulatiory measures on conservation of tigers at national level.

Nipah (Niv) viral infections in wildlife

Wildlife diseases like Nipah viral infections often gains more momentum in the current years due to the complex-linkage with zoonosis, conflicts between wild fauna and homo sapiens in an ascending manner, environmental health care measures etc.All diseases like Nipah virus for which wildlife act as a reservoir have an impact on animal populations (wild and domestic), economies and humans or a combination of all, need extra attention from the international community.

Whenever dealing with wildlife health and diseases in various wild fauna of this country, veterinarians often encounter technical-embarrassment due to the lack of followings.

- Baseline information in assessment of health status in different species of wild fauna are still not up to the mark expected with them due to multifaceted etiological factors and this situation exists often, regardless of whether the wild animals are reared in captive or in free ranging regions
- Adequate technical information related to the various features of diseases among the wild animals are lacking in many countries, including India.

Facts on nipah viral infections

- Nipah Virus is a disease listed in the World Organisation for Animal Health (OIE) Terrestrial Animal Health Code and must be reported to the OIE (OIE Terrestrial Animal Health Code)."OIE-Listed diseases, infections and infestations" (in force during 2018) included the Nipah virus encephalitis.
- Nipah virus been quoted as another product from the Asian "virus factory" (quote from a Swedish article, 2005).
- NiV infection in humans has a range of clinical presentations, from asymptomatic infection to acute respiratory syndrome and fatal encephalitis. NiV is also capable of causing disease in pigs and other domestic animals. There is no vaccine for either humans or animals, in general. The primary treatment for human cases is intensive supportive care.

International scenery of NiV

Nipah virus (NiV) and *Hendra virus* (HeV) - the only known members of the genus *Henipavirus,* are the two emerging Paramyxo viruses that are highly pathogenic in a variety of vertebrate animals, including humans (The Nipah virus has two strains, as revealed in India, ie) Malaysia (NiVM) and Bangladesh (NiVB) strains and both the strains have high fatality rates, between 60% and 85%). Bangladesh strain of Nipah virus is more pathogenic than the Malaysia strain of Nipah virus.NiP is closely related to Hendra virus (Hendra virus, is formerly known as equine morbillivirus pneumonia or acute equine respiratory syndrome, which is an acute, viral respiratory infection of horses and humans that has been reported in Australia). NiV has been earlier documented in Malaysia, Singapore and Bangladesh (near-annual frequency was documented in Bangladesh), Nepal, Philipines, Cambodia,Thailand, Madagascar and evidences have been documented even in China. NiV was first identified during an outbreak of disease that took place in Kampung Sungai Nipah, Malaysia in 1998. However, the pigs were found to be the intermediate hosts in Bangladesh. In the year-2004, strong evidences revealed that humans became infected with NiVHuman cases have been documented in India (Kerala state) in May, 2018 with human-casualty but without apparent related domestic animal.

- The incubation period (interval from infection to the onset of symptoms) is believed to range from 4 to 18 days. However, an incubation period as long as 45 days has been documented.
- Followings are the risk factors associated with prevalence of NiV.
    - Fear complex among public
    - Unrest among public

    - Social consequences
    - Technical dilemmas among scientists
    - Economic consequences (loss of domestic pigs)
    - Conservation-problems of wild fauna (Wild pigs as prey base for carnivore like Tiger & Fruit bats, assisting the pollination in wildlife regions to a great extent)

- Although a small minority of infected patients transmit Nipah virus, more than half of the identified cases were found to result from person-to-person transmission **(Nosocomial infections are very significant in case of NiV).**
- In 62 (51%) Nipah virus-infected patients, illness developed 5-15 days after close contact with another Nipah case-patient and the Nipah case-patients having the difficulty in breathing were more likely to transmit Nipah, than those without respiratory difficulties.
- There is no effective treatment for Nipah virus disease, but ribavarin may alleviate the symptoms of nausea, vomiting, and convulsions. The treatment is mostly focused on managing fever and the neurological symptoms. However, the severely ill individuals need to be hospitalized and may require the use of a ventilator.

Transmission of NiV among fruit bats

Fruit bats of the genus Pteropus have been identified as natural reservoirs of NiV. A seroepidemiologic study in Malaysia implicated four fruit bat species, *Pteropus hypomelanus, P. vampyrus, Cynopterus brachyotis, Eonycteris spelaea*, in addition to the insectivorous bat, Scotophiluskuhlii, in the year 1998. As a result of consuming date palm sap that had been contaminated by infected fruit bats, humans were infected with NiV during the year 2004, in Bangladesh.in Malaysia and Infective NiV has also been isolated from environmental samples of bat urine and partially-eaten fruit in Malaysia (Nipah virus has been isolated from the brain and spinal fluid of victims, in Malaysia).

Transmission of NiV among wild pigs

Droppings / body fluids of fruit bats over the feeding sites / habitats of wild pigs (or stalls of domestic pigs) lead to the transmission of the Nipah viral infections among the swines. Though the transmission shall occur through the bites, it seems to be rare and however, consumption of dead or injured fruit bats by wild pigs, in the wildlife regions also may lead to the transmission of this deadly viral infection in swines.

Clinical symptoms of NiV in pigs

(Synonyms for NiV in pigs: Porcine respiratory and neurologic syndrome / Porcine respiratory and encephalitic syndrome (PRES)/Barking pig syndrome (BPS).

NiV affected febrile respiratory disease with a severe cough and dyspnoea (Predominantly the respiratory signs. Affected pigs may also have encephalitis, revealing the nervous signs that include twitching, trembling, muscle fasciculation, spasms, muscle weakness, convulsions & death. However, some animals may remain asymptomatic. Has high mortality among piglets than in case of adults but morbidity is high regardless of the age group.

Clinical Symptoms of NiV in Fruit Bats

Fruit bats are indeed, encroaching livestock areas and the species identified could be a potential source of infection to susceptible livestock but the symptomatology in the infected Fruit bats are not much revealed in literatures. Carrier status without any apparent symptoms needs to be investigated with Fruit bats, in this regard.

Clinical symptoms of NiV in homosapiens (often, acute in nature)

- Fever / Headache
- Nausea / Vomiting / Fatigue
- Fainting / Epilepsy
- Some patients may slip into a coma within two days after the initial symptoms Understanding about the biology of fruit bats as well as wild swines is a must prior to knowing technical information on Nipah viral infections which are highly zoonotic in nature.

Plan of action for tackling the nipah viral infections esp. related to the wild animals

- Requesting of permission from the state forest department and national biodiversity authority of india for zoonotic disease related surveillance in national parks, sanctuaries, reserve forests etc. associating the wild pigs as well as fruit bats towards the collection of biological samples after trapping-techniques.
- Equipping of Veterinary Research Centers located in Veterinary Institutions with modern diagnostic gadgets for effective diagnosis of zoonotic diseases among wild fauna, as the case with Nipah viral infections.
- Stress indicators among the wild fauna (wild pigs and fruit bats in particular) shall be estimated like cortisol to frame concepts on probable occurrence of viral infections like Nipah virus among them.

- Usage of Personal-Protective Equipment (PPE) by persons exposed to potentially infected pigs is highly recommended.
- Improvement of swine-husbandry practices.
- Undertaking of intensified research on development of vaccines (attempts were by Australia and France) and biological research on wild pigs to prevent the straying of wild pigs into non-forest regions from the forest regions.
- Burial sites of affected patients (whether animal or man) should be applied with chlorinated lime (or) sodium hypochlorite (bleach).
- Moving patients (animal/man) to other locations could result in the spreading of the virus since it is a transmittable disease, esp. during episodes of outbreaks either among wild or domestic fauna or homo sapiens (Minimum mobility is hence often suggested).
- Ban on transportof domestic or wild pigs within the countries affected, during the episodes
- Temporarily ban on pig production in the regions affected.
- Direct contact with live, potentially infected pigs should be minimized to prevent transmission of this potentially fatal zoonosis to humans.
- Netting of specific. area of Bat-habitat (night time-roosting sites).
- Keep the wells and other water sources closed and clean.
- Treated water should be used for body sanitization and cleaning.
- Boiled water shall be consumed for drinking purposes.
- Strengthen the measures to reduce the likelihood of the bat reservoir coming into contact with pig production facilities.
- Conducting of Awareness programmes (Education) on Nipah viral infections
- Culling of either fruit bats or wild pigs shall not the solution in the event of outbreak. Wild pigs are the important links in the food chain of carnivores and are at the bottom of ecological pyramid in the wildlife scenery. Similarly, pollination is highly assisted naturally by fruit bats, leading to the growth of highly diversified vegetation. Indiscriminate killing of the species could lead to dwindling of its population (Prey Base for Carnivores in the Wild) and this will surely upset the food chain, which would lead to ecological imbalances.
- According to the WILDLIFE PROTECTION ACT, 1972, the Fruit bats are placed in Schedule I & Wild pigs in Schedule III; however, the Ministry of Environment, Forest and Climate Change shall shift the wild pigs from Schedule III to Schedule V of the ACT, subsequent to the representation

from the concerned state-forest departments in India (This happened in Uttarakhand, Bihar, Karnataka states etc.)

Note

- In 2012, the OIE launched an updated version of WAHIS (OIE World Animal Health Information System) integrating a new section for wildlife disease notification. WAHIS now allows Member-Countries to complement compulsory information on OIE-listed diseases of wild species, but also to notify, on a voluntary basis specific wildlife diseases that are not officially included in that list. Information received and processed through both systems will be made public and released on the website of the OIE.
- The 2018 review of the WHO list of Blueprint priority diseases indicates that there is an urgent need for accelerated research and development for the Nipah virus.

Hog cholera (Classical Swine Fever)

It is a disease-caused by highly contagious viral agent and this viral agent may survive in refrigerated meat for several months. The virus survives in frozen carcasses for long periods of time. Pigs and wild boar are the natural reservoirs. The pig is the only natural host. The virus is spread from infected or carrier pigs via discharges from the nose, mouth, urine and faeces or infected semen and it is highly contagious. The high prevalence of CSFV antibodies suggests that the disease is endemic in this country.

Avian influenza

This refers to the disease caused by infection with avian influenza (flu) Type A viruses and is basically a disease of birds caused by influenza viruses that are closely related to human influenza viruses. These viruses occur naturally among wild aquatic birds worldwide and can infect domestic poultry and other birds. Avian flu may often cause little or no disease in wild waterfowl but many times get associated with the occurrence of large outbreaks with high mortality in case of poultry. In these instances the term 'highly pathogenic avian influenza' (HPAI) is associated. Transmission to humans in close contact with poultry or other birds occurs rarely and only with some strains of avian influenza. In China, low pathogenic strain of avian influenza virus was associated with OBR recently.

Crimean - congo haemorrhagic fever (CCHF)

It is a zoonotic disease and is a widespread tick-borne viral disease and outbreaks are commonly encountered. This disease is endemic in Asia, Africa, Middle

East, Balkans etc. and the wide range of domestic as well as wild animals. Animals become infected by the bite of infected ticks and the virus remains in their bloodstream for about one week after infection, allowing the tick-animal-tick cycle to continue when another tick bites. Many birds are resistant to infection, but ostriches are susceptible and may show a high prevalence of infection in endemic areas, where they have been at the origin of human cases.

New castle disease (Ranikhet disease)

Free ranging aviary species are more susceptible to this viral disease and the affected birds may reveal signs like watery droppings, dullness etc.

11

Parasitic Diseases in Wild Animals

Natural areas in tropical and sub tropical climates are more likely to enhance development of parasitic loads because of the fact that there are variations in climates of these areas in addition to the variations in the type of vegetations and species of wild fauna. The parasitic diseases have caused serious problems in captive animals and it is to be accepted that some of the diseases bear Zoonotic significance. Hence, treatment and prevention against parasites gain significance always in the wild animal health and disease management.

In non–human primates, the following parasites are more commonly encountered, i.e. Strongyles, *Strongyloides* spp., *Trichuris* spp., *Entamoeba* spp. and *Balantidium* spp. which are zoonotically also important ones.

In carnivores, especially in felids, the parasites are numerous leading to harmful features to different systems in the body and depending on the load and pathogenesis, animals suffer, in general. The common internal parasites in felids are *Toxocara cati, Ancylostoma* spp., *Taenia* spp., *Dirofilaria immitis*, *Spirocerca lupi* and the common blood protozoa parasites that are often encountered comprise *Toxoplasma gondii* and *Hepatozoa* spp. Similarly, fleas like *Ctenocephalides* spp and the ticks are also more common.

Strongyloidosis and hymenolepsis in non-human primates

These parasitic conditions are encountered mainly in non–human primates like bonnet macaques in south India. The cestode that is considered to have the potential zoonotic significance from species belonging to the non-human primates is *Hymenolepsis nana.* This tapeworm causes catarrhal enteritis.

Spirometra in carnivores

Adult *spriometra* are encountered in wild carnivores especially the tigers and canids. The life cycle of this parasite problem is similar to that of *Diphyllobothrium latum.* Persons involved with handling of wide variety of wild animals may get infected and the zoonotic condition is termed as sparganosis.

Hydatidosis and fasciolosis

Larval stages of *Echinococcus* species (hydatid cysts) were revealed in many ruminants. Hydatid cysts have been documented in squirrels, elephants, non-human primates etc. and fasciolosis was documented in elephants etc. Triclabendazole is the drug of choice for fasciolosis in captive wild ruminants.

Giardosis and amoebosis

The protozoal problems like giardosis and amoebosis are commonly encountered in non-human primates and other wild animals. Random examination of fecal samples is highly required even in case of free ranging non-human primates to understand about the various parasitic fauna including the protozoal infections. Metronidazole and related compounds are useful for the treatment.

Hook worm problem

These are commonly encountered in case of felids and canids in particular. Haemorrhagic diarrhea may occur in the affected carnivores. Fecal examination may help to rule out these parasitic problems as in case with multiple parasitic problems. Broad spectrum antibiotic like albendazole, fenbendazole and pyrantel pamoate are generally the chosen anthelmintic drugs against the hook worms in captive wild animals esp. carnivores.

Malaria

Wild mammals are also susceptible to infection by *plasmodium falciparum* that causes human malaria. Plasmodium species has been documented in *Presbytis entellus* in South India and in captive aviary species.

Trypanosomosis

Trypanosoma evansi affects multiple species of wild animals. In free ranging areas, the tryps affected carcases when eaten by predator species like tigers etc. may cause the spread of this infection. Insects form the vectors associated with this haemo-parasitic infections. Camels and felids appear to get mostly affected by this disease condition. Documentations are available for its incidences in hyaena, wild dog, tiger and lion. Quinapyramine sulphate and chloride are useful in therapy against trypanosomosis.

Spirurosis

Spirocerca lupi was encountered in the thoracic cavity of lion at Banarghatta national park and animal was found to have aneurysm in thoracic cavity and spirura species was documented in stomach region of mongoose.

Filaroid infections

Diseases caused by *Indofilaria pattabhiramani* were documented in elephants that revealed haemorrhagic nodules in different parts of body.

Toxocara canis and *Toxocara cati* in wild canids and felids

These parasitic conditions are mainly involved in zoonotic problems and in this condition, a long standing granulomatous lesions occur in the internal organs especially the liver, lungs or brain due to the migrating larvae of this parasite. The eye lesions caused by these larvae often may resemble retinoblastoma.

The eggs of *Toxocara canis* are extremely resistant to the environmental changes.The nematode, *Toxocara canis* occurs in small intestine of wild canids like wild dogs, jackals, foxes etc. *Toxocara cati* and *Toxascaris leonina are* the most commonly encountered parasitic problem in case of lions, tigers, panthers, jungle cats etc. in various zoos. Rodents play an important role as the paratenic host and upon the ingestion of rodents in the premises of cage, the felids like panther, lions etc. get infected.

The trematodes like *Fasciola hepatica* and *Fasciola jacksoni* have been reported in Asian elephants, where as *Protofasciola robusta* was reported in African elephants. There are numerous nematode parasites in the elephant like ascarids, oxyurids, strongylids, paraphistomes, ancylostomes, syngamids and filarids. Cestodes like *Anoplocephala manubriuta* are also reported. The protozoan disease like Trypanosomosis is a serious problem in Asian elephant caused by *Trypanasoma evansi*. Flea and tick infestations are more common in elephants. *Amblyomma tholloni* ticks (elephant tick) are found through out the body. *Haematomyzus elephantis* (elephant louse) are generally found in the base of the tail and behind the ears.

Internalparasitres are more common in wild ruminatnts also. The common parasites are *Haemonchus* spp, *Ostertagia* spp, *Trichostrongylus* spp, *Oesophagostomum* spp.

Strongyloides spp, *Trichuris* spp, *Taenia* spp, *Ascaris* spp, *Eimeria* spp, *Fasciola* spp, and protozoan diseases like *Babesia* spp, *Theileria* spp, *Trypanasoma* spp etc. are more common in wild ruminants. External parasites mange and tick ingestion are also common. *Psoroptes* spp, *Sarcoptes* spp and *demodex* spp are caused mange infestation in wild ruminants.

In case of reptiles like snakes, tick infestation is more common. The common ticks are *Aponomma* spp, *Amblyomma* spp, and *Hyalomma* spp. Internal parasites like *Capillaria* spp, *Rhabdius* spp. *Ophidascaris* spp, *Isospora* spp, *Eimeria* spp, *Kalicephalus* spp, *Polydephis* spp are similarly encountered in them.

Fungal diseases

Particularly, the non-human primates get affected by ring worm caused by *Trichophyton mentagrophytes* causing skin lesions. There are many fungal infections that affect the captive wild animals, causing severe hair loss and also pruritus, in many cases. Fungal infecions are also common in wild animals.

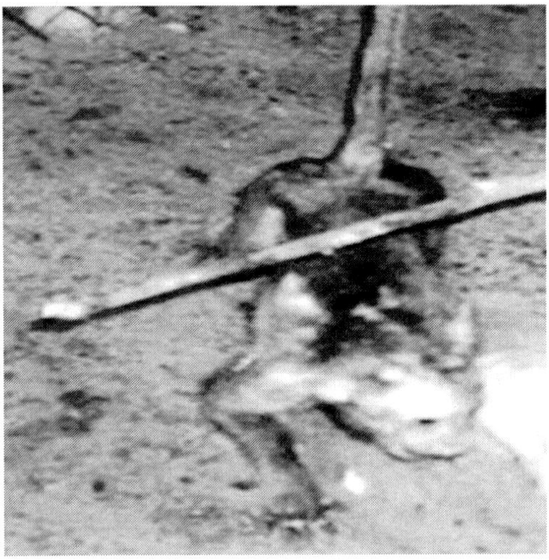

Fig. 1. Patchy distribution of hairless patches in Bonnet macaque

External parasites: Similar to domestic fauna, the wild fauna are also affected.

Prevention and control

- Captive animals need to be periodically examined for presence of external parasites and treatment is to be carried out accordingly.
- Similarly evidences of internal parasitism are to be examined by periodical investigation of faecal samples and anthelmintic therapy is to be initiated.
- Vector control measures need to be undertaken in parasitic diseases related to the vector-based transmissions.
- Endemicity of parasitism in that area needs to be assessed by liasoning with animal disease intelligence units of animal husbandry department of the concerned state.

12

Field Based Identification of Evidences on Different Parasitic Fauna in Captive Wild Animals

Ancylostoma sp. egg (oval, thin-shell, segmented yolk containing usually 8 cells)

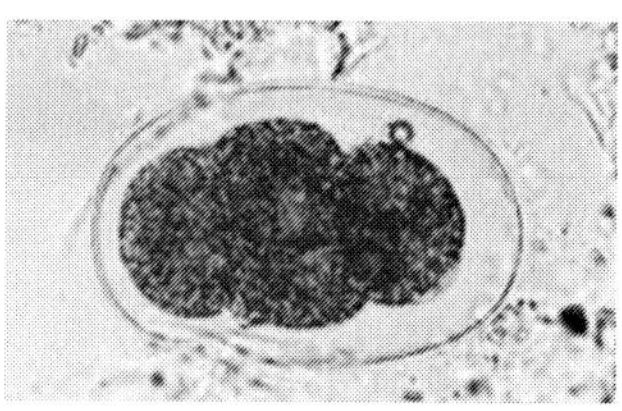

Spirocerca sp. egg (thick shelled and gelatin shape with fully developed larvae inside).

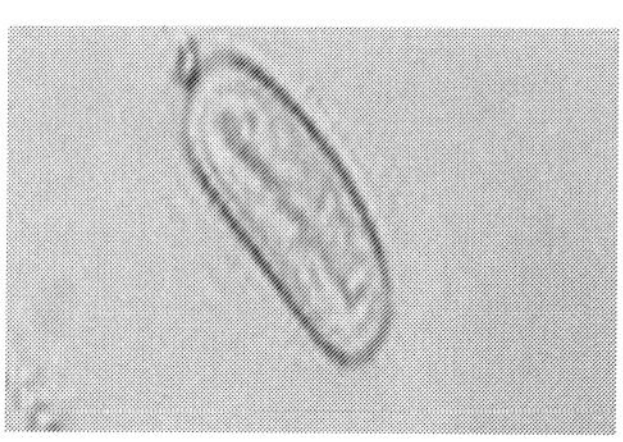

Paragonimus sp.egg (yellowish brow with operculum & shell thickened at opposite pole).

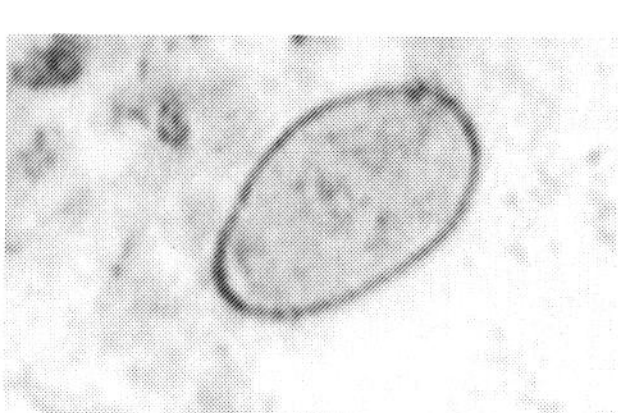

Dipylidium sp. egg (thick plain shell with hexacanth embryo).

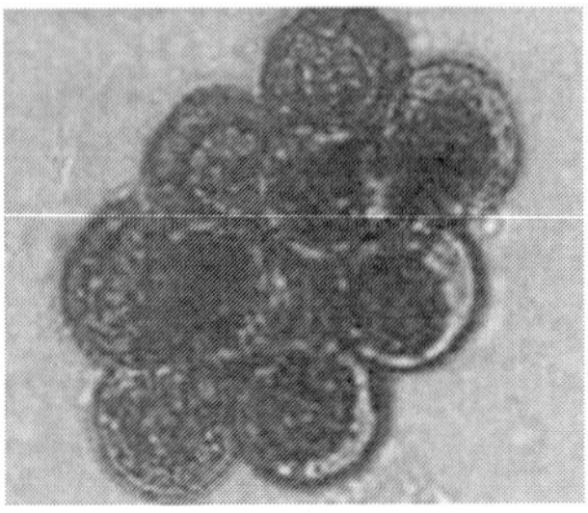

Spirometra sp. egg (yellowish brown, both ends are pointed, presence of operculum and contains yolk cells).

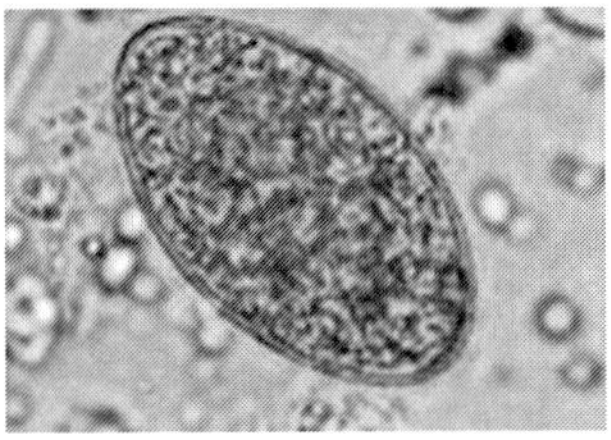

Echnococcus sp. egg (typical taenid egg, circular, thick shelled with radial striations, yellow tinted and hexacanth embryo).

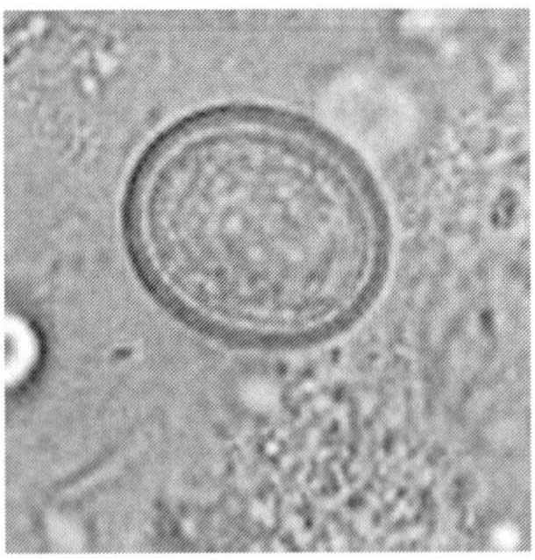

Diphyllobothrium sp. egg (oval shape, yellowish brown, rounded ends, operculum & contains yolk cells).

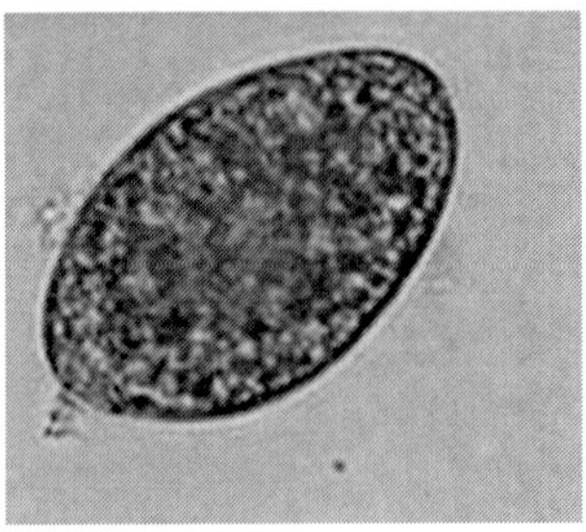

Toxocara canis egg (thick and finely pitted shell with compact yolk inside and egg of *Toxocara cati*is also similar to this).

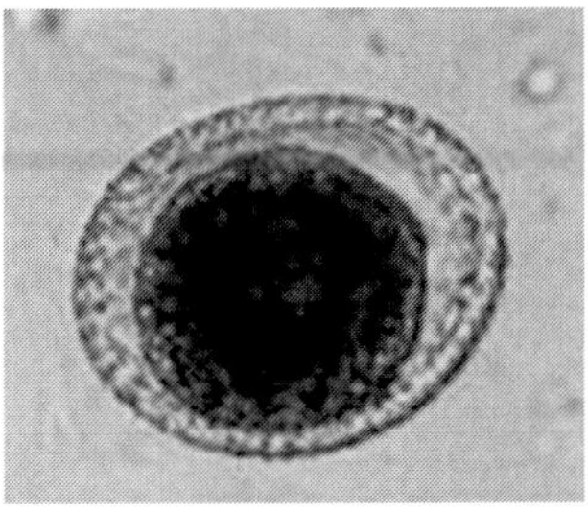

Toxocara leonina egg (mildly oval with thick & smooth shell).

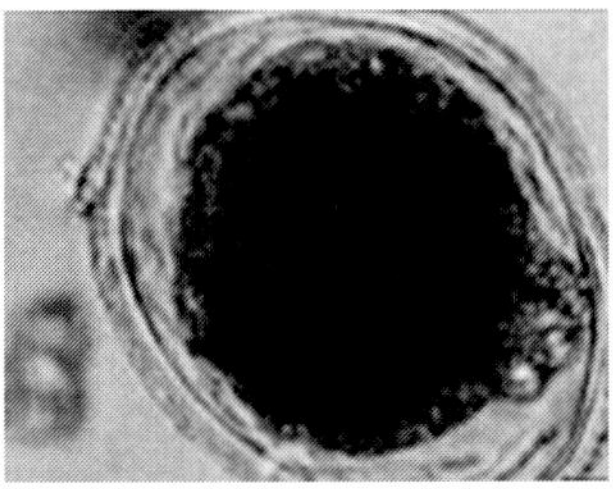

Microfilaria of (***Dirofilaria*** sp.) in blood smear(elongate with a straight tail and tapered head).

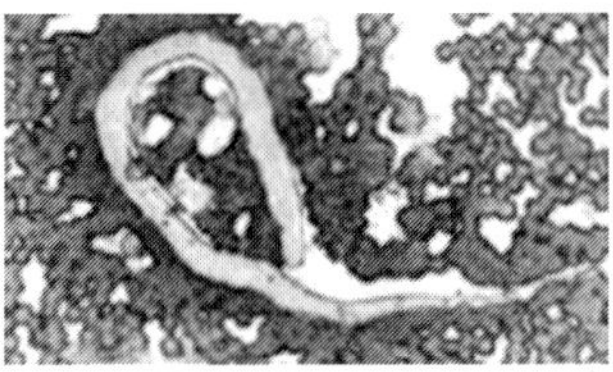

Physaloptera sp.

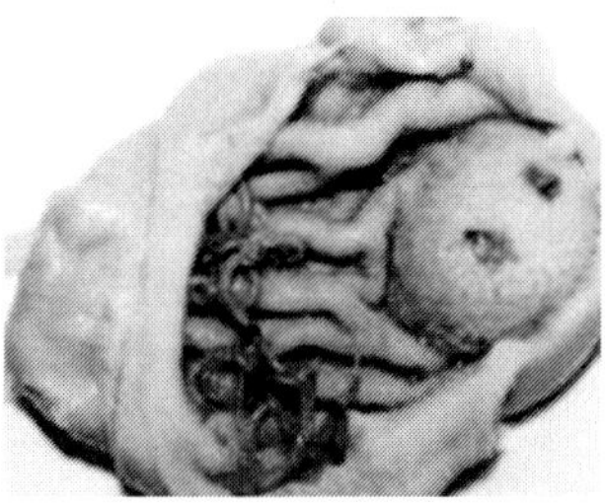

Trichuris sp. egg (brownish, transparent plug at either pole, with unsegmented embryo inside)

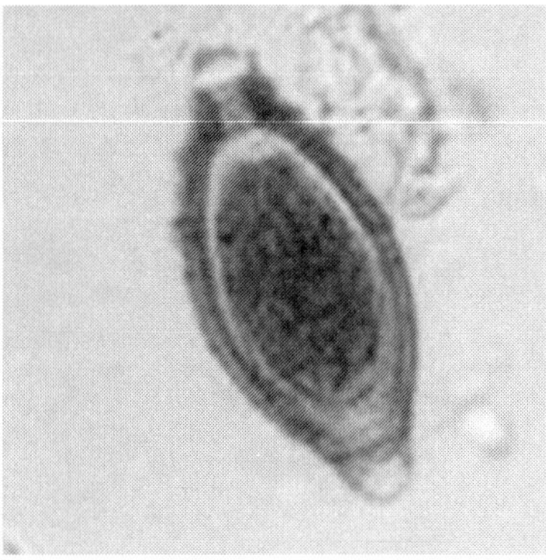

Babesia canis *in blood smear* (Merozoite inside RBC with pyriform bodies lying at an angle to one another but the merozoite of B. gibsoni in the RBC is annular or oval or signet ring form).

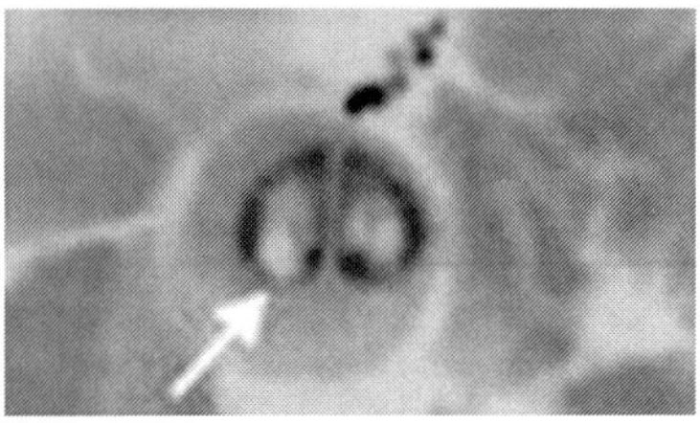

Trypanosoma evansi in blood smear (Free flagella and well developed undulating membrane).

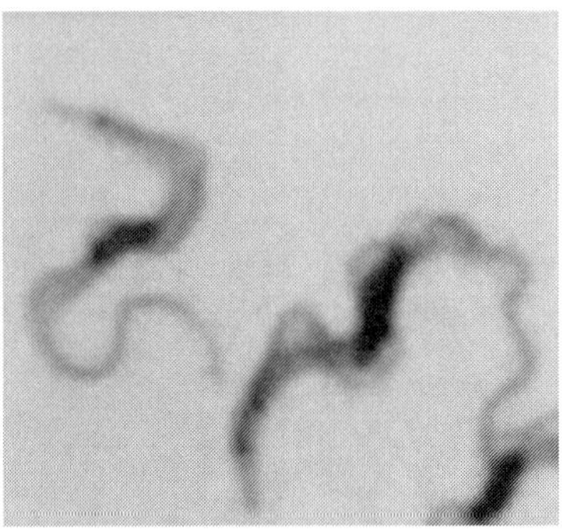

Hepatozoon canis in blood smear(garments commonly occur in leukocytes, gelatin globule shape, dark reddish purple nucleus with horse-shoe shaped chromatin usually at one end).

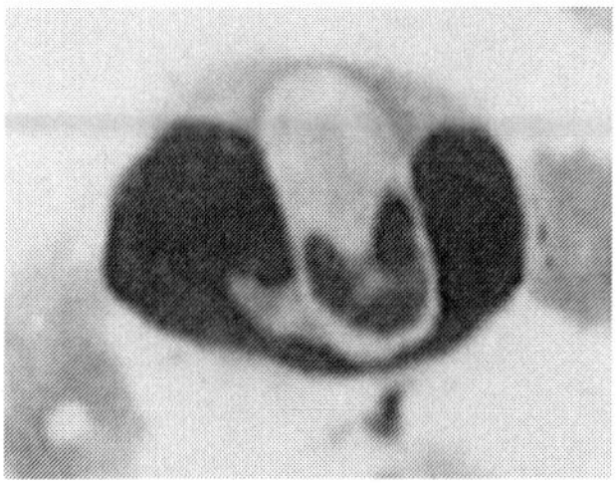

Ehrlichia canis in blood smear (single or compact colonies of inclusion bodies ie. morulae, as intracytoplasmic forms in the circulating WBCs).

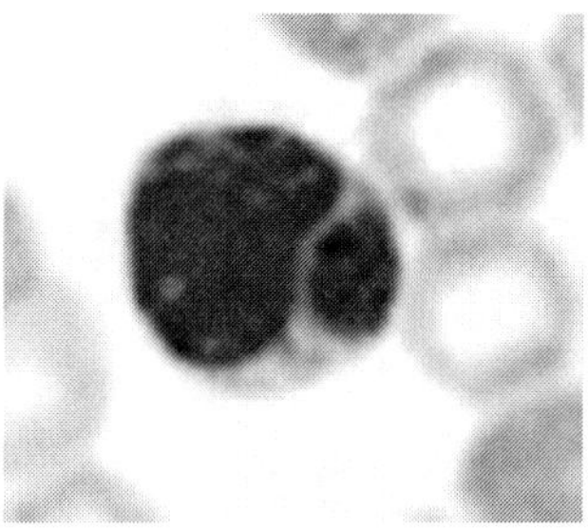

Isospora felis (ovoid and sporulated oocyst with 2 sporocyst and each sporocyst with 4 sporozoites).

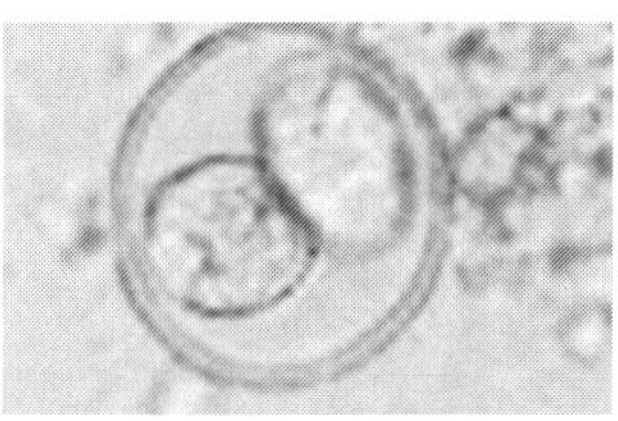

Toxoplasma gondii (spherical and sporulated oocyst with 2 sporocysts and each sporocyst with 4 sporozoites).

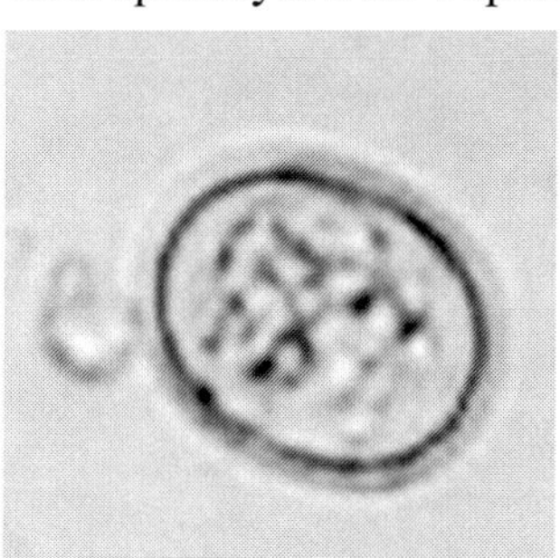

Fasciola gigantica egg (large, oval and yellowish with indistinct operculum and contains yolk cells and germ cells).

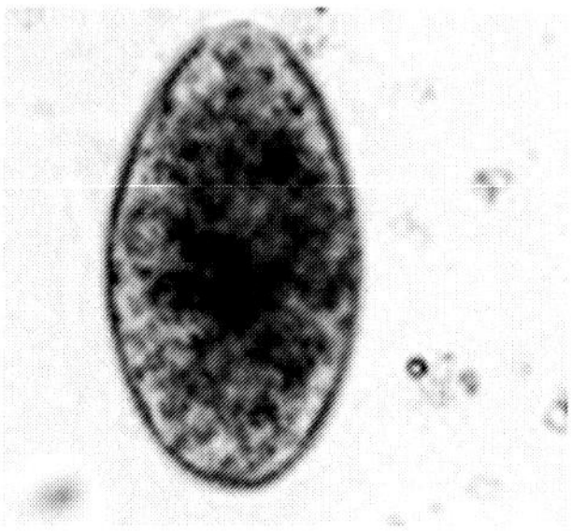

Amphistome egg (clear and pearly in appearance ie. non-tinted and distinct operculum and contains yolk cells and germ cells).

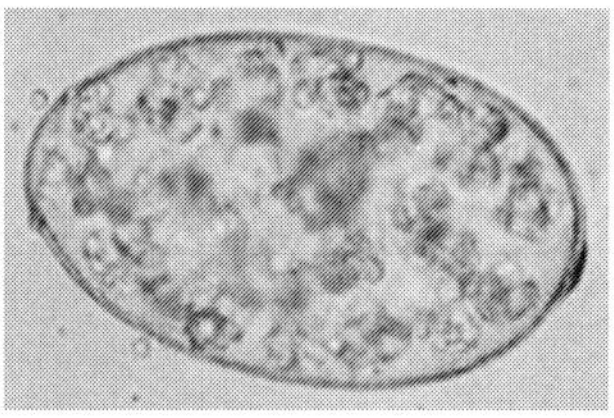

Amphistomes in wall of rumen.

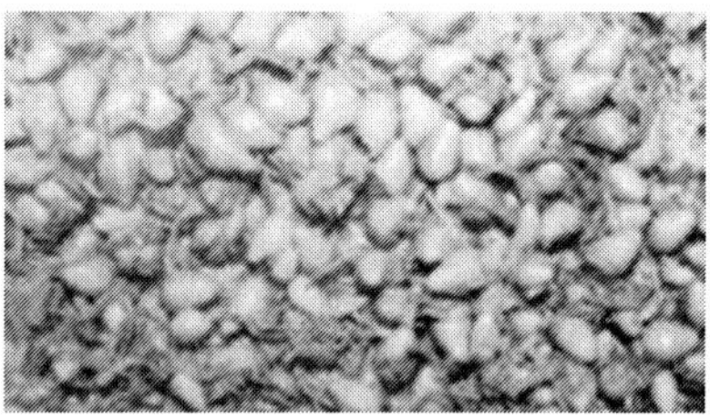

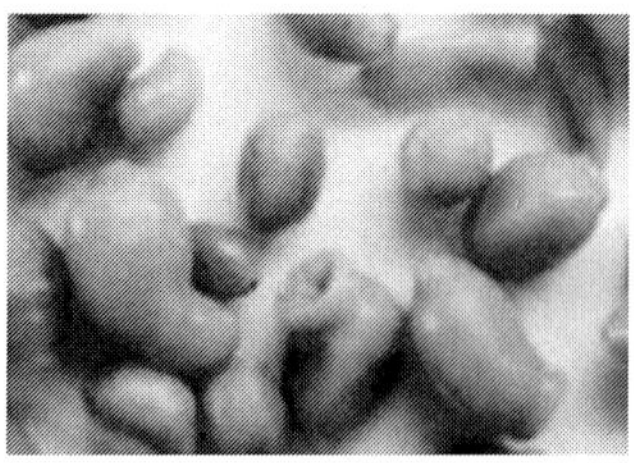

Moniezia spp. (Triangular or squarish shape with well developed pyriform apparatus and contains hexacanth embryo).

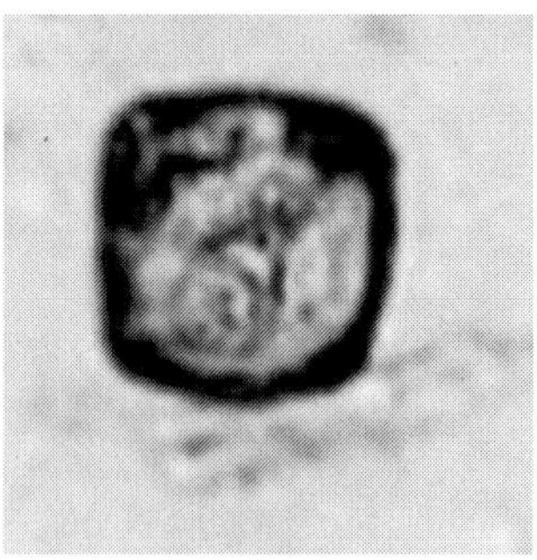

Anoplocephala sp. worm (in small intestine of elephant / rhinoceros).

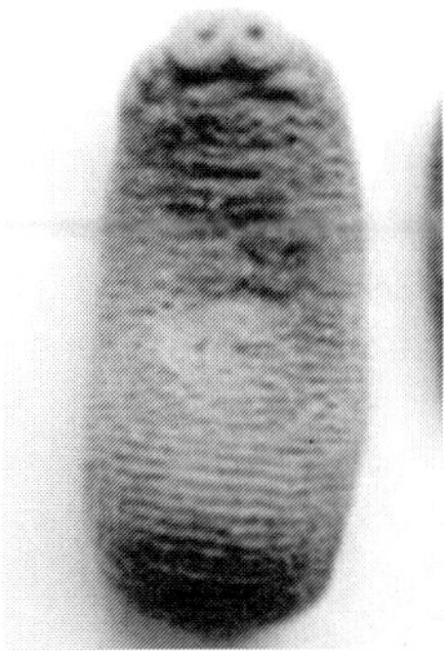

Hydatid cyst (liver)

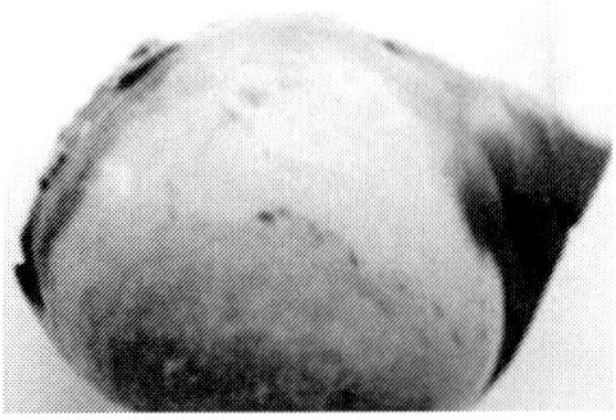

Protoscolices from the hydatid cyst- fluid

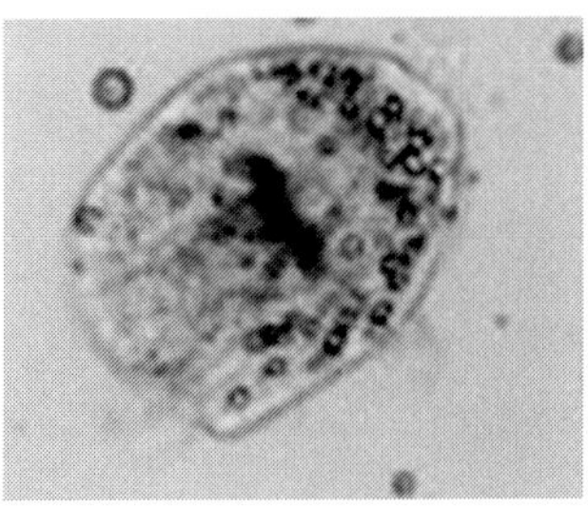

Cyst in Cysticercosis due to ***Cysticercus tenuicollis***
This is associated with the tape worm-*Taenia hydatigena* and the cyst is fluid filled and is about 5 cm in diameter, attached to various organs on the peritoneal surface.

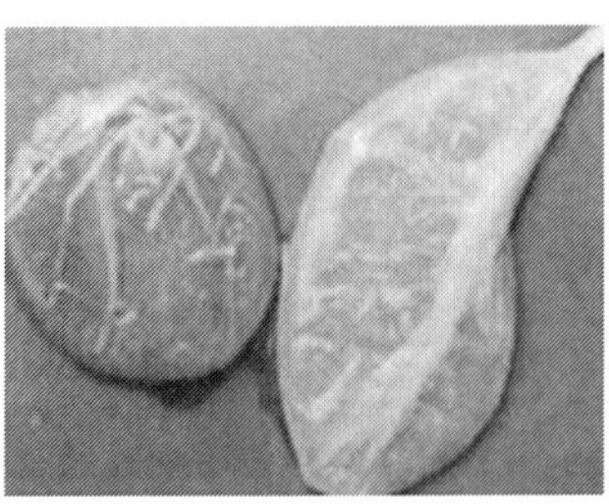

Ascaris suum **egg** (ovoid, thick shelled with prominent projections and brownish yellow and the unsegmented yolk seen as a compact mass).

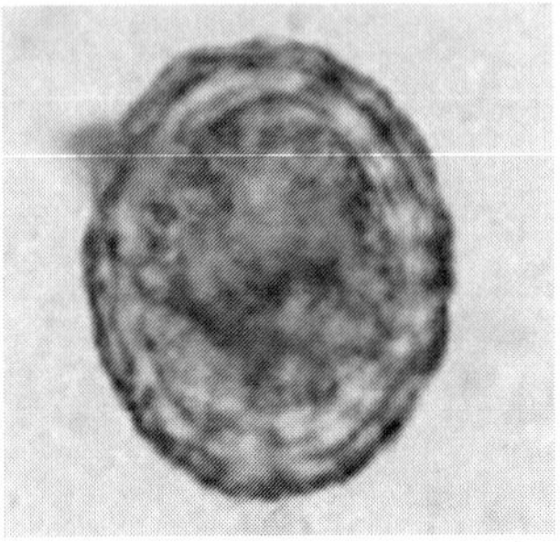

Toxocara vitulorum egg (subglobular, finely pitted albuminous layer and thick shelled with compact yolk).

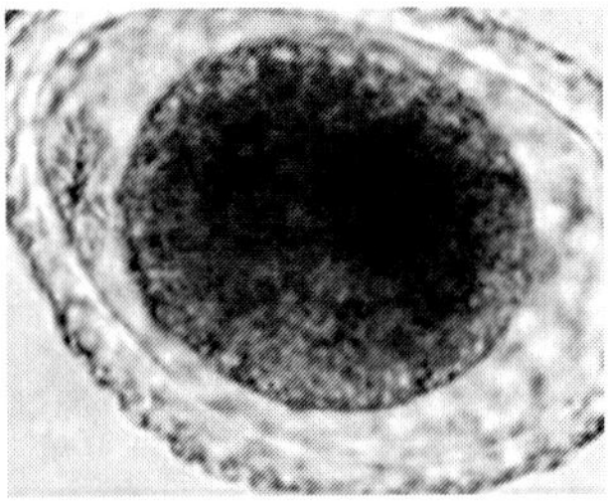

Strongyle egg (eg. *Haemonchus* sp. and *Bunostomum* sp.): oval, thin shelled and segmented yolk inside).

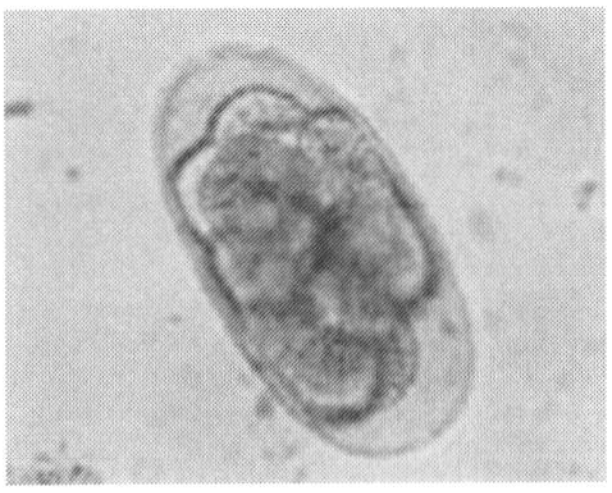

Strongyloides spp. egg (thick shell with both ends blunt and well developed embryo inside the egg).

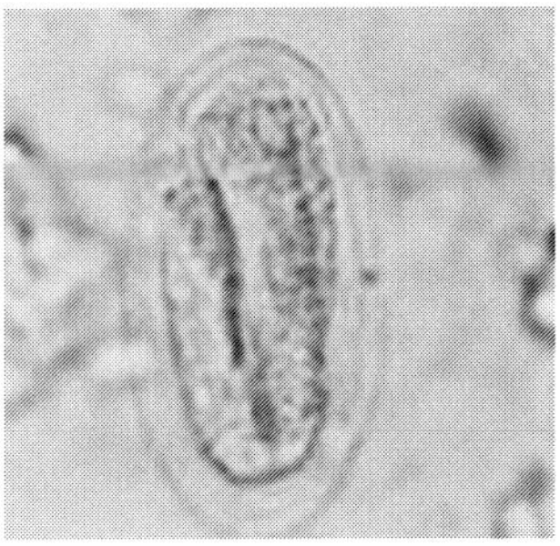

Trichuris sp. egg (brownish, barrel shaped, transparent plug at either pole and contains unsegmented embryo).

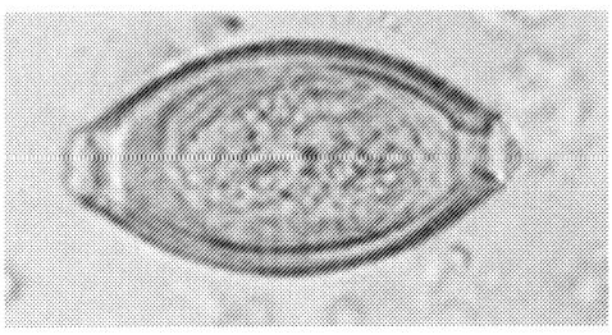

Oxyuris equi egg (creamy colored masses of eggs, flattened one side and presence of plug at one pole; egg in enterobiosis ie. pinworm infection, caused by *enterobius vermicularis* is also similar to egg of *Oxyuris equi*).

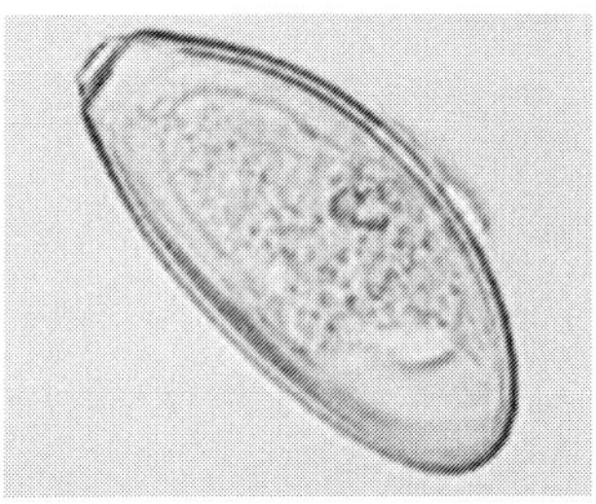

Theileria spp. (merozoites of multiple shapes ie. round, oval, comma or shaped, within the RBCs and schizonts called as Kochs blue bodies as irregularly oval or rounded matrix with numerous chromatin particles in the cytoplasm of the lymphocytes).

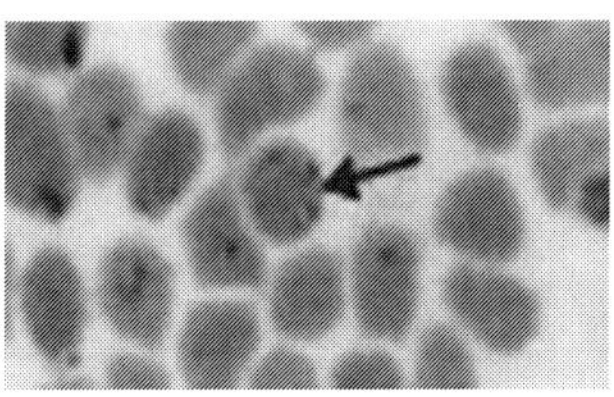

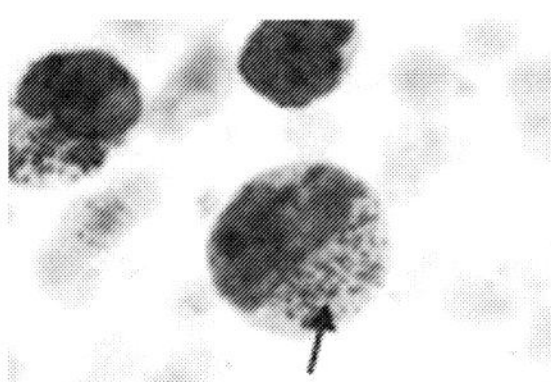

Anaplasma marginale (small spherical red to dark red bodies in the margin of RBCs).

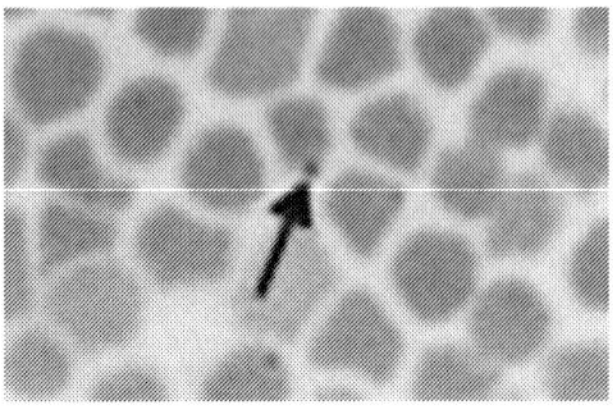

Cysts of ***Entamoeba histolytica*** (round shape with 4 distinct nuclei and chromatoid bodies).

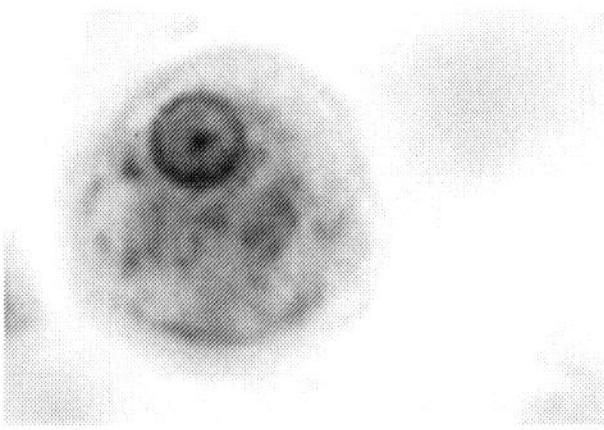

Cysts of ***Giardia lamblia*** (ellipsoidal, bilarterally symmetrical resembling a pear that is cut in half longitudinally) and anterior end is broad and round, while the posterior end is drawn out and presence of two or four nuclei).

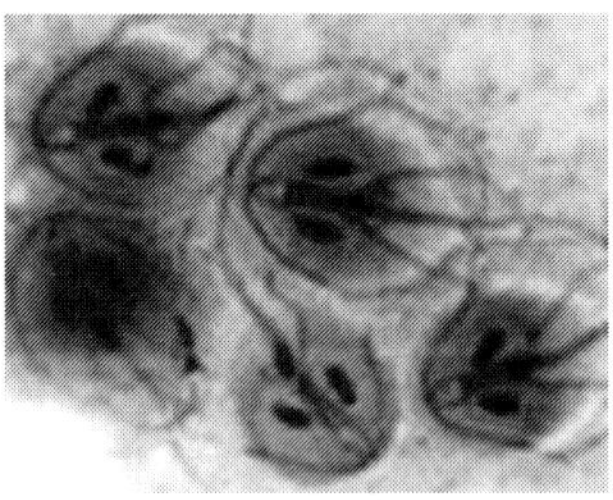

Coccidial oocyst (presence of sporocysts containing sporozoites within the oocyst).

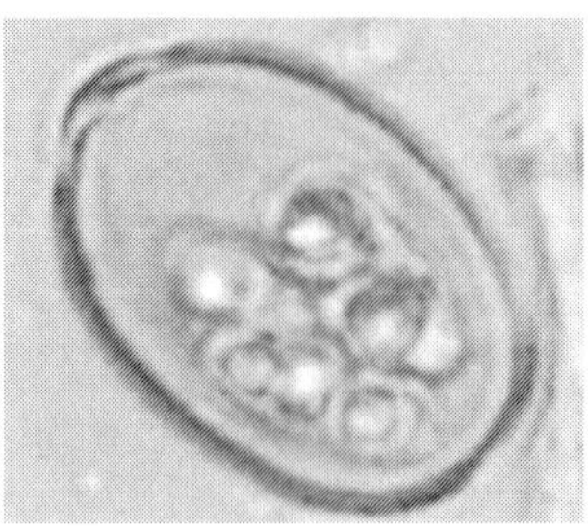

Cyst of ***Balantidium coli*** (ovoid or spherical and is faintly yellowish or greenish with presence of macronucleus and the cyst wall has 2 membranes).

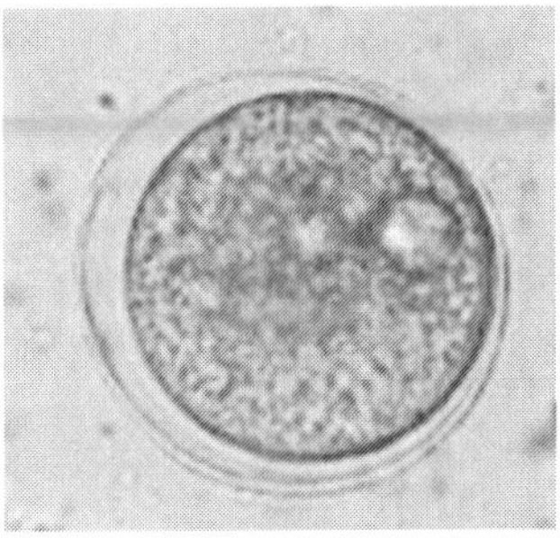

Cobboldia cobboldi maggot (in stomach of elephant).

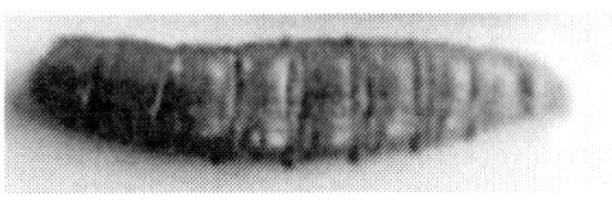

Ctenocephalides felis (flea)

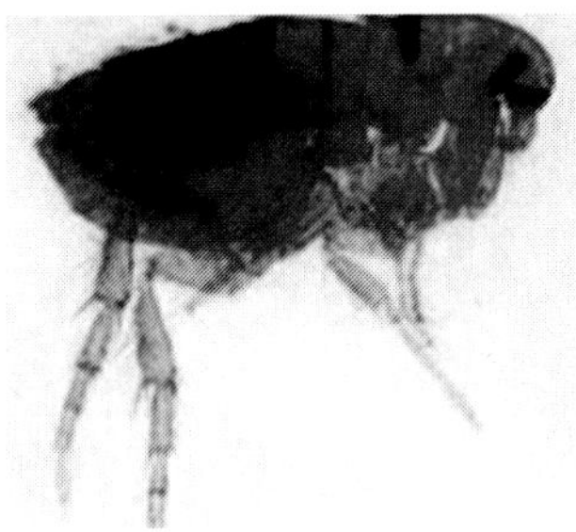

Rhipicephalus sanguineus (tick)

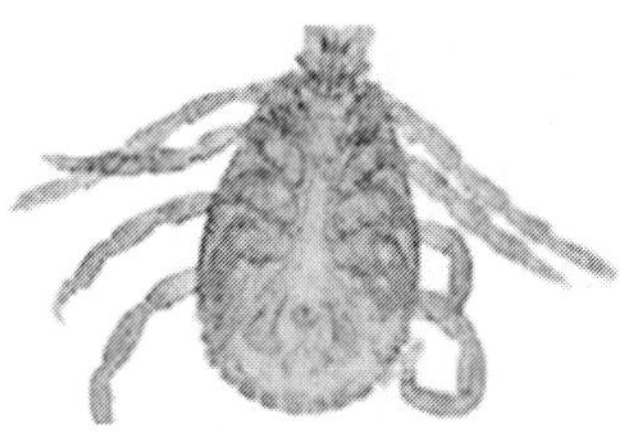

Nits (egg of lice)

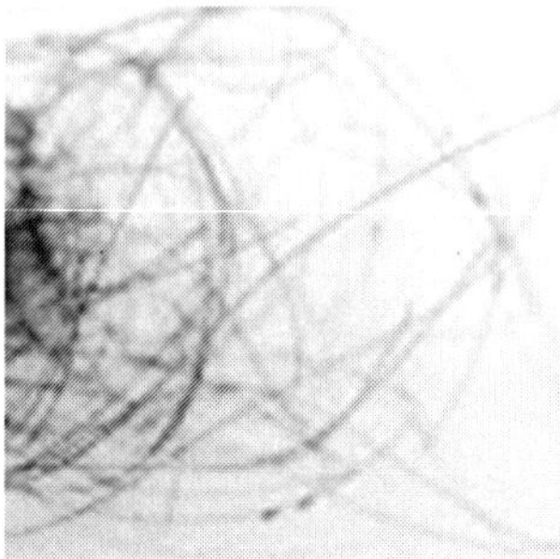

Demodex sp. (burrowing mite)

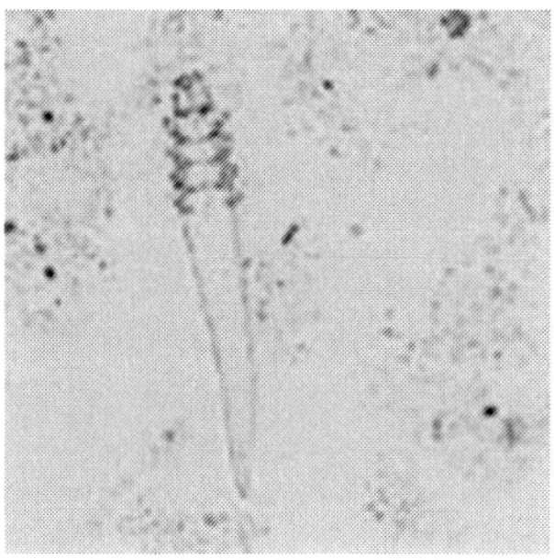

Sarcoptes sp. (mite)

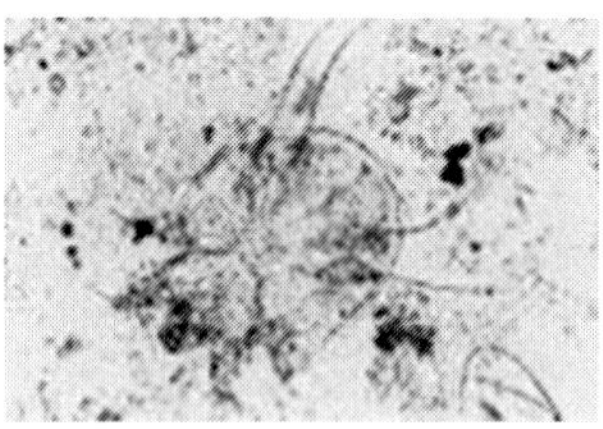

13

Metabolic and Nutritional Diseases in Wild Animals

"Metabolic Diseases" mean the diseases that occur due to the "imbalance between the rate of input of dietary nutrients and the "output of products" (product like new born, milk for young one etc.) and lead to the occurrence of metabolic derangements in the affected wild animal species.

Rickets and osteoporosis

- Rickets occurs due to malformation of the growing bone (bowing of limbs/ curving in limbs) due to lack of vitamin D_3 and there is a failure of hardening of bone.
- In case of rickets, the mineralization and mineral absorption are not in a match.
- Osteoporosis occurs in both the adults and juveniles (but may be frequent in senile female reptiles), where the already hardened bones become weakened by the withdrawal of calcium for metabolic purposes and the wild animals become more prone for the development of fractures.
- This is a condition of bone wherein there is more resorption of osteoid than the deposition of new tissue.
- Hence, there is reduction in the organic matrix of bone. Protein deficiency also may have some influencing effect on the occurrence of osteoporosis.

Osteomalacia and fibrous osteodystrophy

- These disorders are often seen in the young hatchlings of crocodiles which subsequently reveal failure of hardening of bones due to lack of calcium.
- Among mammals, bone eaters (eg. hyaena) if deprived of bones during feeding (like hyaenas) will end up in metabolic bone diseases.

Etiology

- Feeding diet with less calcium (provision of mince with liver and heart without bone or with less bones)
- Failure in proper absorption of calcium (diseases of GI tract / excessive phosphorus in diet)
- Insufficient calcium supplement and hormonal imbalances due to multiple causes
- Lack of vitamin D esp. in indoor-kept wild animals.
- Prolonged storage of ration leads to less vitamin D_3.

Clinical signs

Crocodiles get often affected by the metabolic bone diseases. The signs are:

- Persisting of kyphokoliosis (hunch backed appearance) esp. in subadults and adult crocodiles.
- Weakness of hatchling to walk on land while they still can move freely if in water or can swim freely in water.
- Falling of teeth and poor calcification of teeth.
- Jaw bones become more pliable as evidenced in case of hatchlings (rubber jaws).
- Weakness in hatchlings along with sluggish movements.
- Teeth become diaphanous like shards of glass (glassy teeth).
- In chelonians, lump like appearance of carapace (compare with normal nearby chelonian).

Diagnosis

Serum estimation of calcium and phosphorus in addition to the radiographical examination and clinical signs and history of feeding and management.

Note

In this context, it is to be remembered that especially in the periods of production of egg shells, the calcium mobilization from bones is at peak and hence, the reptiles when hypocalcemic during these periods will have difficulties in maintaining muscular tonicity and as a result, prolapse of uterus may occur in crocodiles.

Prevention, Control and Therapy of Metabolic Bone Diseases

- Hence, whenever prolapse occurs in crocodiles or any reptiles, correlation with the metabolic derangements of calcium need to be paid attention.
- Adequate basking is to be provided.
- Calcium supplements shall be provided as prophylactic measure if events of metabolic bone diseases are encountered in few of individual species.
- Serum level monitoring of calcium is to be carried out in a periodical manner.

METABOLIC BONE DISEASE IN CAPTIVE AVIARY SPECIES

Rickets

Rickets is encountered in growing birds esp. in birds which have long or large legs and is caused by Ca and P. Imbalance and deficiency of vitamin D. But osteomalacia is a disease of adult birds and causes are same as the previous ones.

Clinical signs

- Weakness, anorexia, polydipsia, intermittent loose droppings
- Poor feather growth and chewing at plumage
- Hunch backed appearance if thoracic cage reveals collapse.
- Upper and lower beaks may not oppose each other properly and prehension of food is faulty.
- Hyperaesthetic and reveal muscle spasms
- Improper calcification of eggs (eggs become more soft)
- Retention of eggs without laying due to lack of calcium

Gout in wild fauna

- This condition is more common in captive birds and reptiles in particular.
- Among the aviary species, especially raptors like hawks, eagles, kites, vultures, falcons are highly susceptible in addition to ostrich, cassowary, peafowls, budgerigars, love birds, parakeets, cormorant, goose, duck etc.
- Broader classification and the specific classification of gout should be known for a good understanding about this disorder.

Broader classification

True gout

Deposition of monosodium urate crystals

Pseudo gout

This is formed by deposition of any crystal other than sodium urate.

Visceral gout *(usually occurs as acute form):* Deposition of whitish urate or uric acid crystals (end products of nitrogenous metabolism or protein metabolism) in case of reptiles and birds (urate crystals are deposited as white coloured powder or foci often on epicardium and liver mainly and also on kidney and some times on peritoneum).

NOTE: Localization of urate crystals may vary from individual to individual.

Articular gout or synovial gout (usually occurs as chronic form)

- Urate deposition in and around the joints.
- Deposition of urate crystals form in joints form small white nodules called as tophi or tophus which is clearly visible to the unaided eyes.

Etiology

- *Renal problems* (infection/inflammation/renal lesions due to nephrotoxic substances like gentamicin and anti-inflammatory drugs like salicylates, probenecids, phenylbutazone etc.) are the basic cause because liver and esp.the renal tissues are involved in production of urate crystals.
- *Nutrition* (increased protein intake with provision of water, increased protein intake without provision of water or incorrect balance of aminoacids in the feed).
- *Stress leading to dehydration or dehydration* due to diseases all lead ultimately reduced renal blood flow and thereby renal efficiency is lots and ultimately gout occurs.
- *Congenital causes* might be the causal factors as documented in case of nile crocodile hatchlings.

Clinical signs and diagnosis

- Elevated serum uric acid helps the diagnosis in general, in addition to the specific examination for urate crystals in joints.
- In crocodiles or lizards or chelonians affected by gout, general depression is there but antemortem-diagnosis is difficult in visceral gout.
- Inarticular gout, the affected leg joints become painful and the animal is reluctant to move.

Hypothyroidism in captive mammals

- This may occur in any species of wild mammals.
- *Clinical signs:* Obesity, alopecia, dullness with lethargic movements and lowered serum cholesterol are the major features in this hypothyroidism.

HYPOTHYROIDISM IN CAPTIVE AVIARY SPECIES

(Documented in budgerigars etc.)

- Goiter in birds due to iodine deficiency may lead to hypothyroidism because the iodine is a must for the development of thyroid gland.
- Due to iodine deficiency, there may be hypertrophy of thyroid gland resulting in goiter.
- *Clinical signs.*
  - The affected birds will reveal change of voice i.e. a respiratory noise heard as a characteristic „click and this is due to the pressure of the enlarged thyroid on syrinx and the lower trachea.
  - In addition to the obesity and dullness, there may be ruffled feathers in the affected bird.

Diabetes mellitus in mammals and birds

- Differentiate insulin dependent diabetes mellitus from non-insulin dependent diabetes. Mostly, insulin dependent diabetes mellitus occurs. This condition is recorded in non-human primates in particular. (polyuria, polydipsia, polyphagia and glycosuria in addition to the dullness, anorexia, unconsciousness in extreme stages and staggering may be noticed in the affected animals).
- Other mammals may also get affected by this condition. However, this needs a more detailed but a specific study esp. in case of aged wild animal species.
- Further, this condition has been documented in case of captive birds also (ruffled feathers, polyuria, polydipsia, polyphagia, glycosuria and weakness are the consistent clinical signs in the affected birds).

Fatty liver in mammals and birds

This may occur in captive mammals (herbivores, carnivores and omnivores) and aviary species like budgerigars (male budgerigars especially have increased incidences of fatty liver and multiple metabolic causes might be assigned as etiological factors.

Neonatal hypoglycemia in wild animals

- This occurs mainly due to in-sufficient intake of colostrums or milk from mother due to multiple reasons and this causes metabolic derangements and hypoglycemia occurs in the affected wild animal species.
- Pale skin, weakness, recumbency, hypothermia, incoordination with terminal convulsions are the clinical signs revealed.
- Monitoring the infant for proper feeding (ensure for proper energy intake) and monitoring of the mother on proper nursing may help for the prevention of this problem in case of wild animals.

Ketosis (Acetonemia) in wild ruminants

- In ruminants whether it is domestic or wild (giraffe, deer, antelope, wild goat, wild sheep and wild bovid), the dietary carbohydrates are fermented in the rumen to short chain fatty acids (acetate in majority amount, propionate in moderate amount and butyrate in lesser amount).
- Hence, the glucose needs in these animal species are largely met by gluconeogenesis and it is to be understood that propionate and aminoacids are the major precursors for gluconeogenesis.

Clinical signs

In wasting form: Woody appearance of the animal due to apparent wasting and loss of cutaneous elasticity

In nervous form (rule out rabies): Animal walks in circles, head-pushing, apparent blindness, aimless walking, vigorous licking of objects and skin, depraved appetite, chewing movements with salivation.

Lactation tetany in wild equids

- This can be anticipated in case of wild equids reared under captive conditions. Zebras, wild asses and wild horses may get affected by this condition and often, it occurs in the lactating equids, either at about 10th day, after giving birth or 1 to 2 days after the weaning of the young one for management reasons.
- Even after the prolonged transport or after the severe exertion, this condition may occur.

Clinical signs

- Stiff gait and the tail may be raised.
- Incoordination and tetany.

- Sweating in profuse manner
- Rapid and labored respiration with wide dilatation of pupils which may be accompanied by a distinct thumping sound from the thorax due to spasmodic contraction of the diaphragm.
- Muscular fibrillation esp. of the masseter and shoulder region and trismus without prolapse of membrananictitans unlike in tetanus disease.
- Reduced peristalsis and suspended urination and defecation.
- May attempt to drink but unable to swallow.
- Lowered calcium diet during the pre-stress period may help to avoid the excess gastro-intestinal absorption of calcium.

Parturitient paresis (Milk fever) in wild ruminants

- Though there is no systematic study of this disease condition in wild cervids, this condition can be anticipated in the newly fawned deer or antelopes that have given birth. Especially when there are twin births, this can be anticipated. However, this can affect surely the gaur, mithun etc.
- This condition commonly occurs within two days of parturition and this may also occur few weeks before or after the parturition.

Clinical signs

- Hypothermia, dilated pupils, dry muzzle, suspended urination and defecation along with lethargic movements or dullness.
- Weak heart sounds (rule out immobilization effects) and anorexia.

Diagnosis: Serum estimation of calcium helps to diagnose the condition.

Calcium relates metabolic derangements in wild birds

- Other than bone related disease, some abnormalities are encountered in captive birds due to deranged calcium metabolism and are furnished below
- *Egg binding* is commonly encountered in many aviary species and along with other causes, calcium deficiency due to multiple metabolic derangements play a significant role. Hence, in egg bound aviary species, calcium borogluconate is given by I/V or S/C route and this helps in the improvement of the tonicity of the musculatures and helps in the rapid expulsion of egg · *Malformed egg* esp. shell less egg or partially shelled egg or soft shelled egg may be laid by multiple aviary species reared under captive conditions. In addition to the salpingitis, the etiological factor for this might be the existence of imbalance in calcium and phosphorus levels.

- An imbalance in calcium, phosphorus and vitamin D is commonly encountered in parrots and the problem arises as a result of their customary diet of high oil-bearing foods such as sunflower and peanuts. This in addition to the metabolic derangements produce a variety of clinical expressions in the affected wild birds reared in captivity.
- Provide shell grits as preventive measures.

Colic as a result of metabolic derangment

- Colic is more commonly encountered in case of elephants in severe metabolic
- Derangements like acidosis.
- Feeding of unaccustomed food material, excess feeding of the routine food materials, obstruction anywhere in the gastro-intestinal tract and lesser exercise with non-provision of adequate amounts of water for the drinking purposes- all may precipitate the colic condition, in general.

Signs of colic

- Restlessness
- Constipation
- Depression
- Disobedience/ aggression
- Absence of signs of health, in general.

Acute abdomen

Acute abdomen is a non-infectious clinical condition (disorder) that can affect any wild animal species, in general. However, this problem is more encountered in case of llamas. Camelids often experience this problem, in addition to the equids, elephants etc.

Clinical signs

- Dullness
- Temperature may be normal to sub-normal
- Anorexia
- Increased pulse and pain due to colic
- Normal to cyanotic mucosa
- Decreased defecation
- Decreased motility of stomach
- Increased respiration

Note

Gastric dilatation and volvulus (GDV) shall be anticipated esp. in carnivores and is an acute condition, often; surgical intervention is the remedy for this, as carried out in domestic canines.

Wounds, abscesses and injuries

- These are very common among wild animal species esp. the captive ones. In-fighting is the common cause often.
- Abscesses may occur if immediate treatment is not done due to multifaceted causes.
- Long time persisting wounds are common among elephants in particular and routinetreatment protocol needs to be adapted in all these cases.
- In many captive animals, wounds may get further complicated by affections with maggots.

14

Colic in Elephants

Colic is a general term that implies abdominal pain and is one of the major causes of death in animals including elephants, camelids etc.

Types of colic in Elephants

- Spasmodic colic (MOST COMMOM).
- Obstructive colic (IMPACTION is the cause for this often).

Cause

Colic results mainly from conditions affecting the GI tract but occasionally could be due to conditions involving organs of other systems within the abdominal cavity. The anatomical disposition of the gastrointestinal tract of the elephants and horse, the nature of digestion, and management practices imposed by man are among the main multifactorial predisposing factors for colic in these species.

Hydration plays a huge role in preventing colic

- Reduced drinking (Often as a predisposing factor)
- Watering and feeding immediately after heavy work/a long walk in the heat of the day may precipitate impaction.
- Feeding of excessive quantities of very fibrous feedstuffs
- Feeding of moldy lucerne or any other long time stocked feeds
- Choking related causes (Large sized fruits eg. Big oranges/apples/onion/ potatoes
- Dehydrated status
- Tooth problems leading to improper chewing (Molar maldevelopment and Malocclusion in elephants)
- Feed type (unaccustomed feed types)
- Elephants eating too much after prolonged work (e.g. ceremonial parades) has led to a period of fasting and stress.

- Intestinal parasites
- Liver fluke problems
- Liver diseases
- Inability of animal to digest and pass the digesta (transit) due to digestive.system disorders in particular and other painful disease or disorder condtions.

Obstructive colic occurs in following instances

- Excessive intake of sand, particularly the **clay** material from earthern – floor (GEOPHAGY – the normally observed habit in free ranging elephants; sodium presence is the major stimulating cause for soil consumption in addition to vitamin and mineral deficiency, in general.
- Excessive intake of high fiber feeds / unaccustomed feeds / large sized barks etc.

Pathogenesis

An elephant's inability to effectively digest what she consumes creates pain and distress. The lack of sufficient water intake slows the transit time of the consumed matter. When the digestive progress comes to a screeching halt, with little eaten and nothing eliminated, the elephant is in trouble. Dehydration/Peritonitis/ Intussception/volvulus/Intestinal ulceration /Intestinal rupture.

Clinical symptoms of colic

- Body temperature may be increased.
- Excessive thirst
- Restlessness.
- Constipation / Absence of passage of feces.
- Signs of abdominal discomfort (biting of trunk tip/ leaning on tree or wall or nearby solid objects/ frequent sitting and standing/ excessive movements of body/ unnatural postures/ stretching posture-frequently/ groaning/
- General dullness and depression
- No faeces are passed, or small, fibrous and dry faeces may be passed.
- Tenesmus (frequent or recurrent desire to defecate, with little or no evacuation of faeces resulting) ie) straining as if trying to defecate.
- Anorexia or disinterest in feeding
- Dehydration

- Excessive thirst may be seen or there may be reduced water intake
- Frequent lying down and getting up again, an anxious expression,
- Rubbing the abdomen on solid objects.
- Bloat.
- Gastric fluid may be vomited with anterior obstruction. Mild jaundice may be noted.
- Mild jaundice

Treatment: The key principles in the treatment of colic are:-

- Pain management
- Decompression of the gastrointestinal tract
- Correcting biochemical and fluid imbalances,
- Stimulation and maintenance of gastrointestinal motility
- Reduction of gastrointestinal inflammation (Where pain is severe and non-responsive to medical treatment, immediate surgical intervention is indicated but very difficult)

In addition to pain, other significant indicators of critical cases of colic include heart rate, gastrointestinal borborygmi and signs of hypovolemia

Antibiotics administration: Enrofoxacin / Amoxycillin-caluvulinate

Racking:

Enema administration: 3 gallons of soapy water enema (1 gallon=3.79 litres) by rectum (pass the hose pipe till u get resistance).

Lubricants usage: If the elephant eliminated the blockage and survived, animal shall be administered gallons of oil (vegetable oils like GN oil etc.) or mineral oil/ lubricant like liquid paraffin) that literally lubricates the blockage, so it could be passed or even lactulose-the inert disachharide shall be used (Dose: titrable to the effect).

Purgatives

- Osmotics or irritants should **not** be given until there is proof of at least some matter being passed through the intestinal tract, or the problem may be made worse.
- Epsom salt-Mag sulph (up to 2 lb; 453.6 gm=1 lb).

Dose: Upto 1 Kg may be given orally as a laxative/ 3-7 Kg as purgative (titrated to the effect).

- It was found that combined administration of **psyllium** and **$MgSO_4$** through nasogastric tube once a day for 4 days consecutively was more effective treatment in resolving the impaction than either of them alone.

Antibiotic usage in elephants

Amoxicillin	11 mg/kg q24 hrs
Enrofloxacin	2.5 to 5.0 mg/kg q 12 hrs Oral, I/MSide effects: Young animals / GI stress
Ceftiofur	2.2 mg/kg (to be reconstituted in lesser volume of water than prescribed) I/M & I/V once a day or 1.1 q 12 hrs I/M & I/V (renal and hepatic toxicity)
Doxycycline	10 mg/kg q 12 hrs
Sulfonamides	22 mg/kg (TMP-SMZ) (renal toxicity and watering)
Metronidazole	15 mg/kg, rectally q 24 hrs PO

Antiinflammatory drugs

- Flunixin meglumine by IM. (1.1 mg/kg, IM, PO, Per-rectal daily for 5 days).
- Meloxicam IM. (0.6 mg/kg, daily for a week).

Antispasmodics

BUSCOPAN (butylscopolamine): The antispasmodic drug which works byy relaxing the muscles in the stomach and intestines and is much useful in abdominal cramping; oral medications and injections are available in the market.It is the anticholinergic drug which has majority- the peripheral action and minority-the central action and these anticholinergic drugs will not cross the blood brain barrier (hence, the minimal central action against the muscarinic receptors.

Dose in horses: 0.02-0.04 mg/kg s/c OR im (By IV: 0.2-0.3 mg/kg single dose only) for analgestic effects but effects lost only for 30 minutes.

Used for the control of abdominal pain (colic) associated with spasmodic colic, flatulent colic and simple impactions in horses (and elephants).

As the only FDA-approved antispasmodic for use in horses, Buscopan works to relax the gastrointestinal smooth muscles and control pain associated with spasmodic colic.

Buscopan is known for its ability to relax smooth muscle and is useful in managing and diagnosing abdominal pain (colic) and shall be used prior to the rectal examination (Veterinarians often use the drug to reduce the risk of rectal tear during palpation and when performing a variety of obstetrical procedures including twin reduction and dystocia (difficult birth) management).

Anecdotally, Buscopan has been reported effective in relieving meconium (the first manure a foal produces) and ileal impactions.

For Pain Relief

Butorphanol, which is a partial agonist and antagonist opioid provide the best pain relief with least adverse effects. It can be used alone or in combination with xylazine or detomidine. The dosage range is 0.05-0.1 mg/kg BW, IV depending on the severity of colic (0.2 mg/Kg by IV is optimal for horses for analgesic effects.

Alpha-2 adrenergic agonists such as xylazine, romifidine, and detomidine are sedatives that have both analgesic and muscle relaxant effects, and hence have been useful for control of abdominal pain in horses (and elephants). Xylazine shall be used but bradycardia is the unwanted side effect of xylazine.

Spasmolytic drugs provide analgesia by reducing spasms of the intestine. Hyoscine-N-butylbromide is an anticholinergic that acts centrally and peripherally. It is a widely used spasmolytic for management of abdominal pain in horses but has a shorter duration of pharmacological effect on the intestine relative to other anticholinergics such as atropine. Combination of hyoscine N-butylbromide and para-aminophenol derivative (dipyrone) has been used in the treatment of spasmodic colic as well as impaction colic.

Decompression of stomach

Nasogastric intubation helps to relieve gastric tympany or remove gastrointestinal reflux that is due to small intestinal obstruction or ileus (Pharyngeal pouch is the demerit in elephants for passage of stomach or nasogastric tube).

Fluids: 50 Dextrose and RL

Calcium injections in colic: Administration of calcium borogluconate by IV and calcium pantothenate by IM route.

Metaclopromide and ranitidine shall be used.

Neostigmine use in elephants

Synthetic quaternary ammonium **parasympathomimetic agents**, neostigmine bromide and neostigmine methylsulfate both occur as odorless, bitter-tasting, white, crys-talline powders that are very soluble in wate.

Pharmacology: Neostigmine competes with acetylcholine for acetyl-cholinesterase. As the neostigmine-acetylcholinesterase complex is hydrolyzed at a slower rate than that of the acetylcholine-enzyme complex, acetylcholine will accumulate with a resultant exag-geration and prolongation of its effects. These effects can include increased tone of in-testinal and skeletal musculature, stimulation of salivary and sweat glands, bronchocon - striction, ureter constriction, miosis and bradycardia. Neostigmine also has a direct choli - nomimetic effect on skeletal muscle.

Uses/Indications

Used in elephants for non-obstructive colic for stimulation of defecation (Neostigmine is indicated for rumen atony, initiating peristalsis, emptying the bladder and stimulating skeletal muscle contractions in cattle, horses, sheep and swine. It has also been used in the diagnosis and treatment of myasthenia gravis and in treating non-depolarizing neuromus-cular blocking agents (curare-type) overdoses in dogs).

Contraindications of neostigmine in animals

Neostigmine is contraindicated in patients with peritoni-tis, mechanical intestinal or urinary tract obstructions, late stages of pregnancy, in animals hypersensitive to this class of compounds or treated with other cholinesterase inhibitors.

Use neostigmine with caution in patients with epilepsy, peptic ulcer disease, bronchial asthma, cardiac arrhythmias, hyperthyroidism, vagotonia or megacolon.

Dose of neostigmine in elephants

4-5 mg/animal, IM as a purgative in impactions; author's clinical experience.

Horses

For treatment of paralytic ileus of large colon: 2-4 mg SQ q2h. Use after correction of large bowel displacement; discontinue when GI motility returns. May cause increased secretion into GI Tract

Human approved products: Neostigmine Tablets 15 mg are available.

Neostigmine Methylsulfate Injection 1:1000 (1 mg/ml), 1:2000 (0.5 mg/ml), 1:4000 (0.25 mg/ml) in 1 ml amps and 10 ml vials are available.

Clinical caution with neostigmine

Corticosteroids may decrease the anticholinesterase activity of neostigmine. After stop-ping corticosteroid therapy, neostigmine may cause increased anticholinesterase activity.

Preventive steps of Colic

- Provision of good quality feeds.
- Provision of drinking water *ad-libitum.*
- Provision of supplemental minerals to the feed materials.
- Periodic deworming esp. against the liver flukes.

15

Felid Medicine

Felid medicine needs to be well understood by the veterinarians in zoos or in any other captive wild animal places. Severe toxic reactions occur by usage of paracetamol in felids. Methaemoglobinaemia is the toxic sign noticed in felids. Hence, the zoo veterinarian can use either meloxicam or ketoprofen, in general. Tetracyclines are the drugs of choice for *Ehrlichia canis* and *Rickettsia rickettsii* in feline as well as in canine medicine. Tetracyclines are the most widely used bacteriostatic antibiotics with a blood-spectrum of activity. Felids are more susceptible than any other spp. to the tetracycline- induced hepatotoxicosis, owing to their unique protein metabolism and metabolism. (Increased ALT activity, ptyalism and anorexia including hepatic lipidosis have been documented in felids that were administered with tetracyclines).

The fungistatic drug like Griseofulvin is generally used for the treatment of dermatophycosis in canids and felids esp. with fungal infections caused by *Trichophyton* and *Microsporum* spp. This drug has no effect on other fungi. Avoid usage of this drug in the felids of neonatal-age group. Bone marrow suppression (usually manifested as neutropenia) may occur as an idiosyncratic reaction *esp.* in neonates. (The recommended dose rate is 20-50 mg/Kg/day P.O. It may be given in divided doses and needs to be administered with a fatty meal to enhance the drug- absorption).

Ketaconazole is an azole- antifungal drug that inhibits the biosynthesis of fungal lipids, *esp.* the ergosterol in cell membranes. In contrast to the effect in canids, the ketaconazole does not alter the production of cortisol, testosterone and progesteronein felids. However, in felids, the dose– related (Recommended dose is 5-10 mg/Kg P.O. at 8-12 hours) gastro-intestinal side effects like anorexia and vomiting are common.

Lignocaine is the commonly used drug in canids to treat life-threatening ventricular arrhythmias but seizures occur commonly due to lignocaine in case of felids than the canids and hence this drug must be used, cautiously in felids. (In felids, the initial dose is 0.25-0.75 mg/Kg I/V, followed by an infusion administered at 10-40 μg/kg per minute). Enrofloxacin is a fluoroquinalone bactericidal antimicrobial agent especially against gram-negative bacteria as well as *Brucella, Mycoplasma, Chlamydia* and *Mycobacterium* infections. However, retinal deformation and development of temporary blindness have been documented due to its usage in felids. The dose rates may be selected at lower range in case of felids.

Felids are more sensitive to frusemide than canids and the recommended dose rate in felids is 1-2 mg/Kg b.i.d. Frusemide-the loop diuretic inhibits sodium chloride (NaCl) re-absorption at the thick ascending loop of Henle by actively blocking sodium-potassium-chloride co-transport. Because of the large NaCl absorption-capacity of this segment, diuretics (like frusemide) that act at this site produce diuretic effect much greater than other classes of diuretics.

Digoxin is a positive inotropic and negative chronotropic drug used, frequently in the successful management of cardiac problem. Felids are more sensitive than canids to digitalis-induced toxicosis and hence, the dose needs to be reduced in the felids when compared to the canids and further, the dose needs to be reduced if given concurrently with frusemide and aspirin. (Dose: In jungle cat weighing > 6 Kg, 0.0312 mg at 12 hours).

Doxorubicin is an anthracycline-antibiotic which penetrates cells and is a potent agent against a range of tumors and is the most common single agent used for solid tumors. The dose should be reduced in felids, when compared to dogs (Recommended dose rate in felids is 1 mg/Kg). Felids are relatively resistant to developing doxorubicin-induced cardiomyopathy.

Aspirin is a non-steroidal anti-inflammatory drug (NSAID) used in felids for the management of osteoarthritis and for the prevention of thromboemboli in felids with hypertrophic cardiomyopathy. In felids, the half-life of salicylate is approximately four times longer than in case of canids and further, the felids are relatively deficient in glucuronyltransferase, which is responsible for conjugating salicylate with glucuronic acid and hence the hepatic clearance in felids is very prolonged and the clinical signs of toxicity include hypernoea, hypersensitivity and hyperthermia. (The recommended dose rate in felids is 10-20 mg/Kg at 48 hours). Felids are deficient in glucoronidase.

Chloramphenicol is preferred drug in ophthalmic infections and in meningitis. Felids have reduced capacity to glucuronidate drugs. Hence, more cautions are required during usage of this drug in felids. Organophosphates are used widely in control of ectoparasites but the felids are more sensitive to the effects of organophosphates and the toxicity (chronic or delayed) occur as paresis or paralysis, which may or may not be reversible. Toxic-epidermal necrolysis has been reported in felids that are topically treated with organophosphate- based flea rinses.

16

Disease Management in Rabbits/ Hares

All lagomorphs (meaning "hare-shaped") are small to medium-sized terrestrial herbivores. They superficially resemble rodents and in older classifications were even included in the order Rodentia, as both possess a set of continuously growing incisor teeth. It is now recognized that these two orders have long separate evolutionary histories.

There are no rabbits in Indian forests in general but hares are available in forests.

In wildlife science, one should know the differences between rabbit and hares and the variations are furnished below.

Hare	Rabbit
Larger in size and faster than rabbits	Small size and short hind limbs
Have long and strong hind limbs	Short hind limbs
Longer ears	Shorter ears
Solitary and difficult to tame	Gregarious and social in nature
Have black markings on fur	No such markings on fur
Precocial in nature (baby rabbits are born with hair and are able to see)	Altricial (babby hares are born blind and hairless)
Young hare is called as leveret	Young rabbit is called as bunny or kit or kitten
Eats harder food like bark and twigs	Prefers soft grasses and vegetables
Hares nests above ground	Rabbit's live burrows underground (Exception: Cottontail rabbits live in nests above ground like hares!)
Genus: Lepus	**Genus:** Pentalagus, Bunolagus, Nesolagus, Romerolagus, Brachylagus, Sylvilagus, Oryctolagus, Poelagus.

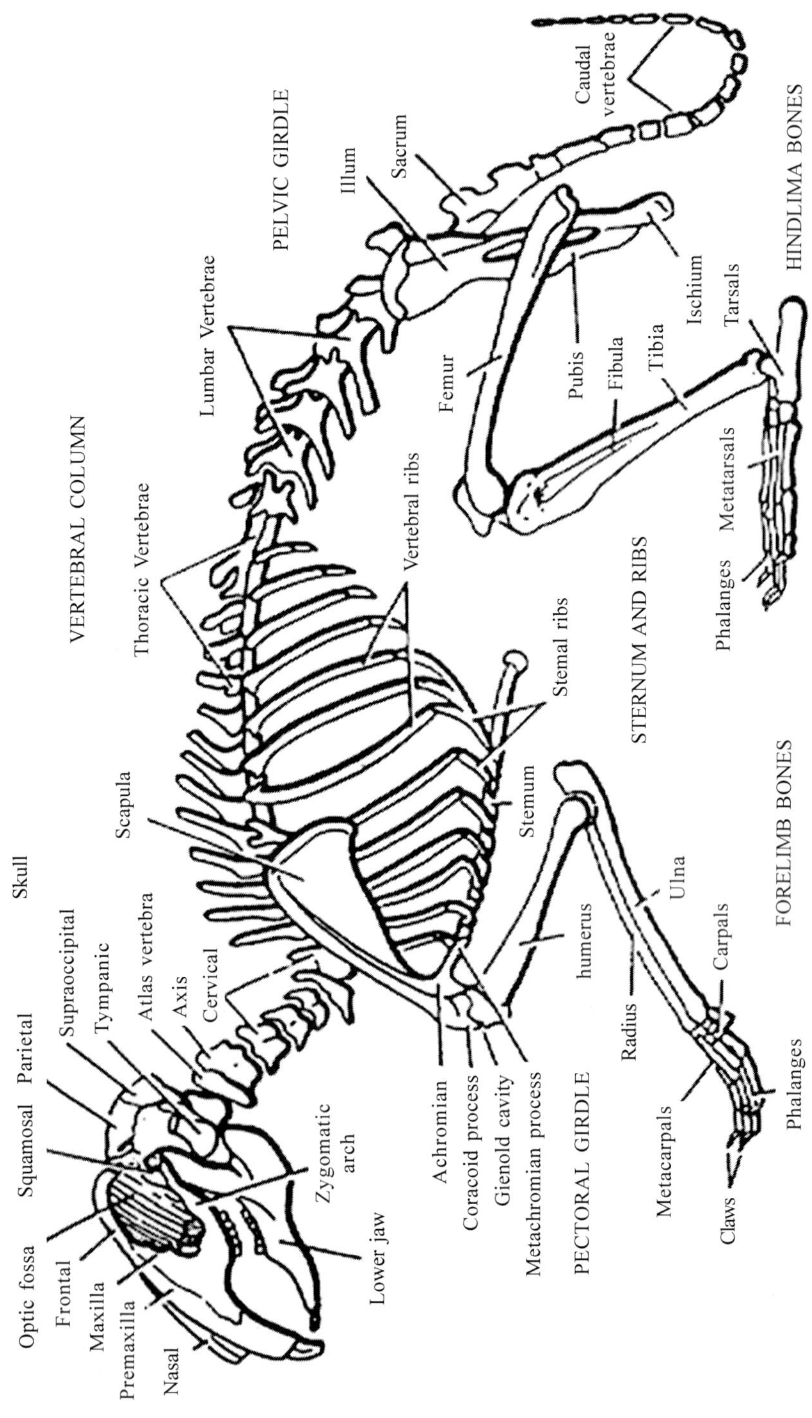

Fig. 1. (Skeleton of Rabbit)

Teeth-structures in Rabbit: Dental formula: I 2/1 **C** 0/0 **PM** 3/2 **M** 3/3

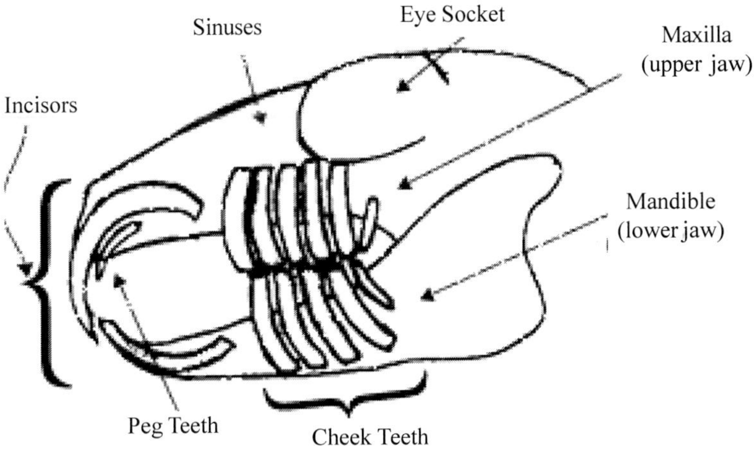

Fig. 2. Teeth and related structures

Note: Rabbits have two sets of incisor teeth in upper jaw, one behind the other. This way they can be distinguished from rodents.

Sexing of Rabbits

Male	Female
Protrude penis by manipulating skin of prepuce.	There is a common orifice for both the vagina and urethra.(like dogs and cats).
Palpate for testicles.	No structure like penis can be protruded from the urogenital orifice.
Anogenital distance is longer.	Anogenital distance is shorter.

Haematological values in Rabbits

Measurement	Normal values
PCV (%)	30-50
Hgb (g/dl)	8-17.5
RBC (10^6 /μL)	4-8
MCV (fL)	58-75
MCH (pg)	17.5-23.5
MCHC (g/dL)	29-37
Reticulocytes (%)	2-4
Platelets (10^3 /μL)	290-650
WBC (10^3 /μL)	5-12
Differential countm	
Neutrophils (%)	35-55

Lymphocytes (%)	25-60
Monocytes (%)	2-10
Eosinophils (%)	0-5
Basophils (%)	28

Serum biochemistry in Rabbits

Measurement	Normal values
ALP (U/L)	Apr-70
ALT (U/L)	14-80
AST(U/L)	14-113
Bicarbonate (mEq/L)	16.2-31.8
Bile acids (μ mol/L)	< 40
Bilirubin total (mg/dL)	0-0.75
Calcium (mg/dL)	8-14.8
Chloride (mEq/L)	92-112
Cholesterol (mg/dL)	12-116
Creatinine (mg/dL)	0.5-2.6
Glucose (mg/dL)	75-150
LDH (U/L)	34-129
Phosphorus (mg/dL)	2.3-6.9
Potassium (mEq/L)	3.5-7
Protein total (g/dL)	5.4-7.5
Albumin (g/dL)	2.5-5
Globulin (g/dL)	1.5-3.5
Sodium (mEq/L)	138-155
Triglycerides (mg/dL)	124-156
Urea nitrogen (mg/dL)	**15-50**

BIOLOGICAL AND PHYSIOLOGICAL FEATURES IN RABBITS

Normal values

Adult body weight: male (buck)	:	1.5-5 kg
Adult body weight: female (doe)	:	1.5-6 kg
Birth weight	:	30-80 g
Respiratory rate	:	30-60 breaths/min
Tidal volume	:	4-6 mL/kg
Heart rate	:	130-325 beats /min

Rectal temperature	:	38.5-40 0 C (101.3-104 0 F)
Life span	:	5-6 years (up to 15 years)
Food consumption	:	50 g/kg/day
Water consumption	:	100 mL/kg/day
Gastrointestinal transit time	:	4-5 hours
Breeding onset, male	:	6-10 months
Breeding onset, female	:	4-9 months
Breeding life of female	:	4 months to 3.75 years
Reproductive cycle	:	Induced ovulation
Gestation period	:	29-35 days
Litter size	:	4-10
Weaning age	:	4-6 weeks

Terms used in rabbits

Rabbitry: A place where domestic rabbits are kept and bred

Barn: A place for housing rabbits

Warren: Rabbits live in burrows below ground. A group of burrows is called aswarren.

Kit/ Bunny /kitten: Babby rabbit

Leveret: Young hare is called as leveret and sometimes, this term is informatllyapplied to a young rabbit as well.

Buck: Male rabbit

Doe: Female rabbit

Dam: A female rabbit which produced an offspring.

Kindling: Giving birth to young

Herd /Colony: Group of rabbits

Hutch: A term used to refer a cage in which a rabbit is housed. (Rabbit-cage).

Fostering: It is a process of placing rabbit kits from one litter in with another doe.

Intra-venous drug administration

The marginal ear veins shall be selected due to their prominence and easy access and 1.5" 22 gz needles shall be used in general. Ears are larger with more surface area and are highly vascular in nature.

Increase the visibility and dilatation of the vein by gentle rubbing, application of heat as done with heat-lamp, alcohol and / or xylene. Always administer the IV drug slowly, titrated to effects and preferably given as dilute solutions.

Treatment of Mite / Flea infestations

- Ivermectin at dose rate of 0.4 mg/kg, SC q 7-14 days for 3 treatments
- Selamectin at dose rate of 10-20 mg/kg, topically at base of neck or ear q 2-4 wks for 1-3 treatments.

Note: In rabbits, selamectin is rapidly metabolized and hence has minimum half life that in dog and cats. All these warrant the frequent usage of selamectin every 7 days in case of rabbits but in dog and cat, it is every 30 days.

- The 10% spot-on topical formulation (skin at the base of neck) of imidacloprid needs application of 0.4 ml in rabbits weighing less than 4 Kg and 0.8ml for rabbits weighing more than 4 kg.
- Meloxicam at thez dose rate of 0.2 mg/kg PO once or twice per day may be given for 5 days to reduce pain and inflammation.
- Don't debride the aural crusts in mite infestations.
- Never use fipronil in rabbits (The frontline plus®-product has fipronil which kills adult ticks and fleas and S-methoprene which attacks flea eggs and larvae).

Scabies (Sarcoptic Mange) in rabbits

Mange infestation caused by mites belonging to the species: *Sarcoptes scabiei* is common in rabbits, which is characterized by presence or absence of pruritis, specific morphology of mite and pattern of lesion distribution.

Sarcoptes scabiei is a burrowing mite, and spends most of its life-span in tunnels set under the host's skin, i.e., at the stratum granulosum of the epidermis. When infection occurs, it usually presents with several signs such as seborrheic dermatitis, erythematous papules, hyperemia and partial alopecia at the beginning. The condition is also associated with crusting, thickening of the skin, wrinkled, extensive hyperkeratosis, loss of hair, and even death at the chronic stage.

Human scabies also show similar clinical signs, but if the mites originated from another animal host the infections are mostly self-limited and short-lived.

Generally, the lesions (whitish, thickening of the skin ie. the whitish crusts) were distributed in the ear margins, nose, face and legs. The affected rabbits reveal often intensive itching on legs, eyes, tail and ears. The microscopic examination of skin scrapping reveals usually the high density of adult *Sarcoptes scabiei,* along with eggs.

Scabiosis is still hard to control. So many variants that influence include geographic factors playing an intensive role towards occurrence of these parasitic diseases.

Treatment of scabies in rabbits

Control of scabies has been by way of drug delivery. Using injectable macrocyclic lactones like Ivermectin, doramectin, and moxidectin instead of dips have many advantages like they are quicker and safer, cause the least stress to the rabbit, does not require any special handling facilities and they are also having broad spectrum anthelminthic activity.

Subcutaneous administration of Ivermectin is effective in mixed mange infestation involving Sarcoptes, Notoedres, and Psoroptes in rabbits. Several authors have used parentral Ivermectin at different dose rates for the treatment of mange in rabbit and among them, most of the treatment protocols involves a 7 day gap between subsequent injections of ivermectin.

The ivermectin- injection shall be given to the affected rabbits @ 400 μg/kg body weight (ie. 0.4 mg/kg) using the sub-cutaneous route, every 7th day for 3 or 4 occasions.

Long acting injectable Ivermectin (3.15% w/v) preparations are superior to that of conventional Ivermectin preparations (1% w/v) in managing the commonly occurring sarcoptic mange-infestations in rabbits. The single dose regimen of long acting Ivermectin will additionally be helpful in reducing the stress associated with multiple subcutaneous injection of 1% w/v Ivermectin treatment regimen. Further, the slow release and prolonged presence of Ivermectin in the circulation helps to prevent toxicity and also provide prolonged biological activity against the mites. By reducing the number of doses, the high cost of treatment due to multiple dosing can be considerably reduced making the single dose regimen the most economic treatment protocol against *Sarcoptes scabiei* in rabbits. Both Ivermectin and eprinomectin are highly effective in managing the sarcoptic mange infestation, when used topically. All the rabbits shall be expected to have complete recovery four weeks confirming efficacy. Malathion application as well as permethrine cream shall also be used externally. a single dose of long acting injectable Ivermectin (3.15% w/v) formulation at a dose rate of 700 mcg/kg bodyweightthrough subcutaneous route is sufficient in completely eliminating *Sarcoptes scabiei* mites in naturally infested rabbits.

The control related method requires high costs because of the fact that the scabies infections can occur repeatedly, if the surrounding environment is not treated or attended promptly.

Cestodiasis in rabbits

Similarly, lagomorphs like rabbits acts as intermediate host for tape worm *Multiceps serialis* (adult form occurs in definitive host like dogs and cats). In rabbits the elongated cysts of *Multiceps serialis* found in subcutaneous muscle and muscle mass. The parasitic worm is also called as *Taenia serialis.*

Treatment consists of oral administration of praziquantel at the rate of. 5-10 mg/kg bwt.

Myxomatosis

- Myxomatosis is an important disease of rabbits caused by a poxvirus called the Myxoma virus (MV). MV causes a very mild disease in its original host native to South America, but in some species of rabbits and hares, especially the European rabbits it causes a severe disease with high mortality. Myxomatosis is a highly contagious viral disease in rabbits that is usually fatal.
- Biting insects such as fleas, mites and mosquitoes spread the illness.
- Vaccination is the only way to protect the rabbit against myxomatosis.
- The virus only affects rabbits and poses no public health risk.

Myxomatosis (sometimes referred to as myxi) is caused by the myxoma virus which is a kind of pox virus that only affects rabbits. There are also different strains of the virus which vary in their virulence (basically the ability to cause disease) but both the wild and the domesticated rabbits can contract the disease.

Myxomatosis is called "big head" and is characterized by mucinous skin lesions or myxedema of the head. Wild rabbits such as the cottontail (*Sylvilagus*) and jackrabbits (*Lepus*) are quite resistant.

Transmission

The virus is spread by blood sucking insects (fleas, mosquitoes, mites, lice, and flies) in most cases. The rabbit flea is usually the reason for myxomatosis in our pet rabbits.

Symptoms

Myxomatosis, sometimes referred to as myxi, is a serious condition that can appear with several different kinds of clinical symptoms.

Depending on the strain of the virus, it can take up to 14 days for an infected rabbit to begin to show symptoms. During the incubation period, a rabbit's behaviour and eating habits may change. When the virus takes hold, the eyes, nose and genitals are usually the first parts of the body to be affected. Symptoms include.

- Swelling, redness and/or ulcers.
- Nasal and eye discharge.
- Blindness caused by inflammation of the eyes.\
- Respiratory problems.
- Loss of appetite.
- Lethargy
- Most rabbits die within 14 days of the onset of symptoms. In more chronic cases (and depending on the strain of the virus and immunity of the rabbit), lumps and nodules (myxomas) may develop on the body.
- Rabbits with this form of myxomatosis may survive and become immuned to myxomatosis virus and it is commonly seen in wild cottontail rabbits. This seems to be a less likely course of disease in domestic rabbits (*Oryctolagus cuniculus*) since most that are diagnosed with the disease end up suffering from the acute forms with eventual death. Domestic rabbits tend to be very susceptible to the virus and tend to suffer a long and painful death.
- Few characteristic gross lesions are found at necropsy in the acute form of the disease. The spleen is occasionally enlarged and is almost always devoid of lymphocytes when examined histologically. In rabbits that survive longer, subcutaneous edema and nodular skin tumors are seen. The seasonal incidence of the disease, clinical signs (especially the swollen genitalia), and high mortality are all of diagnostic significance. Large, eosinophilic, cytoplasmic inclusion bodies in the conjunctival epithelial cells are also helpful in diagnosis.

Treatment

There is no specific treatment for myxomatosis unfortunately so only supportive care (fluids, antibiotics to prevent secondary infections, etc.) can be offered.

Prevention

- Keep your rabbit indoors and away from mosquito infested areas and use mosquitoe nets on rabbit-cage/enclosure.
- Quarantine period is 14 days.

- Use a safe flea preventative like selamectin (Revolution) for pet rabbits (discuss this with your exotics vet since you will need a prescription) even if your rabbit never goes outside.
- The vaccine can be given to rabbits once they are six weeks old (immunity develops within 14 days), and repeated yearly, or every six months where myxomatosis is common.

DERMATOMYCOSIS

For individual rabbit

- Grieseofulvin at dose rate of 15-25 mg/kg bwt, PO daily or divided q 12 hrs for a month.
- For ultramicronized grieseofulvin, reduce the dose rate to 50% and administer with a high fat meal for better absorption.

Note: Grieseofulvin is teratogenic and should not be given to the pregnant Does.

- Itraconazole 5-10 mg/kg bwt, PO daily.
- Terbinafine 10 mg/kg bwt PO daily.

For massive nos. of rabbits

- A 2-3% lime sulfur solution is to be sprayed on large no.of infected rabbits weekly for 4 weeks.

flea infestations

Ctenocephalides canis and *Ctenocephalides felis* affect rabbits also.

- Ivermectin is one of the drugs used for external parasitism in rabbits.
- Selamectin (Revolution®-Pfizer) at dose rate of 20 mg kg^{-1} topically at base of neck or ear q 7 days for 1-3 treatments.
- Topical application of 0.4 ml of 10% imidacloprid (Advantage®-Bayer) as spot-on formulation shall be carried out as a single topical application onto the skin of the dorsal mid-line behind the base of the skull, in rabbits.

Pin worms in rabbits

Passalurus ambiguus, is the commonly encountered rabbit pinworm and *Passalurus nonanulatus* is another sp. of pin worms found in rabbits. The adult worm lives in the cecum or anterior colon.

Treatment of Pinworms (Passalurus ambiguus)

- Clean piworms from the perianal regions.

- Fenbendazole at dose rate of 10-20 mg/kg PO and repeat after 10-14 days.
- Alternatively use Piperazine dose rate of 200 mg/kg PO and repeat after 14 days. Piperazine citrates in the water (3 g/L) for alternating 2-wk periods or fenbendazole (50 ppm in feed for 5 days) are effective treatments.

  Rabbit pinworms are not transmissible to people.

Giardiasis

Metronidazole is the drug of choice (20 mg/kg bwt, PO twice/day).

Encephalitozoonosis

Encephalitozoon cuniculi is a widespread protozoal (microsporidian) infection of rabbits and occasionally of mice, guinea pigs, rats, and dogs.

Encephalitozoonosis is an emerging disease of immunodeficient people.Usually, no clinical signs are seen, but a few rabbits develop mild, chronic renal disease.

Some develop brain lesions that may result in convulsions, tremors, or head tilt. Head tilt is often caused by bacterial infection with *Pasteurella multocida*; this can be difficult to distinguish from head tilt associated with *E cuniculi* infection, because both infections are common and can occur together.

Treatment of *Encephalitozoon cuniculi(Encephalitozoonosis).*

Fenbendazole	20 mg/kg bwt, PO once daily for 5-28 days.
Albendazole	20-30 mg/kg bwt, PO once daily for 30 days and reduce to 15 mg/kg once daily PO for 30 days.
Oxybendazole	20 mg/kg bwt, PO once daily for 7-14 days, then reduced to 15 mg/kg bwt, once daily for 30-60 days.
Praziquantel	5-10 mg/kg bwt, PO and repeat in 10 days.

Barbering (OR) hair pulling (OR) self mutilation

If no treatment is available, to stop the self mutilation, administer haloperidol (0.2-0.4 mg/kg PO twice daily).

Coccidiosis

There are two anatomic forms: hepatic, caused by *Eimeria stiedae*, and intestinal, caused by *E magna*, *E irresidua*, *E media*, *E perforans*, *E flavescens*, *E intestinalis*, or other *Eimeria* spp. Transmission of both the hepatic and intestinal forms is by ingestion of the sporulated oocysts, usually in contaminated feed or water.

Hepatic coccidiosis

- This is most often sub-clinical in nature and young rabbits are mostly affected. Small yellowish nodules were found through hepatic parenchyma and in early stages, the lesions have a milky content and the older lesions have more cheese like consistency.
- Microscopically, the nodules have hypertrophied bile duct or gall bladder.
- Impression-smears over the liver and examination under light microscopy often reveal oocysts.

Intestinal coccidiosis

- Rough coat, dullness, decreased appetite, dehydration and weight loss occur, abdominal pain, diarrhea and faces with blood or mucus.
- Generally the lesions of hepatic and intestinal coccidiosis are similar.

Treatment of Coccidiosis

- Amprolium 9.6% in drinking water (0.5 ml per half litre water).
- Trimethoprim-sulfamethoxazole at dose rate of 30 mg/kg PO twice daily for 10 days.
- Sulfadimethoxine at dose rate of 15 mg/kg PO twice daily for 10 days.
- Toltrazuril (Baycox®), 2.5 to 5 mg/kg (higher doses cause anorexia and decrease in size of fecal droppings), twice, repeat after 5 days.

For massive nos. of rabbits

Sulfadimethoxine is to be added to the diet to ensure intake of 75 mg/kg for 7 days or 0.02% sulfamerazine sodium to the drinking water is efficacious for treatment of group of rabbits.

Very few products are licensed for use in rabbits, leading to extra-label use of drug therapies approved for use in other species. Particular caution must be exercised in use of antibiotics that suppress normal GI microflora and result in enteric dysbiosis and/or enterotoxemia. This has been called "antibiotic toxicity."

Antibiotics contraindicated in rabbits include clindamycin, lincomycin, erythromycin, ampicillin, amoxicillin/clavulanic acid, and cephalosporins. The flea treatment fipronil is contraindicated in rabbits because of severe toxic reactions in some individuals.

Supportive care for rabbits often includes aggressive IV fluid support. The maintenance fluid rate for rabbits (120 mL/kg/day) is much higher than that for dogs and cats. Hospitalized rabbits often require doubling of maintenance rates, or 10 mL/kg/hr.

In addition to fluid support, pain control is also commonly needed. NSAIDs and opioids are often used in synergy. The dosage of meloxicam in rabbits is 1 mg/ kg/day, which is also significantly higher than that in dogs and cats.

Opioids such as oxymorphone or hydromorphine can readily be used and have not been shown to cause GI stasis. In most cases, additional force feeding is not required, and the rabbit should be offered food after fluid and pain management has been initiated. Syringe-assisted feeding can be offered to see whether the rabbit is interested in food intake.

In rare cases in which the rabbit refuses to eat, eg, cases of severe hepatic lipidosis, active feeding is necessary; treatment may require aggressive nutritional support via syringe feeding, nasogastric tube (3–5 French), or pharyngostomy tube (soft esophagostomy tube designed for cats). The least invasive method is often the most successful approach. Various commercial products for assisted feeding of rabbits are available.

Restraint related medicaments for use in rabbits

Rabbits have a high body surface area to body weight despite the existence of heavy fur and hence, the rabbits are often predisposed to hypothermia. Hence, monitoring the respiratory rate and body temperature is a must during usage of any immobilizing agent in case of rabbits.

In general

- Body temperature of rabbits: 37.8^{0}C (100-104^{0}F).
- Respiratory rate: 33-36 breaths/minute.

DRUGS	DOSE RATE	TECHNICAL POINTS
Atropine (this anticholinergic agent is generally required to counteract salivation and bronchial secretion (during usage of ketamine) and bradycardia (during usage of xylazine)	0.8-3 mg/kg bwt, SC, IM	High levels of endogenous atropinase are present in 30-50% of all rabbits and hence the use of atropine in rabbits as a standard premedication is a controversial one. Glycopyrrolate is a better choice than atropine in case of rabbits due to its longer duration of action.
Glycopyrrolate	0.01-0.1 mg/kg bwt, SC	It is an anticholinergic preanaesthetic agent.
Xylazine	4-5 mg/kg bwt, IM	Sedation, some analgesia, cardiac dysarrhthmias and respiratory depression.
Ketamine	25 mg/kg bwt, IM	Sedation but muscle rigidity and muscle necrosis and tissue irritation

		and seizures. Hence, better to combine with benzodiazepines, preferably or with xylazine.
Diazepam	4-10 mg/Kg bwt, IM	Good sedation and muscle relaxation but no analgesia.
	2 mg/Kg bwt, IV	Broad therapeutic index (if vein is inaccessible, rectal administration shall be carried out).
Midazolam	4 mg/Kg bwt, IM 2 mg/Kg bwt, IV	Similar to diazepam.
Butorphanol	0.1-0.5 mg/Kg bwt, IM, IV q 4-6 hrs	Analgesia and sedation
Acepromazine	0.5-2 mg/Kg bwt, IM	Moderate sedation, tranquilization; no analgesia; hypotensive and hypothermic effects.
Chlorpromazine	20-25 mg/Kg bwt, IM	
Propofol	8-12 mg/Kg bwt, slow IV	Respiratory depressions dependent on the speed of injection and dose.
		Hypotensive Induction and recovery are free of excitement.
Thiopental	30-45 mg/Kg bwt slow IV	Transient apnea is possible; abnormal bronchial and salivary secretions.

17

Therapeutic Management of Significant Captive Wild Animal Diseases & Disorders

Due to the paucity of clinical data, therapeutic management measures available with domestic animal-practice needs to be extrapolated for due usage in case of captive wild animals reared in zoos, zoological parks and zoological gardens.

Trypanosomosis

- The affected wild animal is to be treated with diminazene aceturate (curative) at rate of 3.5 mg/kg body weight by deep IM, for 5 days along with supportive therapy; sometimes, treatment by SC route with diminazene aceturate at rate of 7 mg/kg on the first day and 3.5 to 7 mg/kg on the following day also may yield success. A total of 5–8 sezrial injections with diminazene aceturate at 3.5 mg/kg bw at a 2-3 week interval by IM is also recommended. Melarsomine dihydrocholoride (which is generally used against heart worms of carnivores both for treatment and prophylaxis) shall be used at a rate of 1-2 mg/kg wt by IM, in general.
- Quinapyramine sulphate and chloride (3.5 mg/kg bwt, SC) shall be used in dogs and this drug is meant for both the curative and prophylactic purposes..
- Meloxicam shall be given by IM at dose rate of 0.5 mg/kg bwt and anemia is to be corrected appropriately.

Babesiosis

Imidocarb dipropionate: 1 to 1.2 mg/kg SC or even IM. Sometimes, up to 3 mg/kg is also given and it gives protection up to four weeks and also it helps to eliminate both B. bigemina and B. bovis in carrier animals also. For prophylaxis purposes, this drug shall be used temporarily to protect the bovids.

In bovids

Diminazene aceturate (7%) shall be administered by IM route at dose of 3.5 mg/kg for two successive days (or) 12 mg/kg as single dose by IM. Supportive therapy with blood transfusion is to be undertaken additionally. Quinoronium-sulphate (5%) shall also be given.

In equids: Imidocarbdipropionate: 4.4mg/kg once IM.

In canids

Diminazene aceturate (or) preferably the Imidocarb dipropionate @ 6.6 mg/kg in canids and 5mg/kg in felids, by IM route and in these animals totally 2 doses are to be given, 14 days apart. For B.gibsoniof carnivores, marshal protocol (Metronidazole + doxycycline+clindamycin) shall be used (or) atavaquone, with azithromycin shall be given (or) buparvaquone with azithromycin shall be given and it appears better to administer dexamethasone (or) other steroids as needed, concurrently.

Theileriosis in ruminants

Buparvaquone (@ 2.5 mg/kg, IM) or oxytetracycline @10mg/kg IM/IV or long acting oxytetracycline at the dose rate of 20 mg/kg b.wt. IM orhalofuginone (treatment with halofuginone administered orally, which is the typical treatment for cryptosporidium in neonatal animals) are effective in ruminants. Frusemide also shall be given along with the Parvaquone in the theilieriosis affected animals revealing pulmonary system-derangement related clinical symptoms.

Ehrlichiosis and anaplasmosis

Both of these conditions have similar clinical manifestations in general with high fever and haematologic abnormalities.

In carnivores: Doxycycline: Dose rate is 5-10 mg/kg/day, PO or IV, for 10-21 /28 days (drug of choice); Doxycycline is the most commonly used antibiotic. Other antibiotic options are tetracycline (or) minocycline.

Note: For both Anaplasmosis and Ehrlichiosis, the doxycycline (one of the tetrayclines which has a merit of low renal toxicity) is the drug of choice because of it's superior intracellular penetration and bacteriostatic properties against the rickettsiae; further, the doxycycline is recommended for canids of all ages.

- Tetracycline: Dose rate is 22 mg/kg, PO, three times a day (≥2 weeks, acute cases, 1–2 months, chronic cases)
- Imidocarbdiproprionate: 2 doses, 5–7 mg/kg, IM, 2 weeks apart (also effective for some strains of babesiosis)
- NSAIDs and appropriate fluid therapy (isotonic saline in pyrexia-cases) are to be additionally given.

In ruminants

Generally, oxytetracycline at dose level of 10 mg/kg body weight for 5 days was found to be effective. If neonatal ruminants are affected, oxytetracycline (10 mg/kg/day, IM) or doxycycline (@ 2 mg/kg/day) shall be given and this will usually affect a cure, if administered early in the course of ehrlichiosis. A higher dosage of oxytetracycline (20 mg/kg) is usually required if treatment begins late during the febrile reaction (or) when clinical signs are evident. In such cases, the first treatment should preferably be given slowly IV. A minimum of 3 daily doses should be given regardless of temperature; if fever persists, oxytetracycline treatment should continue for a fourth and fifth day. If the fever still does not abate, a potentiated sulfonamide (15 mg/kg/day, IM) shall be given. Corticosteroids have been used as supportive therapy (prednisolone 1 mg/kg, IM), although there is debate as to the effectiveness and rationale for their use.

Hepatozoonosis

- Imidocarb dipropionate IM 5-7 mg/kg imqt 14 days till there is no organism found out in blood smear.
- Doxycycline @ 10 mg/kg, PO daily for 24 days.
- Many times, Doxycycline is given along with the Imidacarbdipropionate.
- Meloxicam @ 0.5mg/kg bwt, IM daily for 3-5 days.
- Haematinics, PO daily for few weeks.

Thelaziasis (Eye worm infestations in conjunctiva)

Thelazia species related infections have been successfully eliminated from carnivores with administration of ivermectin at 0.2 mg/kg, SC (or) milbemycin oxime at a minimum dosage of 0.5 mg/kg, PO (two treatments 1 week apart improved efficacy) or spot-on treatment with 2.5% moxidectin. Additionally, eye drops containing ciprofloxacin in combination with dexamethasone shall be used every 8 hours for bovids and equids for about five days.

For canids and felids, macrocyclic lactones are available (mostly tablets eg. Ivermectin, Milbemycinoxime and Moxidectin) or injectables (e.g. moxidectin) or spot-ons (e.g. selamectin) shall be used. Ocular drops (e.g. moxidectin+ levamisole) shall also be used against thelaziasis.

For large and small ruminants, the macrocyclic lactones shall be used and additionally the pour-ons or drenches (e.g. abamectin, doramectin, ivermectin, moxidectin) shall also be used.

Slow-release boluses also shall be used, in this regard.

Setariasis (Eye worm infestation, esp. in equids)

Ivermectin is the most advocated drug for ocular equine setariasis, but long term tying of medicinal should be avoided and surgery should be advocated. The standard antifilarial drug, diethylcarbamazine citrate (DEC) has generally given inconsistent results only. However, the medical treatment has not been considered suitable because of the slow absorption of dead parasites and the attendant antigenicity.

Surgical measures using 21 gz needle for paracentesis-procedure involving affected eye. Needle paracentesis at 3 O' clock and nick incision at 12 O' clock position are most commonly used surgical procedure. Both the techniques give satisfactory results (A slightly modified technique of using a 21 gauge needle attached with the syringe to aspirate the worm into the syringe also gives satisfactory result). Remember that corneal opacity is the most common post-operative complication and post-surgical use of placentrex has also been advocated to enhance healing and to resolve the corneal opacity, in general.

Subsequent to surgical interventions, antibiotic related eye-drops need to be used to avoid bacterial infections.

Heart worms in carnivores

Melarsomine dihydrochloride is to be used.2.5 mg/Kg by deep IM at lumbar-epaxial muscles i.e. muscles lying dorsally at the level of 3rd to 5th lumbar vertebrae in the affected carnivore.

The goal of treatment is to kill all adult heartworms with minimal drug toxicity and a tolerable degree of pulmonary thromboembolism caused by the dying worms. Microfilaria should be eliminated, but it is not necessary to administer a rapid-kill microfilaricide such as Interceptor. Gradual elimination of microfilaria over a period of 6 to 8 months with monthly macrolide administration is acceptable and shall be adapted in general.

As microfilaricide, one can use Avermectins/ Milbemycin (Like Melarsomine, the Milbemycin also be used for prevention of heart worms) but they may not have effect on the adult heart worms.

Doxycycline (or) preferably the minocycline shall also be used additionally to treat Wolbachia - an organism that infects heartworms, in general (*Wolbachia* is a genus of intracellular bacteria that infects mainly arthropod species, including a high proportion of insects and also some nematodes).

HELMINTHIASIS IN GENERAL

Ivermectin

200 mg/kg, SC (or 0.2 mg/kg, SC) in all species.

300 to 400 mg/kg PO in all species.

Fenbendazole dose

Large and small ruminants and swines: 5 to 15 mg/kg bodyweight

Swines: 3 to 6 mg/kg, PO

Canids and felids: 50 mg/kg, PO

Albendazole dose

Large and small ruminants and swines: 5mg/kg bodyweight, PO

Canids and felids: 10 to 25mg/kg bodyweight, PO

Levamisole dose

Canids (5mg/kg SC, IM or 7.5 to 16 mg/kg, PO)

Felids (8mg/kg SC, IM or 7.5 to 25 mg/kg, PO)

Bovids (5mg/kg,IM or 7.5 mg/kg, SC or 7.5 to 12 mg/kg, PO)

Equids (5 to 10 mg/kg, SC or 7.5 to 15 mg/kg, PO)

Swines (5mg/kg SC, IM or 7.5 to 10 mg/kg, PO)

Praziquantel dose

5 mg/kg (general) or even 10 mg/kg, PO in all species except the equids in which the dose is 1 to 2.5 mg/kg, PO but in swines for C.tenuicollis: 10 mg/kg, daily for 10 days, PO.

Demodicosis

The generalized form requires more aggressive treatment using special shampoos and dips, along with oral medication. Carnivores with secondary infection, excessive scale/exudate or with numerous comedones should be shampooed with 2.5% benzyl peroxide before each amitraz dip; benzyl peroxide has disinfectant, astringent and keratolytic properties and has the capacity to flush debris from hair follicles, facilitating the entry of amitraz.

Use 0.05–0.1% amitraz solution twice weekly in canids and 0.0125% to 0.025% in felids. Adapt long term chemical immobilization, to avoid licking of Amitraz dip solution applied all over the body and suitable Elizabethan collar shall be used in animals to avoid licking of medication applied on the body. Effective treatment for generaliseddemodicosis as a weekly wash at a concentration of 500ppm.

A new spot-on Amitraz- formulation containing metaflumizone and amitraz shall also is used as a topical bi-monthly treatment for generalized demodicosis.

Lime Sulfur dips can be used for demodicosis and are particularly effective in the earlier phases of treatment of very severe cases of generalized demodicosis with severe furuncolosis forming deep pyoderma. Dose for external application of the lime sulfur dip solution is 1.6% to 2% once (or) twice-weekly, in carnivores.

The gold standard of treatment is to reach two negative skin scrapings from previously affected sites within a 30 day interval.

Endectocides (or) macrocycliclactones are veterinary parasiticides used globally to control nematodes and arthropods. Use Ivermectin (Injection / oral tab / Pour-on-preparations)

Ivermectin is found to be the ideal drug in the treatment of demodicosis in domestic as well as wild animals.

Dose of ivermectin in animals

Injection: 0.2 mg/kg bwt by sc injection / oral tab: 0.4mg/kg bwt. PO / Pour-on-preparations, daily for about 28 days or even more if required), in general.

In captive swines, ivermectin at a daily oral dose of 0.45g/kg of feed, for a week.

Eprinomectin (Pour-on solutions) shall also be used against the external parasitic conditions in animals.

Moxidectin at dose of 0.2 to 0.5 mg/kg shall also be used by oral route by concealing in meat pieces offered for the affected carnivores once in a day.

Milbemycin, like ivermectin is an oral avermectin registered for heartworm prevention in dogs and when used at a dose rate of 1–2 mg/kg PO once in 24 hrs, this drug is very effective in the treatment of canine demodicosis.

Merits of Milbemycin

- Milbemycin is better tolerated.
- Much fewer side effects than with ivermectin.

Fluralaner belongs to isoxazoline group of drugs and is the potent inhibitors of NS of arthropods.

Dose of fluralaner : 25mg/kg, PO once in 8 to 12 weeks.

Scabies/ lice infestations & fleainfestations

Lime-sulfur, Ivermectin, Milbemycin, Doramectin, Amitraz and Fipronil spray. Moxidectin-Imidoclopridare etc. are generally used against the scabies.

Leptospirosis

Doxycycline (5 mg/kg PO q12h or 10 mg/kg PO q24h, PO, for a total period of 14 days.

Following drugs are also used

- Penicillin G 25,000–40,000 U/kg IV q6–8h.
- Ampicillin 20–30 mg/kg IV q6–8h.

Supportive measures for acute kidney injury and liver disease (fluid therapy, with electrolyte supplementation, correction of acid-base disorders; antiemetics; phosphate binders; hepatic support medications (or) appetite stimulants) also need to be given to the leptospirosis affected animals. Intermittent hemodialysis or continuous renal replacement therapy also need to be given priority if severe oluguria or anuria is evident in the leptospirosis affected carnivores.

Haemorrhagic septicaemia (HS) in wild animals

Mammals esp. small and large ruminants, elephants, birds esp. aquatic and semi-aquatic aviary species etc. are generally affected frequently by HS, particularly in monsoon periods. Tetracycline by oral route or by injection (IV) shall be used or preferably enrofloxacin shall be used at appropriate dose rate.

Tetanus in non - human primates, cervids etc

Tetanus anti-serum shall be given and sub-cutaneous injection of mag sulph shall also be given and in the event of convulsions if any, diazepam shall be given by IV route at rate of 0.3 to 0.8 mg/kg bwt by IV and in severe cases, xylazine shall be given with caution like prior carrying out of atropinization of the animal. Tetanus toxoid is to be given for prophylaxis esp. before carrying out the surgical interventions.

Immune mediated haemolyticanaemia (IMHA) and immune thrombocytopenia (ITP) in captive carnivores

Treatment of IMHA may involve dealing with any underlying diseases that may have caused the IMHA (RICKETTSIA, MYCOPLASMA etc). NOTE: Babesia infections have a wide range of severity: they can be very mild (or) very severe, sometimes even fatal. The severity depends mainly on the strain of Babesia involved but also on the immune system of the carnivores. In ITP, prednisolone shall be used at rate of 1mg/kg bwt, orally on daily basis till platelets get increased to a desirable level. Similar dose shall be used in IMHA cases also and tapering dose of steroid is to be followed as in case of domestic animals.Therapy with prednisolone preferably with Vincristine shall be considered as the first line of therapy in immune mediated diseases and the second line of therapy includes use of cyclosporine esp. if the immune mediated diseases become refractory to prednisolone therapy shall be adapted, either by using prednisolone in combination with Cyclosporine-a costly drug or Cyclosporine alone (Dose of Cyclosporine: 2.5 mg/kg BID orally initially and later on modification in dose shall be adapted depending on clinical response). Azathioprine (initially 2 mg/kg SID orally) shall also be used like the prednisolone as an immune-suppressant drug, like the cyclosporine.

Intravenous human immunoglobulin (IVIG) also shall be used at dose rate of 0.5 to1g/kg IV, once) but this is costly. Anaemia in these immune mediated diseases shall have to be corrected by blood transfusion as in IMHA and preferably by platelet transfusion in ITP affecting the animals and the precise-cause needs to be however concurrently addressed in a fast manner.

Colloids i.e. the blood volume expanders (hetastarch, dextranetc, which are comparatively better than crystalloids like Isotonicsaline/5% DNS/5% Dextrose/ Ringers lactate etc.) shall be used for fluid therapy in animals with autoimmune diseases, in order to stabilize the immune mediated diseases. In totally refractory cases for these treatments, splenectomy shall be considered, taking other care related measures.

Congestive heart failure of carnivores

Digoxin (with loading and maintenance dose) or preferably, the Pimobendan (0.2 to 0.6 mg/kg PO, IV, daily &this is to be divided bid/day) shall be used as a positive inotropic drug of choice by oral route or if it is emergency, it is to be used by IV route. Diuretics like frusemide (2 mg/kg, IV / PO) or Spiranolactone (Canids: 1-2 mg/kg once in 24 hrs and Felids: 1 mig/kg once in 24 hrs) shall be used esp. in cases with any type of oedema or fluid accumulation as in pulmonary tissue-infiltration with fluid-secretions, in addition to the usage of ACE inhibitors like enalapril with the dose of 0.25 to 0.5 mg/kg, PO in carnivores esp. the canids that are identified with clinical symptoms pertaining to the hypertension.

For bradycardia, atropine sulphate (0.04 mg/kg) shall be used along with slow fluid therapy using blood volume expanders. Dopamine at dose rate of 5-15 mcg/kg/min IV (medium dose) given along with fluid therapy using esp. the blood volume expanders like dextrans or preferably the hetastarch IV infusions. Such measures may often result in increase of the renal blood flow, cardiac output, heart rate, and cardiac contractility.

HYPOCALCAEMIA

Carnivores

In eclampsia affected carnivores infuse by IV the calcium gluconate (or) calcium borogluconate solution. Calcium borogluconate is the drug of choice and is available as 25 % solution (1 ml / Kg of 25 % Calcium borogluconate solution by IM or SC; if the quantity is more, SC route is preferred). If 10% Calcium gluconate is available, 1 ml / Kg of this 10% solution by slow IV may be given. When the condition becomes stable in the female canids, then the strength of calcium gluconate may be reduced with equal volume of 0.9% Na Cl and this should be given by SC route, twice daily.

Herbivores esp. ruminants:

Usually 20% calcium borogluconate solution is being used for IV purpose (350 to 450 ml; 50% by slowIV and 50% by SC route), in the treatment of the milk fever in ruminants. It is better to administer the Calcium-Magnesium-borogluconate combination solution at the dose rate of 200 to 350 ml IV, followed by SC for rest of dose. Single injection of 8 mg of Vitamin D_3 (ie. Cholecalciferol) 3 to 10days before calving in bovids generally can reduce the rate of occurrence of milk fever without producing any clinical signs of hypervitaminosis D. Calcium propionate in propylene glycol gel (or) powdered calcium propionate (0.5 kg dissolved in 8–16 L water) shall be given orally.

In non-ruminants like pigs, 100 ml of 20% calcium borogluconate shall be given by slow IV or 25 ml by IM in four sites.

Hypomagnesemia in ruminants

Animals showing clinical signs require treatment immediately with combined solutions of calcium and Mg, preferably given slowly IV while monitoring the heart. The response to treatment is slower in animals with hypomagnesemic tetany than in animals with hypocalcemia alone, because of the time it takes to restore Mg in the CSF. The animal should not be stimulated during treatment, because this could trigger fatal convulsions. Additional Mg sulfate (200 mL of a 50% solution/cow) can be given SC. After treatment; cows should be left to respond without stimulation and then moved off the tetany-prone pasture, if possible. Animals must be provided with hay treated with 2 oz (60 g) of Mg oxide daily; if this is not done, the condition can recur within 36 hr after initial therapy.

KETOSIS IN RUMINANTS

The treatment of ketosis mainlycomprises the intra-venous infusion of 50% dextrose solution (about 500 ml in 400kg ruminant) in a slow manner and avoid SC injection of hypertonic solutions due to possibility of the tissue irritations at the sub-cutaneous regions. Concurrently, by oral route, about 300 ml of propylene glycol, BID/day in a 400 kg ruminant, for five days shall be given to hasten the recovery from ketotic condition and also, the ammonium lactate which is highly glucogenic shall be given at the rate of 200 gm per day for five days, by oral route in ruminants with ketosis.

Similarly, 40 mg of dexamethasone sodium phosphate or 5 mg of flumethasone has to be concurrently given to produce the hyperglycemic state in a fast manner in ketosis affected ruminants. Cyanocobalamine dose rate of 1 to 4 mg by IV, daily shall be given, preferably in combination with butaphosphan. Cysteamine which is a precursor of coenzyme A shall be given at dose rate of 750 mg by IV for 3 doses at one to three days intervals.

Capature myopathy in equids

Injection of Vitamin E (1 to 2 IU/kg bwt, IM / IV and in a wild horse or other equids like zebra, 800 to 900 IU shall be administered in a 500 kg equid and thiamine HCl (Vitamin B1) shall be given at rate of0.5 to 1 gm, IM followed by 100 to 200 gm thrice daily by oral route. Corticosteroid like prednisolone shall be given at a larger dose rate (1 to 2 mg/kg bwt, IM). Hot and cold fomentations/ applications shall be carried out over the muscles esp. muscular regions of the hind limbs. If the pain is severe, diazepam shall be used at rate of 0.5 to 1 mg/kg bwt, IM (or) even IV. Empirical therapy in equids generally consists of auto-haemotherapy by drawing of the same affected animal's blood from jugular vein and giving it by sub-cutaneous route for the same animal.

Dantrolene-the skeletal muscle relaxant shall be used in equids and carnivores with myositis.

Dose of Dantrolene in equids:Preventive: 500 mg BID daily for 3 to 4 days.

Curative: 4 mg/kg, PO, daily via NG tube (2 mg/kg if by IV)

Dantrolene is used in case of malignant hyperthermia affected canids or even in other carnivores:

Dose of Dantrolene canids or even in other carnivores:1.5 mg/kg PO, daily bid for 5 days,in case of malignant hyperthermia and in stress syndromes)

In recumbency related to myositis, frusemide at rate of 1 mg/kg shall be given if pulmonary fluid accumulation is present in them.

Iron deficiency anaemia in captively held wild piglets

Dose of iron in piglet anemia cases is 200mg of iron as total dose / piglet (IM/SC) in first days of life ie.at 3rd day of life (when wt may be abt 1 or < 1 kg) and split dosing shall be given in the first few months of age to promote the weight gain as well as to take care of anaemicproblems in the piglets. The IM injections are to be given to the captive pigletsdeep into the muscle with a relatively long needle - up to 20 mm.

Demerits of iron-dextran injection

1. Narrow safety index (common is the iron-toxicity related reactions); hence, administer parenterally the dexamethasone on safe side at rate of 0.3 to 0.5 mg/kg bwt.
2. Iron dextran can stain the tissues at the site of injections
3. Injection is painful, in general.

Combination of ferrous sulphate (25 mg) and copper sulphate (5 mg) shall be given daily in feed/water to the piglets. Iron licks (or) blocks shall be used in the concerned enclosure of the pregnant sows. Oral supplementation of mineral mixtures and tablets containing iron shall be given. Daily painting of iron sulphate solution (0.5kg of ferrous sulphate in 10 litres of water) onto the sow's teat shall be carried out if practically possible in a zoo environment though it is difficult most of the times.

Hypoglycaemia esp. in neonatal animals and more particularly in newborn piglets

Administer 5% glucose solution at rate of 10 to 25 ml through intra-peritoneal route and the injection shall be repeated at 4 to 6 hours interval till the condition reveals the improvement and piglets can suckle their mother and also attempts need to be made to keep the affected piglets in a warm environment.

Rhino diseases in general and treatment

Parasitic diseases encountered generally include the roundworms, flat worms, protozoa and miscellaneous parasites of large ungulates with Anaplacephalidae, Plagiotaenia, Schistosoma, Fasciolidae, Paramphistomidae, Stomach botfly larvae, Trichostrongylus, Oesophagostomoma, Strongyloidae, Ophryoscolecidae, Cryptosporidium, Entamoeba, Balantidium, Maggots around the horn base etc.

Blood protozoa in rhinos include trypanosomes, babesia spp. and theileria spp. which are common in free ranging rhinos of Africa.

For the treatment of Paramphistome species, praziquantel at rate of 3mg/kg, PO shall be used.

Pasteurellosis has been documented in rhinos, in addition to the incidences of pox virus.

Similarly, in Sumatran rhinos, during the warner and humid environment, external parasites often associated include ticks, flies and leeches.

Sumatran rhinos have more propensities to develop ocular disorders than the other captive rhinoceros species, like starting with mild corneal odema progressing to severe corneal opacity, uveitis and blindness, which is also followed later by secondary bacterial infections as well as fungal infections. Suspected etiology is the excessive UV exposure or dry conditions of the eye that exists in particular few months of the year. Corneal oedema progresses to anterior uveitis followed by invasions of leukocytes and release of immune mediators from the damaged cells leading to the cyclic damage and reinjury. Hence, the best response to treatment may be achieved using topical cyclosporine ointment as an immunomodulator drug that inhibits the T-lymphocyte proliferation.

Iron overload disorder (or) Haemochromotosis (as noticed often in hill mynahs) has also been documented. The measurements of serum ferritin concentrations and transferrin saturation (the ratio of serum iron to total iron binding capacity i.e. TIBC) provides the least invasive means of assessment of iron status. The inevitable mortality and morbidity arising due to the chronic progressive iron toxicity can be prevented by induction of negative iron balance through periodic phlebotomies, as done even in hereditary haemochromatosis. Correction of nutrition accordingly is also to be taken care concurrently in the rhinos that are reared under the captive conditions.

For immobilization of rhinos

General dose rate: 1.25 - 1.5 mg etorphine + 5 - 6 mg acepromazine.

For Greater one horned rhino: 0.5 - 1.5 mg etorphine.

Therapeutic tips on lameness-management in Giraffe esp. the chronic ones

Chiropractice may help correction of changes in spine or limbs with abnormal distribution of body weight.

Gabantin (Dose rate: 1 to 5 mg/kg bwt, sid, q24 hrs to bid) is particularly useful for Giraffe in cases of suspected spinal injury as well as in chronic lameness.

Similarly, Gabapentin (Dose rate: 12 to 25 mg/kg bwt, q24h) shall also be used in Giraffe with abnormalities in the body posture and in cases of spinal injury.

18

Rescue of Wild Animals in Natural Disasters

Rescue of any wild animal during the occurrence of natural disaster regardless of the habitat / topography is totally difference when compared with any domestic animal species. The person engaging in the rescue activities of wild fauna in regions exposed to natural disasters or calamities need to understand about the general classification of wild fauna as a first step.

Biology of the concerned wild animal species should be understood in nutshell. Before making attempts of rescue in such cases. Evacuees at disaster or natural calamity affected region are generally more concerned with their pet animals only and virtually, there is less coordination existing in rescue of wild fauna in a proper manner during such catastrophic events.

Strategies related to Natural Calamities/Disasters

Catastrophes unite us in our courage, our challenges and our grief. But they also provide a blueprint for our future. Natural calamities include occurrence of hurricanes, opening up of volcanoes, occurrence of tsunamis, earthquakes, floods etc. associating the natural processes of the earth.

There is considerable potential for veterinarians to play a role in responding to natural disasters. The areas of disease control, animal care, animal control, protection of the food supply, disinfection/sterilization, and planning are all areas where veterinarians can take an active part. Inclusion of the veterinarian in the process of planning for and responding to natural disasters will yield significant public health benefits.

Natural disasters or calamites create a multiplicity of complicated problems and hazards ranging from outbreaks of infectious disease to animal control problems. A multidisciplinary response is required to solve such problems.

- Natural calamities may be devastating to wild fauna of different species including the endangered and nearly extinct species of wild fauna. Hence, due to differences between domestic animals and wild animals, approaches always need to be in a strategic manner using maximum kinds of gadgets available for use in wild animals of different species.

- Before engaging any kind of rescue operations, one should first need to plan about the gadgets required for such rescue measures like selection of cage or container or place for temporary confinement in a safe manner. In this regard, safety for the wild animal species under rescue as well as safety for the rescuing personnel associated needs to be ensured, without any problems. Veterinarians in the proximity shall be immediately called, in order to undertake any health related measures that may be required on an emergency basis for the rescued wild animal species. Local veterinarian should be the part of this integral part of these processes of rescue of wild animals affected in areas with natural calamities or disasters. This ensures the survivability of the concerned wild animal species which is under the rescue operation.
- Rescuing a wild animal like a jackal or fox or any carnivore floating or swimming in floods needs adaptation of a safety based strategy, unlike the domestic dog or cat. Nets are of high use in this regard.
- Zoonotic disease related features need to be taken care of during any kind of natural calamities in any region and rabies, brucellosis, anthrax, tuberculosis, salmonellosis, H1N1 viral infection etc. are the examples for the zoonotic diseases. Hence, usage of gloves and proper protective covers or coverall including spectacles need to be emphasized for the rescue personnel associated with relief and rescue operations in such natural calamity affected region.
- Since natural disasters lead to a multiplicity of problems and hazards ranging from occurrence of multiple zoonotic diseases to death related events, trained veterinarians may be the better choice in handling the rescue measures pertaining to wild animals. Medical supplies have to be maintained continuously and adequate containers and safety related gadgets as well as modern communication related gadgets have to be kept ready in such occasions. Veterinarian engaging in rescue operations of wild fauna has important task after a natural disaster also, just like the case with 'before a disaster event'.
- Rescuing an injured wild fauna of large sized one like a wild elephant first requires safety measures to the rescuing personnel as well as to this mega herbivore. Wild elephants are mostly aggressive when the animals are approached at a shorter distance for whatever reasons. It requires a team work rather than an enthusiastic single individual with sincere desire on welfare of the injured wild elephant.
- Rescuing a wild herbivore or carnivore with burn injuries due to natural calamities like volcanoes or extensive fire engulfing wider areas unexpectedly also requires basic precautions to be adapted. The unconscious or

semiconscious wild animal if associated with such burn-injuries, need to be handled gently and rubbing or compressing the blisters arising out of burn injuries need to be avoided and immediate attention on prevention of infections has to be paid by consulting a veterinarian in this regard without wasting much time.

- Rescuing a cobra or vipers or krait in a disaster area may cost your life itself, if you don't protect yourself from the bite due to aggression, thus necessitating the need for understanding about the king cobra esp. its biological features and scientific information about bites or venom of king cobra and the precautions that are required before handling of such highly venous species. Tongs are basically required, in addition to cloth or durable bags with ropes to tie, during the physical restraint of such species of serpentines. One should know that there are four poisonous snakes distributed in our Indian sub-continent and this poisonous group of snakes mostly comprises Indian cobras, Common krait, Russell's viper and Saw scaled viper. Handling of snakes for clinical examination and during snake threats to public. Remember that the restraining of such poisonous snakes during occurrence of natural calamities or disasters in a region is perhaps an art and is a difficult task and little carelessness may lead to loss of life of rescuing personnel associated.
- Equal attention has to be given in removing of wild animal carcase if any is encountered by the rescuing personnel and this may help to avoid many zoonotic diseases affecting homosapiens.
- Post operative measures need to be paid maximum attention as for as concerned with the different species of wild fauna that are under rescue operations, during the occurrence of natural disasters or calamites affecting the whole or part of the regions.
- Strict control on visitors is highly required in order to avoid the capture based myopathy in wild fauna, since many species of wild animals esp. spotted deer, black buck, wild dogs etc. get affected rapidly by capture myopathy and death is more common in such incidences. Hence, if proper attention is not given to avoid excitement related events like allowing of more number of visitors to see the rescued wild animal or making of more sounds near the rescued wild animal species or chasing the wild animal that has been rescued for whatever be the reason within the enclosure or confined place.
- Legal measures need to be paid equally more attention whenever any kind of rescue operations are carried out during occurrence of different kinds of natural calamities in an area(s). Features of wildlife protection act 1972 with amendments made shall be known to the team leader in this aspect.

Affection of wildlife by natural disasters

- After an earthquake, volcanic eruption, hurricane, wild fire or flood there is concern about impacts on wildlife. In some cases, there are few or no wild animal losses.
- Wild animals have evolved to respond to their natural environment, coping with seasonal flooding, wild fires, volcanoes and earthquakes. Most often loss of wildlife in the face of a catastrophic environmental event is a result of changes made to the ecosystem. Habitat fragmentation, in particular, prevents them from responding as they normally would.
- Wild animals are tuned in to their environment. Even domesticated or tamed animals often show a similar flight response in the face of potential environmental disaster. In Sri Lanka, Asian elephants carrying tourists on the beach ran away minutes before the tsunami struck. Many locals spoke of being saved as they chased their dogs that were also running away from the wall of water. This response reduces losses.

Environmental disasters with low impact on Wildlife

- Earthquakes and hurricanes tend to have little effect on wild animals. The animals will naturally move to areas of safety where possible. Most reported damage from earthquakes is to man-made structures and the people inside them. Animals are often aware of the approach of tsunamis, which may follow ocean-based earthquakes, and hurricanes, allowing them to move to safer habitat. In areas where natural vegetation is present, native plants often mitigate the effect of tsunamis and hurricanes on wild animals.
- After a hurricane, earthquake or tsunami, in areas where victims move out into previously undeveloped areas, the habitat fragmentation and loss that results is likely to have a more significant impact on the area's wildlife than the actual natural disaster.
- As with earthquakes, there is plenty of warning of pending volcanic eruptions. Wild animals have plenty of time to avoid the lava flows and may be seen moving out of the area as a volcano becomes more active. Once the volcano has erupted, the animals may move back into the area if suitable habitat is still available.

High impact on wildlife by catastrophic environmental events

- The inability to escape from a natural disaster results in the largest numbers of wild animal losses. The two most common scenarios are seasonal flooding and wild fires. Lightning often ignites true wild fires. The sudden nature of these fires makes it difficult for wildlife to escape, especially if the forest fire is aided by strong winds.

- These fires also result in habitat fragmentation and destruction, which has significant longer-term effects for wildlife. Fires that are accidentally or intentionally set increase the level of damage and reduce the amount of alternative habitat for the animals.
- Flooding is another problem for wildlife, if there is nowhere to move to when the waters rise. Flood damage to wild animal habitat is often the result of human alteration to the environment. Lowland areas prone to flood risk, as was shown after Hurricane Katrina, are best left undeveloped as they serve as a buffer when storms hit.
- The ability to move to safer habitat is key to ensuring wildlife losses are kept to a minimum in the wake of catastrophic environmental events. Wildlife corridors, particularly in flood risk areas and in forests prone to wild fire, will help reduce the impacts of natural disasters on wildlife.

19

Captive Breeding Strategies

Use of modern reproductive biotechnologies or assisted reproductive techniques (ART) include in general artificial insemination, embryo transfer/sexing, *in vitro* fertilization, gamete/embryo micromanipulation, semen sexing, genome resource banking, and somatic cell nuclear transfer (cloning) in conservation programs for endangered mammalian species. The biotechnologies of these kinds generally permit more and more offspring to be obtained from selected parents to ensure genetic diversity and may reduce the interval between generations. However, the application of reproductive biotechnologies for endangered free-living mammals is rarer than for endangered domestic breeds. Captive breeding programme is generally considered as a process of breeding animals in controlled environments within well-defined settings, such as wildlife reserves, zoos and other commercial/ noncommercialconservation facilities. Progress in ART for non-domestic species will continue at a slow pace due to limited resources in addition to the limitations encountered with the management and conservation of the targeted endangered species and whole processes are biologically quite complex. In combination with modem reproductive technologies, there is potential to use frozen and stored germplasm (genetic resource banks) to support conservation measures for the maintenance of genetic diversity in threatened species. However, turning this idea into reality is a complex process, requiring interdisciplinary collaboration and clearly defined goals.

Successful captive breeding programmes carried out

- Reintroduction of Przewalski's horse was successfully reintroduced in the wild after breeding these equids under captivity and these animals are native to Central Asia.y
- Pere David's deer were successfully saved by captive breeding programmesafter almost being hunted to extinction in China.
- De Wild Chettah and Wildlife Centre established in 1971 at South Africa successfully bred cheetahs.
- The Mysore zoo, has also been identified as the participating zoo in the conservation breeding of lion-tailed macaques and Nilgiri langur.

- Successful breeding of Nilgirilangur is being carried out at Arignar Anna Zoological Park, Vandalur.
- The century-old Sri Chamarajendra Zoological Gardens in Mysore, which has the largest collection of Indian bison or gaur, has been identified as the coordinating zoo in the country by the Central Zoo Authority of India (CZA) for carrying out "Coordinated Conservation Breeding" (CCB) of endangered species and is successfully undertaking the captive breeding programmes of gaur-the Indian Bison.

Merits of captive breeding programmes

- Recent advances in molecular biology would contribute towards captive breeding of animals that cannot be saved in the wild.
- The low birth and high mortality rate in many wild fauna (as the case with elephants- the mega herbivores) cause the captive population to decline rapidly, thus leading to the necessity for adaptation of successful and well carefully framed captive breeding programmes related to the different species of wild fauna.

Demerits of captive breeding

- Less expression of natural instincts in captive bred wild fauna.
- Fear complex might be absent leading to succumbing to poaching.
- Lesser foraging abilities unlike the naturally bred wild animals.
- Absence of fully learned natural escape mechanisms unlike the natural ones.
- Inbreeding resulting in more heterozygosity/compromised immunity/disease occurrences.
- Re-introduction related field-problems.

Factors associated with captive breeding strategies

- Environment
- Enrichment in the captive breeding places for the targeted wild fauna.
- Social group-availability.
- Knowledge on biology, anatomy and physiological features of the concerned wild fauna undergoing the captive breeding programmes.
- Assistance from the Animal keepers, mahouts and other care-takers including the authorities.
- Technical assistance from the nearby veterinary institutions.
- Huge funds.

Types of captive breeding strategies

- Conventional approach of planned breeding
- Modern approaches like cloning of endangered species, establishment of gene banks by cryopreservation of semen, eggs and embryos of endangered species, and resurrection of extinct and endangered species by cloning with the assistance related to the frozen genetic material.

Captive wild animal places in India carrying out captive breeding programmes

- Zoo
- Zoological park
- Zoological garden
- Elephant camps
- Wildlife reserves
- Specific breeding centresmaintained by the forest department.
- NGOs/Trusts etc.
- Research Institutions (Laboratory for the Conservation of Endangered Species or La Cones for short, at Hyderabad is actively involved in captive breeding programmes including development of technology for the cloning of extremely rare species, monitoring of genetic variations, establishment of gene banks, study of semen quality for the selection of animals for breeding purposes & undertaking of *in vitro* fertilization for conservation purposes of various species of wild fauna). Agencies like (CZA) of India are involved in granting permission for transfer of captive wild fauna etc.).

CAPTIVE BREEDING STRATEGIES: ENDANGERED WILD MAMMAL: ELEPHANT-AS A MODEL

Understanding about biological features of elephants

- Body weight:About 5000 Kg (Males may weigh more in general and elephants have largest brain among land-animals.
- Sexual maturity: At the age of 15-16 years in females & it are at 12 years of age in males and the males have fertile sperms, when they are 18-20 years old.
- Oestrus cyçle:About 15 to 19 weeks (About 4 months).
- Gestation period: 20-22 months (Females can continue to breed to the age of 55-60 years).

- Raising of young one:Because males play no part in raising the young and are not needed to protect the mother or baby, their role appears to be purely reproductive.
- Longevity of elephant: About 75 years (Captive elephants live longer than the wild due to intense care related measures adapted for rearing of elephants under the captivity).

Phases of oesturs cycle in elephants

- Follicular phase (ovulatory or non-luteal phase) lasts for 4 to 6 weeks and this phase is concluded by two, precisely spaced and timed, LH surges. In general, the first, anovulatory LH surge occurs exactly 19-21 days before the second, ovulatory surge. ie) during the follicular phase, approximately 18-20 days prior to ovulation, a 1-day LH-peak concentration can be distinguished, which may result in a temporary rise of progesterone. A second LH peak occurs just prior to ovulation; normally, a single follicle is ovulated. However, beside a corpus luteum (CL) forming on the site of ovulation, multiple accessory CLs can be found on the ovaries. Follicular phase is followed by luteal phase.
- Luteal phase-non follicular phase (lasts for about 6 to 12 weeks or 8-11) appears to be longer than the follicular phase. Progesterone increases 1-3 days after ovulation, indicating the start of the luteal phase. Elephant's ovaries contain multiple corpora lutea.

Merits of Strategy like Artificial Insemination in elephants

- Increases the genetic diversity,
- Increases the number of elephants that can be reproductively active,
- Reduces the need to transport (AI may also be a tool in the future for
- Introduces new genetics into a population ie. increase in the heterozygosity becomes possible leading to decrease in in-breeding among the elephants.
- Range countries through the use of semen collected from wild bulls).
- Reduces the need to disrupt established female social groups.

Understanding about estrus and courtship behavior

A female may perform an "estrous walk," where she walks away from the male with a long gait and her head held high and to the side. The male has to then chase after her and stop her movement with his trunk.

Hormonal assessment related strategy to fix up the time of Artificial Insemination

- Weekly sampling in follicular phase ie. Non-luteal phase (Two surges of LH-incd LH leads to incd progesterone) is necessary as a priority measure.
- Daily sampling in luteal phase is required (LH monitoring daily during the non-luteal phase is necessary for artificial insemination programs. Determination of the post-luteal phase (=first) LH-peak can help predict the first opportunity for (natural) breeding, as the interval between both LH-peaks is rather constant. The fertile period is restricted to the time around the second LH-surge, which occurs immediately prior to the rise in progesterone.
- Further, immediate increase of progesterone/pregnanetriol is suggestive for the right timing for breeding.

Inter-calving period: The inter-calving period should be restricted to maximal 5 years.

Ultrasonography related breeding strategies: Prior sensitization or training of elephant is a "must" for the ultrasonographic interventions.

Utilities of ultrasonography related to breeding

- To follow the follicular development.
- To confirm the site of semen deposition.
- To predict the impending ovulation.
- To confirm the occurrence of ovulation.

Transrectal ultrasonographic examination

Transrectal ultrasonographic examination at 8 - 20 weeks (about 2 to 4 months) after mating allows visualization of single or twin calves. Between 10 and 20 weeks, the larger mature animal may need to lay down on its side for reliable ultrasonographic examination of the uterus. Uterine vascularization can be visualized to determine viability of the fetus, to exclude embryo absorption and mummification.

Milk accumulation in mammary gland regions can be visualized using transcutaneous ultrasonography several hours prior to parturition.

Transcutaneous ultrasonographic examination

Transcutaneous ultrasonographic examination (both flanks have a "small window" where visualization of fetal movements may be seen) may help to determine the status of the fetus in the last months of pregnancy.

Pregnancy period

Twenty to twenty two months (longest gestational period of any animal on earth, with large sized brain of any animal on earth).

Visual signs of Pregnancy in elephants

Confirmed history of mating, with dates will assist in indulging of diagnosing the signs of pregnancy, in general.

First visual sign is the develop't of mammary gland from the beginning of 6months (increase in consistency-increase in glandular firmness & swollen- appearance). As the pregnancy proceeds, the mammary glands become more obvious, in elephants.

Serum Progesterone for diagnosis of pregnancy in elephants

Weekly progesterone monitoring is better but daily monitoring is best in the last month of pregnancy period. Measurement of circulating progesterone (P) is widely used to confirm and monitor pregnancy in the captive Asian elephant (Consistently elevated progesterone (P) concentrations for a minimum of 12 weeks can be used as a positive indication of pregnancy).

The commercial test kits reveal that the high plasma progesterone levels proved to be the pregnancy attest after 4 months conception (1.01-1.96 ng/ml, n=3). In addition, lowering of plasma progesterone can determine that parturition would take place in a few days (0.06-0.03ng/ml, n=3).

Serum progesterone level in elephants

- Varies from 30 to 700 pg/ml in non-pregnant elephant.
- In pregnant elephant: It rises to the range of 1200-1670 pg/ml (but it rapidly falls to less than 100 pg/ml (falls to 0.10 to 0.15 ng/ml, over a period of one to two days during final days of parturition), prior to parturition, in the last few days.
- Birth occurs in 2- 3 days following the return of serum progesterone level to the base line values (ie. < 0.10 to 0.15 ng/ml, which is the level in non-pregnant cow elephant).

Use of prolactin for diagnosis of pregnancy in elephants

Serum Prolactin can be used to detect pregnancy after 4-7 months of gestation (abt 6 months postbreeding) and the levels still remain elevated until parturition. Prolactin is increased to 50±7ng/ml during pregnancy while the level is 6.9±0.7ng/ml in nonpregnantanimals.

Use of urinary progestagens for diagnosis of pregnancy in elephants

- The technique of detecting urinary progestagen, either EIA or RIA would be very much advantageous to monitor the ovarian cycle, pregnancy diagnosis and also signaled impending parturition. Unlike many other species, the predominant progestagen secreted by luteal tissues is not progesterone, but rather its 5-alpha-reduced metabolites.
- Pregnanetriolwas the major urinary gestagen metabolite enabling the noninvasive monitoring of the reproductive cycle of the Asian elephant.
- Analysis of the ratio of 17 alpha hydroxyl progesterone which is a precursor of Pregnanetriol: Pregnanetriol (17á OHP: P) shall also help in the diagnosis of pregnancy in elephants.
- Continuation of high progesterone/pregnanetriol level continuing for at least 16 weeks after mating is highly suggestive of pregnancy.
- Use of hCG for diagnosis of pregnancy in elephants. The research-reports also reveal that the Asian and African elephant-urine testing to detect pregnancy using a test kit for human chorionic gonadotropin (hCG).

Prediction of parturition in elephants

The parturition can be predicted on the basis of the rapid decrease in progestogens that occurs about 2–5 days before birth.

Care during the pregnancy

- After confirming the pregnancies, the vet should begin to monitor each cow elephant-weight subjected to the captive breeding programmes earlier, very carefully.
- Social grouping is necessary whenever the clinical procedures are over with the targeted elephant (Anti-stress).
- Total wt gain in pregnant elephant should be <250 Kg (Avoid still birth or dystokia). Mothers should not gain a lot of extra weight during pregnancy Elephant calf should not be too big at birth (A baby elephant can weigh 90 to 120 Kg).
- Accelerated fitness programmes need to be designed for the expectant cow elephants (mother elephants) for a safe delivery of elephant calf.

Calving process in elephants

- The normal calving process should take place within 2 hours after rupture of membranes (release of fetal fluids). (If the plasma progesterone level decreases to below base line concentration, calving should take place within

48 hours. However, parturition can take place without a complete drop to base line level).

- Loss of mucous plug (may not be seen in many facilities).
- Pre-and post-parturition ventral edema may be noticed.
- Group members may react differently (vocalizations, restlessness).
- In most cases (75%) rupture of allantois sac and loss of allantois fluid (looks like urine) is seen within 2 hours prior to birth.
- The size of fecal balls may get smaller towards the end of pregnancy.
- Frequency of urination may increase around parturition, resulting in more "watery" consistency of the urine, resembling more like allantois fluid.
- Development of mammary gland and production of milk shortly before birth is often seen, however this may also occur in a much earlier stage of pregnancy.
- Softening of the pelvic ligaments (due to estrogen surge) may result in slightly abnormal locomotion of the hind legs.

ROLE OF VETERINARY MEDICINE DURING THE BREEDING PROGRAMMES

Following drugs shall be kept ready during calving

Calcium borogluconate, Estradiol gel, Oxytocin, Lidocaine, Xylazine, Dexamethasone, Azaperone-butyrophenone compound used for standing sedation in elephants; total dose of azaperone for adult Asian captive elephants is 80-100 mg; up to 140 mg for a largeelephant; induction is in 20-30 minutes; duration is 45-60 minutes. (median dosage = 0.08 mg/kg; total doses ranged from 240-400 mg/animal), Atipamezole, Doxapram, Oxygen, Povidone iodine solution for navel disinfection (umbilical infection is a major cause of perinatal complications) and Lubricant (many liters).

Note

Oxytocin has been associated with the occurrence of a uterus rupture because of insufficient cervix dilatation. It should never be used without ultrasonographic examination of the cervix uteri. The visible presence of the allantois sac as a subcutaneous bulging mass under the tail is not a guarantee for a sufficiently dilated cervix. Dose of oxytocin in elephants during calving is 25-50 IU oxytocin s.c. or i.m. Oxytocin should be used with care, as it may dramatically exhaust the contractibility of the uterus muscles as well as the general condition of the female. There might also be the risk of reduced blood circulation in the umbilical chord, due to the spasms in the myometrium. Oxytocin should be given in intervals of at least 2 hours for a maximum of 12-24 hours under the guidance of ultrasound to evaluate the progress. The dosage of oxytocin may only be increased to 100 I.U. after parts of the calf have entered the pelvic area and progress is clearly observed.

Vaginal vestibulotomyas assisting technology for successful breeding in elephants

If the increased dose of oxytocin does not result in parturition a vaginal vestibulotomy should be performed soon to get better access to the calf. It is a surgical procedure, in which the vertical part of the uro-genital tract (vestibulum vaginae) is exposed by a percutaneous approach.

The amniotic sac that covers the body directly, usually remains intact during the expulsion of the calf and ruptures during the final passage through the birth canal and is actively removed by the dam. NB: a chained dam, may not be in the position to remove these membranes, possibly resulting in suffocation of the calf. If the sac is not removed by cow elephant, help in removal of amniotic sac of the elephant's calf, manually, taking safety-factors, duly.

Current Status and Challenges

Results show that zoos in India concentrate largely either on those species which are at a lower risk of extinction in the wild or on large bodied mammals like Panthera tigris, which are difficult to reintroduce into the wild. This is mostly not much in accordance with the IUCN Policy Statement on captive breeding.

Breeding policies need to adhere even to various invertebrates like the case with butterflies.

Need of prioritisation of Indian taxa for conservation breeding.

Need of payment of more attention on smaller bodied mammals like the rodents and bats, which are easier to reintroduce without compromising on visitor appeal.

There is need of intensified research programmes on re-introduction or introduction of captive bred-wild fauna in the wildlife environment.

Captive breeding of butterflies

Since even the butterflies,termites etc. fall under wildlife category despite their comparatively tiny sizes and it is to be remembered that conserving species like the butterflies will improve our whole environment for wildlife and enrich the lives of people now and in the future.

Around 70% of all food crops are pollinated by insects, according to FAO (They act as a pollinator and as a food source for other species, acting as an important connector in the ecosystem web. Hene, butterfly like invertebrate breeding is to be taken care currently.

Butterflies also provide assistance for genetic variation in the plant species they that they collect nectar from (long distance travel by butterflies & gives them a better chance at survival. Butterflies have a role at lower level of food chain (food for lizards, birds,mice,rat etc. Nearly two thirds of all invertebrates can be connected back to the butterfly on the food chain.

The loss of this seemingly insignificant insect could, potentially, collapse entire ecosystems that rely so heavily on them.Currently, the bee population drop, the role of the butterfly becomes even more vital. Butterfly breeding promotes aesthetic values, as well as the ecotourism leading to more revenues.

Embryo manipulation techniques (Often used in captive felids-breeding programmes)

Subsequent to the oocyte collection, the adaptation of embryo manipulation techniques show promise towards greatly advancing conservation biology.

Zoo researchers employ several techniques for successful embryo manipulation as follows

- Laparoscopic transabdominal oocyte aspiration.
- Oocyte in vitro maturation.
- Oocyte in vitro fertilization (IVF).
- Embryo assessment.
- Embryo transfer (ET).

Embryo manipulation provides specific advantages

- It allows for more efficient use of the genetics of a valuable female that may be physically incapable of reproducing due to injury, disease, or age.
- The genetics from valuable females can be proportionately and rapidly distributed through the population by transfer to recipients from a closely related, yet more abundant species.
- The oocytes can be recovered and utilized following the acute death of an adult or a prepubertal animal.

  Project Tiger: Launched in 1st April, 1973.

20

Reptilian Features

TYPES OF REPTILES

There are four groups or types of reptiles

1. The chelonians (tortoises & turtles)
2. The squamata (lizards and snakes and worm-lizards)
3. The crocodilians (crocodiles and alligators)
4. The tuatara (lizard-like)

Reptiles can be divided into three major groups

Crocodiles, lepidosaurs (snakes and lizards) and turtles.

Metabolic rate of reptiles (low BMR in reptiles)

The metabolic rate of reptiles is lower than for mammals and birds, and consequently the k constant in determining energy expenditure, nutritional requirements and even calculating allometric drug doses are related to the equation: Basal Metabolic Rate (BMR) = K(Wkg0.75) = Kcal/day, where K is the energy constant = 10 in reptiles and Wkg is the animal's weight in kilograms.

Features of Reptiles

- More broadly, reptiles are vertebrate animals, meaning they have backbones, housing spinal cords, which run down the lengths of their bodies-a characteristic they share with birds, fish, mammals, and amphibians.
- In evolutionary terms, reptiles are intermediate between amphibians (which have moist skin and need to stay near bodies of water) and mammals (which have warm-blooded metabolisms and have diversified into every habitat on earth).
- Most of the reptiles are tetrapods (four legged animals). They have claws on their toes. Reptiles such as snakes and some lizards only are legless.

Skin

- The scales of reptiles, which develop from the epidermis (the outermost layer of skin), are small, hard plates made of the protein keratin. Scutes, such as the shells of turtles and the armor of crocodiles, are similar in appearance and function to scales but are bony structures that form in a deeper layer of the skin, the dermis. Scales and scutes provide the reptiles with physical protection, and also prevent water loss; in many species, the shapes and colors of these structures play a role in territorial disputes and courtship displays. Bear in mind that, although all reptiles have scales, this is not a unique reptile characteristic; butterflies, birds, pangolins, and fish all have scales, as well.
- Reptilian skin is usually heavily keratinized and protected by scales, with the chelonian shell composed of both dermal bone plates and epithelium.
- Reptiles do not have extensive skin glands and their skin is essentially dry.
- However, in many species of lizards the mature male will possess a series of pre-femoral pores located on the craniomedial aspect of the hindlimbs (e.g. Eublepharis macularius).
- Some lizards have salt glands (oral or nasal) which excrete excess salt (ie: iguana-nasal glands, crocs-ventral tongue gland).
- Crocodilians have perianal musk and mandibular musk glands which are thought to produce pheromones. Some tortoises (Gopherus sp) have mental glands, which are lobular-alveolar glands similar to sebaceous glands that secrete pheromones.
- Chromatophores are a common component of the skin and enable many species, most notably the Chamaeleonidae, to change color. Bony skin structures, osteoderms, are also encountered in the crocodilians and lizards (e.g. Corytophanes spp).
- Certain species of snakes (vipers and boids) have heat sensitive receptors located around the maxilla (pits) which are used in prey location.
- The parietal eye is an invagination of the thalamus and is connected to the pineal gland via the parietal nerve. It aids in regulation of circadian rhythms and annual rhythms. Skin characteristics (e.g. crests, spines, dewlaps etc) are often used for species identification or gender identification in those species that exhibit dimorphic variation.

ECDYSIS (DYSECDYSIS = DERANGED ECDYSIS)

Ecdysis

Comes from the Greek word ekdusis, which means "put off." It describes the process by which arthropods and insects shed their outer cuticle (exoskeleton), or how reptiles shed their old skin. This process is necessary in order for the organism to grow.

All reptiles shed their skin as they grow, and they continue to shed periodically throughout life. Improper or incomplete shedding may occur because of mites, incorrect humidity or handling, malnutrition, dermatitis or trauma. As the shed begins, the skin appears slightly dull as the separation between old and new skin begins. The eyes turn whitish blue because of lymph like fluid accumulating between old eye covering layer and newly formed layer.

The shedding differs from species to species, the environmental conditions, their nutritional status and their growth rate. Turtles shed in pieces. They will slough skin on their neck and legs as well as old scutes located on top of their top and bottom shell. Lizards too shed their skin in pieces and some lizards eat their sloughed skin. Iguanas shed their skin in pieces on the outside of their bodies except for their eyeballs. In rapidly growing reptiles shedding occurs every 2 weeks.

Snakes shed their skin in one piece except for the giant snakes which may tear their skin. During shedding the snakes are very irritable and temperamental and may strike if handled. Handling during this time damages their new skin. A healthy growing snake sheds at least once a month. Normal shedding is an important process for growth in all the reptiles, which depends on a number of factors like nutritional status of the reptile, the environmental conditions, and the health status of your pet. Malnutrition, bacterial infection, mites and too much handling can all result in improper shedding. So, proper management is an important aspect in case of reptiles.

Autotomy

Also called "Self-amputation" (only in lizards, certain worms, salamanders and spiders).

It is the ability of certain animals to release part of the body that has been grasped by an external agent. A notable example is found among lizards that break off the tail when it is seized by a predator. The cast-off part is sometimes regenerated.

The tails of some lizard species are useful in defense in another way. When captured, some lizards voluntarily shed, or autotomize, their tails, which wriggle violently, temporarily confusing the predator and allowing the lizard to escape.

Each vertebra of the tails of tail-shedding lizards has a fracture plane that can voluntarily split by the appropriate twitch of the tail muscles. Simultaneous stimulation of the nerves in the severed portion keeps it twitching for a few seconds after separation. Usually the tail is broken in only one place, but a few lizards, particularly the so-called glass snakes (*Ophisaurus*), break their tails into several pieces. The stump heals quickly, and a new tail grows; often, however, the regenerated tail is not as long as the original and has simpler scales.

Snakes, turtles, and crocodiles may have their tails bitten off by predators. However, they cannot break them voluntarily or regenerate them. In confrontations with enemies, some snakes use their tails as diversions by raising them and moving them slowly. Species with this habit commonly have thick, blunt, brightly coloured tails. For example, the small African burrowing python (*Calabaria reinhardtii*) waves its tail in the air as it moves slowly away from a threat.

Balling

Many snakes, both harmless and venomous, attempt to hide their heads under coils of their bodies. For most species with this habit, the body may be coiled loosely. However, it may also be tightly coiled so that it forms a compact ball with the head in the centre. Balling, as the latter habit is called, is a characteristic response of *Calabaria* and another African python, *Python regius*. Armadillo and The African armadillo lizard (*Cordylus cataphractus*), a species with heavy scales on its head and hard spiny scales covering its body and tail, rolls on its back and grasps its tail in its mouth to present an imposing ring of hard spines to a predator.

Odours

Some reptiles use musk-secreting glands when other defensive measures fail.

Eg: The water snakes (*Nerodia*), the garter snakes (*Thamnophis*), and the alligator lizards (*Gerrhonotus*) emit a foul-smelling substance from their cloacal glands.

Anassortment of turtles, such as the mud turtle and the musk turtle (Kinosternidae), have glands on the bridge of their shells that excrete a vile-smelling fluid that likely makes them distasteful to many predators.

Ectotherms

Reptiles & amphibians arecold blooded animals(ectodermic vertebrates). They have the capacity to regulate their body temperature according the temperature of the environment. The body temperature of cold-blooded animals is determined by the temperature of their environment; this contrasts with warm-blooded animals (inwhich the body temperature of which is maintained within a small, constant range largely independent of external conditions). Because they are cold-blooded, or ectothermic, reptiles must bask in the sun to increase their internal body temperatures, which in turn allows for a higher level of activity (as a rule, warm lizards run faster than cool lizards). When they overheat, reptiles shelter in the shade to cool back down to a safer temperature, and at night many species are virtually immobile due to the non-availability of energy sources (sun).

Homeotherms and endotherms are synonyms (man or mammals or birds); these are animals (such as humans) that keep their body temperature at a constant level. Poikilotherms, therefore, eat only S! to 1/10 of the food needed by homeotherms to survive.

Respiration

As a general rule, the lungs of reptiles are more advanced than those of amphibians, but less sophisticated than those of birds and mammals.One of the most important characteristics of animals is how efficiently they gather and utilize oxygen, the molecular fuel that powers metabolic processes.

All reptiles, including snakes, turtles, crocodiles, and lizards, are equipped with air-breathing lungs, though different kinds of reptiles employ different means of respiration. Reptiles don't typically breathe the same way as mammals, since many reptiles lack a diaphragm. Reptiles use their axial muscles, the ones attached to their ribs, to expand their ribcage for breathing. During periods of intense activity, reptiles might be forced to hold their breath, as they use those muscles for running away.

To process the oxygen, all snakes have an elongated right lung; many also have a smaller left lung, and a few even have a third lung along the trachea.

Most of reptiles don't have diaphragm (Exception: Crocodiles; Crocodilians use a diaphragm muscle for lung ventilation, but their respiratory system differs from mammals. They use a hepatic piston, a process involving muscular movement of the pelvis and liver rather than the rib cage. This organ movement allows the lungs to expand).

Snakes and lizards don't have diaphragm muscles for lung ventilation: muscles used for locomotion are the same used for their respiratory systems. Contracting and flexing body muscles moves their ribs and fill their lungs. Sea snakes, for example, can take in nearly half of the air they need through their skin.

Most squamate reptiles must hold their breath when they engage in bursts of intense physical activity. Some lizards complement lung ventilation with buccal pumping. This involves using throat muscles to help fill their lungs.

The hard shell that turtles and tortoises have makes lung expansion a bit more difficult. Most must use their limbs for lung ventilation. Some turtle lungs are covered with a sheet of muscle. Pulling their limbs in expels air from the lungs and pushing their limbs out of their shells expands the lungs. The lungs of many turtles attach to both the shell and the internal organs. By contracting and flexing a series of muscles, these turtles can push these organs up and down, contracting and expanding the lungs. Movement of their limbs aids this respiratory process. Some aquatic turtles even have gills on their bodies to assist them in respiration.

Breathing is accomplished by expansion of coelomic cavity by intercostals muscles, pectoral limb movements and smooth muscle contraction of the lungs. Crocs use movement of liver to create some negative pressure. Chelonians use movement of front limbs and viscera. Some reptiles can extract oxygen from water through the skin. Some aquatic turtles can exchange dissolved oxygen through the mucosa of the pharynx and cloaca while being submerged. Crocs posses a gular flap (pharyngeal membrane) which allows breathing while the mouth is full of water or food.Gular movements in chelonians is actually associated with olfaction. The glottis is located at the base of the tongue. Tracheal rings are complete in chelonian and crocodilians; incomplete in lizards and snakes. The trachea bifurcates more cranially in chelonians. The reptile lung is made up of open-ended sacs lined with alveoli-like structures which are supported by smooth muscle. Each sac connects directly to a bronchus or to secondary bronchi. Lungs end in thin walled air sacs, which can be used as a defense mechanism or buoyancy control. Vipers have a tracheal lung (collection of alveolar tissue on dorsal portion of trachea) which allows for gas exchange when prey items compress lungs. In most snakes, the right lung is larger than left.

Hibernation

This is a period of dormancy, marked by a decrease in metabolic rate. This follows an adequate period of recovery after the most taxing activities, such as reproduction. It precedes a period when food resources are scarce, so the GI tract is typically empty at the time of hibernation.

Temperate species require hibernation at 5-10° C for at least 2 months, and usually 3-5 months.

Habitats

Diversified; amphibians and crocs live near water; mammals move near the water sources; Tuataras today are restricted to a few remote islands of New Zealand.

Head

Two-headed snakes are less like the terrifying multi-headed monsters of myth and more like conjoined twins which rarely survive. In crocodiles, the upper jaw is mobile unlike in man. Snakes can expand their jaw muscles by loosened attachment of jaw bones to accommodate even the larger prey species.

Heart

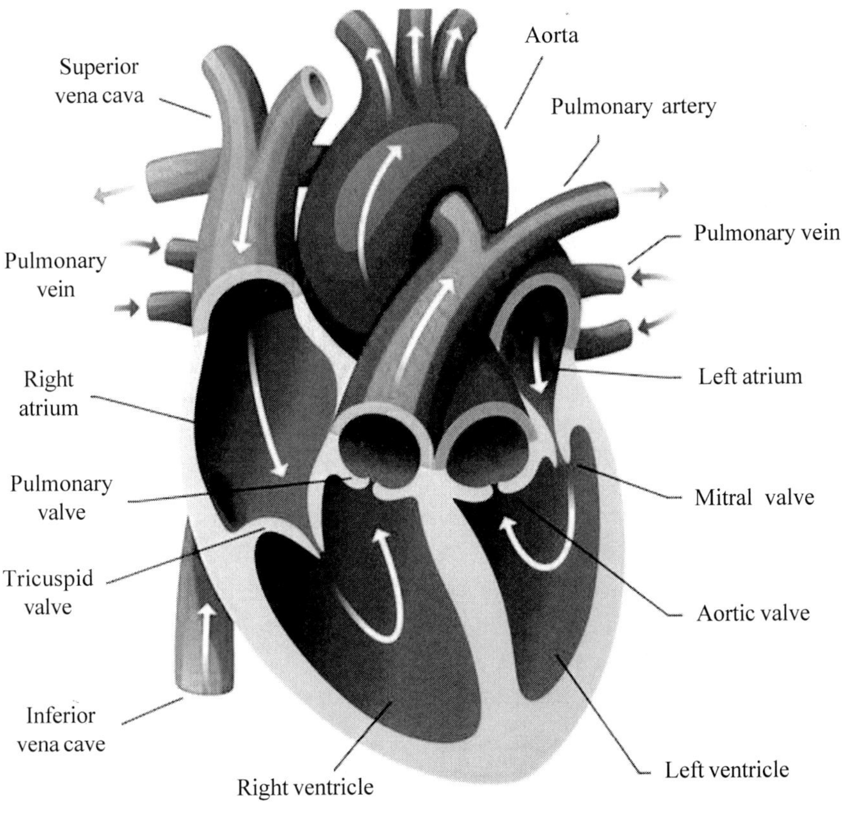

Fig. 1. Normal mammalian heart

Note

In monotremes, the left atrio-ventricular valve is tricuspid.Like homosapients, the heart is four chambered in case of mammals or birds but the airsacs are the special features in aves.

The four chambered heart in crocodilians, birds and mammals has two independent circuits which instead are connected in series. The left and right ventricle pumps the same volume of blood per unit of time.

An advantage of the four chambered heart is that the pressures generated by the two ventricles can be different. The pressure in the pulmonary circulation should not be too high since it is vulnerable to edema formation in the delicate vessels of lungs while it is advantageous to be able to have a higher driving pressure in the systemic circulation in order to be able to increase flow rate and thus oxygen delivery and a high metabolic rate.

Merit of fourchambered heart in crocodilians or alligators

Crocodilians, the reptile family most closely related to birds, have four-chambered hearts, which presumably gives them a much-needed metabolic edge when snapping at prey.

Three chambered cardiac system (two atriums and one ventricle) in snakes & other reptiles, including the amphibians

All reptiles (except crocodile & alligator) including the amphibians contain a three chambered heart that is made of two atria and a single ventricle. In a three chamber heart, there should be a unwanted mixing of oxygenated and de-oxygenated blood because the ventricle is not split completely but due to tiny chambers in ventricle in addition to the movement patterns of the walls of ventricles, such mixing is greatly avoided and the blood flow is in following order:

- The atrium receives deoxygenated blood from the veins. The oxygen has already been used by the body's various organs.
- The left atrium receives oxygenated blood from the lungs and skin. Oxygen can pass through the skin of many amphibians. Thus, the skin of many amphibians serves as a gas exchange organ.
- Both atria empty into the single ventricle. The ventricle is divided into tiny chambers (Syn: Sub-chambers) that helps to prevent the mixing of the oxygenated and deoxygenated blood coming from the two atria (hence, functionally blood circulation is equal to the mammalian cardiac system, despite the presence of three chambered heart) & hence, able to maintain different pressure in pmy and systemic circulations, like mammals or man or birds.
- Contraction of the ventricle sends oxygenated blood to carotid arteries and then the brain.
- Contraction of the ventricle sends deoxygenated blood to pulmocutaneous arteries that takes blood to the skin and lungs in order to become oxygenated.
- Blood that passes through the aortic arches after the heart contracts delivers oxygen to the rest of the body.

In three chambered hearts found in other reptiles, blood is pumped from the undivided ventricle to both the lungs (pulmonary circulation) and the rest of the body (systemic circulation). Both circuits are connected in parallel and this makes it possible to distribute the blood pumped from the heart unevenly between the pulmonary and systemic circulation. Animals with a three chambered heart are able to reduce or even stop the flow to the lungsand yet maintain or even increase blood flow to the systemic circulation. This is believed to be useful in situations when the lungs have no function, such as when the animals dive and hold their breath under water. The disadvantage of this system however, is that a single chamber cannot generate different blood pressures in the two circuits.

Demerit of three chambered heart in reptiles (exception is crocodiles which have 4 chambers like mammals or birds but with foramen of panizza)

- There is a marked disadvantage of having 3 chambered hearts in snakes, lizards & chelonians, whencompared to the four-chambered hearts of birds and mammals. The problem is that three-chambered hearts allow for the mixing of oxygenated and deoxygenated blood, a relatively inefficient way to deliver oxygen to body tissues.
- However, the hearts of snakes, lizards, chelonians contain three chambers-which is an advance over the two-chambered hearts of fish and amphibians.

Cardiac system in Crocodiles & Alligators

Among the reptiles, only the crocodiles (& alligators) have four - chambered heart.

Aorta & Foramen of Panizza in Crocodiles

Crocodiles have two aortas (Pulmonary artery as well as the left aorta leaves the right ventricle and a right aorta leaves from the left ventricle ie) two blood vessels namely the left aorta and the pulmonary artery, exit the right ventricle, whereas man, mammals and other reptiles & amphibians have only one aorta coming out only from the left ventricle. Blood from the right ventricle goes to the lungs through the pulmonary artery in case of crocodiles similar to the case with the mammals and birds. However, in crocodiles, in addition to the regular pulmonary valve, aunique active valve called as the cog-teeth valve is present in the right ventricle which acts as an extra valve between the right ventricle and the pulmonary circulation. This valve system is not only unique in its presence but it is also the only known actively controlled heart valve.

When this unique active valve contracts, pressure in the right ventricle can increase and blood can leave the right ventricle, enter the left aorta, and therefore bypass the pulmonary circulation.

There are two points of communication between the left and right aortas in crocodiles

1. Immediately next to the aortic valves, (but before forming of the aortic arches) called the Foramen of Panizza, described by an Italian anatomist in 1833 and is located.
2. Communication point is found further down in the abdomen, where the left aorta joins with right aorta and is called the "anastomosis".

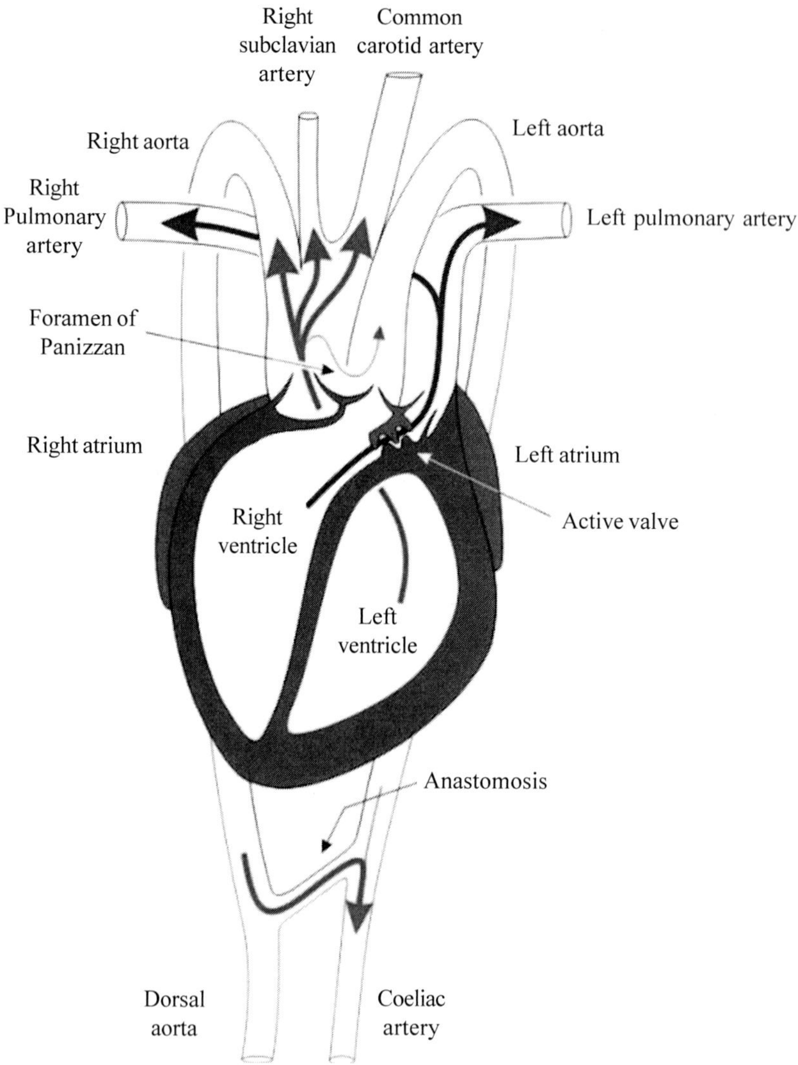

Fig. 2. Blood circulation in crocodile

A number of laboratory-based studies have shown that crocodilians can shift between the bird-mammalian type circulation without any shunting of blood from the right ventricle into the left aorta to a situation were part of the blood in the right ventricle is shunted into the left aorta (back into the body) instead of being pumped into the pulmonary circulation. This shunting can be observed in resting calm animals while in active animals the heart works as in birds and mammals. It is still unclear when and why the crocodiles use this unique capacity to switch from a fully separated circulation to a shunting condition. Several hypotheses have been put forward but it is hard to study this in a laboratory environment since it does not allow the animals to express their natural behavior due to stress induced by the environment itself.

Five chambered heart

Only bees have 5 chambers in their heart. All other species have lesser chambers in their hearts. Human heart has 4 chambers: 2 atria and 2 ventricles. Bees have an open circulation system, unlike us. In such a system, the blood is not enclosed within vessels or tubes, rather it is everywhere inside the body. The heart of a bee is a simple structure and consists of musculated chambers and 5 pairs of openings. The dilation of heart forces the blood into the heart, while its contraction forces the blood to the aorta. The 5 chambered heart is the rarest of rare occurrences in human beings and is a congenital cardiac defect called Cortriatriatum.

Recently an infant boy, in Russia, was reported to have 5 chambers in his heart. Another case has been reported in Nigeria; a human being with a 5 chambered heart is also called as a "bee-baby".

Two chambered heart (one atrium and one ventricle): Eg. Fishes

Lizard Heart (partially inter-connected ventricles at upper portion)

The ventricle of the lizard heart is incompletely partitioned into two subchambers by a muscular ridge that descends from the roof of the heart almost to the floor. The right subchamber is called the right ventricle, or cavumpulmonale; it leads to the lungs. The left subchamber is called the left ventricle, or cavumvenosum; it receives blood from the right atrium and leads to the body. The two subchambers are connected not only beneath the partition but also across its incomplete rearward end.

Resistance to blood flow is lower in the pulmonary (heart-lung) circuit than in the systemic (heart-body) circuit, so that when the ventricles contract, the deoxygenated blood in the right ventricle follows the path of least resistance and proceeds through the pulmonary artery into the lungs. The emptying of the right ventricle causes more deoxygenated blood from the left ventricle to move around the open end of the partition into the right ventricle and to continue on to the lungs. The contraction of the ventricle also brings the partitioning muscular ridge into full contact with the floor of the heart, sealing off any flow from the right ventricle back into the left ventricle.

As the ventricles continue their contraction, the pressure on the blood held within the third subchamber (cavumarteriosum) exerts a reverse force on the valves, opening the passageway between the third subchamber and the left ventricle. The oxygenated blood in the third subchamber now moves into the left ventricle and from there into the aortas leading to the body circulation.

Brain

Brain size usually increases with body size in animals (is positively correlated), i.e. large animals usually have larger brains than smaller animals but this is not true always. Eg: Elephants have a comparatively small brain/body size (1/560), despite being quite intelligent animals.

Animals	Brain to Body ratio
Man and mouse	1/40
Elephant	1/560
Lion	1/550
Horse	1/600
Hippo	1/2789
Sharks	1/2496
Dolphin	1/50
Dog	1/125
Cat	1/100

Cognitive (intelligence) power of species

Carnivores generally need to find and kill their prey, which presumably requires more cognitive power than browsing or grazing eg: The brain size of a wolf is about 30% larger than a similarly sized domestic dog.

Birds generally have lower IQ than mammals, but parrots and particularly the corvids show remarkable complex behaviour and high learning ability (Their brains are at the high end of the bird spectrum, but low compared to mammals. Bird cell size is on the other hand generally smaller than that of mammals, which may mean more brain cells and hence synapses per volume, allowing for more complex behaviour from a smaller brain).

With some exceptions, reptiles are about as smart as one expects; more cognitively advanced than fish and amphibians, about on an intellectual par with birds, but way down on the charts compared to the average mammal.

Vision

Snakes do not see colors, but their eyes are equipped with a combination of light receptors: rods that provide low-light but fuzzy vision, and cones that produce clear images. The complexity of the eyes varies among species because of their different lifestyles. For instance, snakes that live primarily underground have smaller eyes that only process light and dark, but snakes that live above ground and hunt by sight have crystal-clear vision and good depth perception (Some species, specifically boas and pythons, have a second visual tool: Pit organs on their heads see heat sources in their surroundings like infrared goggles-an effective ability for nocturnal hunters of warm-blooded animals). Snakes have infamously poor eyesight, which is why they resort to sticking out their tongues all the time to get a sense of their surroundings. But the creatures may have a way to improve their vision in a pinch.

Smell

Like humans, snakes breathe airborne smells into nasal openings that lead to an olfactory chamber for processing; but snakes have a secondary system, as well. When a snake flicks its tongue, it is gathering odor particles for transfer to two fluid-filled sacs at the roof of the mouth - Jacobson's organs - that lead to a second, smaller olfactory chamber. The tongue is used only to assist in this process; snakes do not have a sense of taste.

Reproducion in reptiles

Lizards: Males are often highly territorial and will fight to the death.

Chelonia: Males are often very virile and will engage in relentless courtship (shell butting, leg biting). In some cases a female may become traumatized and need separating from an amorous male.

Snakes: Many species require multiple males to encourage mock combat and copulation.

Reptiles that lay eggs out (like aves): Most commonexample all members of Colubridae family of snakes&Cobras, mambas, adders, and most other members of the *Elapidae* family.

Oviparous

Reptiles are the first world's amniotes (i.e. laying eggs with amniotic sac). Most reptiles are oviparous, laying hard-shelled eggsie). Most of the Reptiles lay eggs to give birth to the young ones. Oviparous reptiles lay amniotic eggs. Amniotic eggs have a hard shell which protects the embryo, and a special membrane to prevent the embryo from drying out. Most of the reptiles like Turtles, crocodiles, tuatara and fishes and amphibians are all oviparous as are several species of snakes and lizards.

Egg laying and development of embryo

Egg-laying reptiles typically lay their eggs once the embryos are nearly one-third of the way through their development. Viviparity is beneficial in the sense that it keeps predators from eating developing eggs - however, it places a higher physical demand on the female reptile.

Reptiles that give birth to young one: Less common than the oviparous reptiles

Viviparity (Viviparous but lacking of placental tissues but nourished by yolk of egg) of reptiles. Vipers are heavy bodied poisonous snakes with fangs that fold back into the mouth until ready to strike and most of the vipers and all of the rattle snakes, boas, pit vipers and spitting cobras are viviparous.

Viviparous animals give birth to live young; the embryo develops inside the body of the mother, as opposed to outside, in an egg. The more developed form of vivipary is called placental viviparity; mammals are the best example of this. Viviparous offspring live independently and need to eat from birth. Many of the viviparous species feed the growing fetuses through a placenta that is similar to those of mammals.

Histotrophicviviparity: the zygotes develop in the female's oviducts, but find their nutriments by

a) Oophagy (Oophagy sometimes ovophagy, literally "egg eating", is the practice of embryos feeding on eggs produced by the ovary while still inside the mother's uterus.Oophagy is also used to refer to more general egg-eating behaviours such as those practised by some snakes)

b) (Or) Adelphophagy Intrauterine cannibalism is a behaviour called as adelphophagy or embryophagy in which the fetus eats sibling embryos (but in oophagy, it feeds on eggs) in some carnivorous species like sharks and black salamanders etc. in which multiple embryos are created at impregnation, but only one or two are born. The larger or stronger ones consume their less-developed siblings as a source of nutrients.

In Adelphophagy occurs in some marine gastropods (calyptraeids, muricids, vermetids and buccinids) and in some marine annelids (*Boccardia proboscidia* in Spionidae.

Intrauterine cannibalism is known to occur in lamnoid sharks, such as the sand tiger shark, and in black salamander (*Salamandra atra*) and the fire salamander, as well as in some teleost fishes. The Carboniferous period chimaera, Delphyodontos *dacriformes*, is suspected of having practiced intrauterine cannibalism, also, due to the sharp teeth of the recently borneg

Filial cannibalism is a specific type of size-structured cannibalism in which adults eat their own offspring. Although most often thought of as parents eating live young, filial cannibalism includes parental consumption of stillborn infants and miscarried fetuses as well as infertile and still-incubating eggs. Vertebrate examples include pigs, where savaging accounts for a sizable percentage of total piglet deaths, felids, great apes esp. the chimpanzees,hippopotamuses (even though the hippos are herbivores by nature in general), polar bears and tiger salamanders.

Cannibalism: Animal eating the animal of the same species.

- Male consuming the young one example is lions.
- Female consuming the male-mate.

The mating habits of the praying mantis, and several species of spiders, for example, will sometimes involve the female of the pair bite off and consume the head of her mate shortly after becoming inseminated in an effort to nourish herself and prepare her body for gestating offspring.

Mother consuming the young one

Some animal mothers, mainly nesting animals such as rabbits and hamsters,will eat sickly, weak, or dead babies left in the nesting area in an effort to deter predators, who would be lured in by the smell, from entering their domain.

Baby consuming the mother

In a few instances, however, it's the young who turn on their mothers. Known as "Matriphagy", or mother-eating and this occurrence is usually the result of extreme acts of self-sacrifice, in which the mother offers her own body for the sake of the survival of the next generation. Eg) some species of insects, scorpions, nematode worms;Among these are the caecilians-a group of wormlike, legless amphibians that live underground in the tropics.

Spiderlings of the spider (*Stegodyphus lineatus*, which is found in the Mediterranean and Middle East. eat, mom's innards) eat the mom's innards.

1. Hemotrophic viviparity: nutrients are provided by the female, often through some form of placenta. In the frog *Gastrotheca ovifera*, embryos are fed by the mother through specialized gills. The skink *Pseudemoia entrecasteauxii* and most mammals exhibit a hemotrophicviviparity.

2. Placental viviparity is arguably the most highly developed form of viviparity. Placental mammals, including humans, are the best-known example, but adaptations in some other animals also have incorporated this principle or close analogies. Other examples include some species of scorpions and cockroaches, certain genera of sharks and snakes, and velvet worms.
3. Ovoviviparity, a less developed form of viviparity, occurs in most vipers, and in most live-bearing bony fishes (Poeciliidae). However, the term is poorly and inconsistently defined, and may be obsolete.

Ovoviviparous animals give birth to live young eg) anacondas and skinks (In fact, 45% of the skink species are viviparous) and few spp of snakes like garter snakes.

Ovoviviparous (egg inside; hatches out inside ie)inside hatching; then, gives birth of live young): Eg: Anaconda, slow worms.

Ovoviviparous animals are similar to viviparous species in which there is internal fertilization and the young ones are born alive, but differ in that there is no placental connection and the unborn young ones are nourished by egg yolk. Some reptiles give birth to live young, but so do certain species of fish (Most reptiles differ from mammals in that they lack placentas).

Ovoviviparity (aplacental viviparity) is a mode of reproduction (eg. as of various fishes or reptiles, Sharks), in which embryos develop inside eggs that are retained within the mother's body until they are ready to hatch. Ovoviviparous sharks are similar to viviparous species in that there is internal fertilization and the young are born live, but differ in that there is no placental connection and the unborn young are nourished by egg yolk.

Producing eggs that develop within the maternal body and hatchwithin or immediately after release from the parent.

Most of the sea snake species give birth to live young, which means the babies are born alive in the water. But there is one genus, *Laticauda*, which is oviparous.

PARTHENOGENESIS MEANS OF REPRODUCTION IN SELECTIVE REPTILES

(Haploidity or virginal birth or Immaculate Conception)

Reproduction by Parthenogenesis is asexual form of reproduction i.e.without mate). In certain species, haplidity if necessity arises by means of non-availability of males or routine reproduction may happen.

Haplodiploidy is a phenomenon that appears in two insect orders, hymenopterans (bees, ants and wasps) and thysanopterans (thrips or stormbugs).

Most reptiles of the squamatan order (lizards and snakes) reproduce sexually, but parthenogenesis based reproduction ie) without sexual partner or male occurs naturally in certain species of whiptails, some geckos, rock lizards, Komodo dragons and snakes. Parthenogenesis occurs naturally in some species including mostlower plants, invertebrates such as water fleas, aphids, and some bees. Parthenogenesis has also been observed in vertebrates such as some reptiles and sharks.

Parthenogenesis is a form of asexual reproductionin several species of geckos and other lizards. Parthenogenesis is an asexual form of reproduction found in females where growth and development of an egg into an embryo occurs without fertilization by males. In parthenogenesis, the offspring comes from a non-fertilized ovum. Without fertilization (union of the oocyte's and the sperm's genetic material) the offspring won't have any part of the father's DNA (if there is a father). The resulting babies will be genetic copies (clones) of their motherand by parthenogenesis females are born

However, when no male anacondas are available to provide offspring facultative parthenogenesis is possible ie) in anacondas, reproduction by mate as well as when needed parthenogenesis based reproduction ie) asexual form of reproduction also occurs naturally.

As with all types of asexual reproduction, there are both costs (low genetic diversity) and benefits (reproduction without the need for a male) associated with parthenogenesis. The offspring produced by parthenogenesis are always female in species where the sex of the offspring is determined by the sperm (XY chromosome system), and they are male in species where the sex of the offspring is determined by the egg (as in the ZW chromosome system).

Most mammals have the XY chromosome system. XX individuals are female, and XY individuals are male. Other organisms, such as birds & butterflies, have the ZW chromosome system. ZW individuals are female, & ZZ are males. Sex can also be determined by the environment; for example, the sex of crocodilians and turtles are dependent on the incubation temperatures of the eggs.

Renal System of reptiles

Terrestrial reptiles excrete uric acid (uricotelic). Aquatic reptiles either excrete ammonia (ammonotelic), urea (ureotelic), or uric acid.

Some examples: sea turtles excrete mostly ammonia or urea; semi-aquatic turtles excrete 50% urea, 50% uric acid; desert tortoises excrete >90% uric acid. No loop of Henle→onlyisosthenuric urine possible.

Uric acid is extremely insolubleand thus in extreme dehydration, urates can precipate in the nephron leading to obstruction. Right kidney is cranial to left in snakes.

Some reptiles (geckos, skinks, iguanas, snakes) have a sexual segment of their kidneys, which means that cells lining the distal convoluted tubule hypertrophy during breeding season and excrete eosinophilic granules into the tubules. These granules can be found in the vas deferens. Since there are no accessory glands, the sexual segment provides seminal fluid.

Some reptiles have bladders-mostly terrestrial chelonians and some lizards (iguanas do, monitors do not). Water is resorbed in the bladder. Isosthenuric urine flows from kidney'!ureter'!cloaca'!bladder'!cloaca'!outside. Those without bladders retroflux urine from cloaca into distal colon for water resorption. Salt is also resorbed in this way.

Feeding

Mostly carnivorous. Only herbivorous reptiles are turtles and iguanas.

Some marine reptiles (like saltwater crocodiles) have also been known toswallow rocks, which weigh down their bodies and act as ballast, so they can surprise prey by leaping out of the water. Pebbles or stones are commonly noticed in stomach of crocodilian species.

Differences between Alligators and Crocodilians

- In crocodiles and alligators, upper jaw is mobile unlike humans
- Alligators possess a broad, U-shaped snout and have an "overbite"- that is, all the teeth of the lower jaw fit within (lingual to) the teeth of the upper jaw. The large fourth tooth on each side of the alligator's lower jaw fits into a socket in the upper jaw. Usually, no lower teeth are visible when the mouth is closed. In contrast, crocodiles have a narrow, V-shaped snout and the large fourth tooth on each side of the crocodile's lower jaw projects outside the snout when the mouth is closed.
- The cecum or distal colons are highly developed in herbivorous reptiles but caecum is absent in case of crocodiles and snakes.
- The liver of most reptiles has melanin aggregates. Most reptiles have gallbladders.
- Pancreas located between ascending/descending portion of duodenum in chelonia and lizards. In snakes, located caudal to pylorus near gall bladder and spleen, in some snake spp, it is fused with spleen = splenopancreas.

Sexing in reptiles

Temperature dependent sex determination (TSD): High temperature ofenvirontment = females.

Temperature-dependent sex determination (TSD) is a type of environmental sex determination in which the temperatures experienced during embryonic/ larval development determine the sex of the offspring. It is only observed in reptiles and teleost fish.

Reptiles and fishes are the only vertebrates to exhibit "temperature-depend sex determination": the ambient temperature outside the egg, during the development of the embryo, can determine a hatchling's sex. TSD differs from the chromosomal sex-determination systems common among vertebrates. The eggs are affected by the temperature at which they are incubated during the middle one-third of embryonic development. This critical period of incubation is known as the thermosensitive period (TSP).

SNAKES

Invisible Hemipenes

Male snakes have a pair of tube-shaped hemipenes (sex organs) that normally sit inside their bodies. They are basically two small penises that are kept safe inside the snake's tail. Female snakes do not have hemipenes.

The hemipenes are located just below the cloacal (vent) opening and down along the tail on either side of the snake's midline.

Since these sex organs are housed inside the male snake, they may not be obvious, in general.

Visual differentiation of sex

Male snakes have longer and thicker tails at base, than in the females.

OOPHIPROBE FOR SEXING IN SNAKES

Males (more length in cloaca) and Females (less length in cloaca)

Probing a snake involves inserting a thin metal rod (called a snake probe) into the cloacal vent of the snake while it is awake. This special probe can be inserted further in males since they have a hemipenis on either side of the vent. The probe will drop down into one of these spaces that point towards the tip of the tail.

Basically probing is meant to find one of the hemipenes. Keepers insert the blunt rod inside the organ while it's at rest in a male's tail base. If the probe enters and descends toward the tail tip more than two or three subcaudal scale widths behind the cloaca, it has entered one of the hemipenes' prongs. On most adult colubrids 3 to 5 feet long, each side is roughly 1½ to 3 or more inches deep.

If the oophi-probe only goes in a half-inch or less, it's a female ie) when probing a female snake, the probe will not drop down into the vent very far.

- If it is a female, the probe will only drop in an average of one to three scales.
- If it is a male, it will drop in an average of nine to fifteen scales.

Spurs in both sexes of Boas & Pythons including Indian Rock Python (*Python molurus*) but in males, it is longer. Pelvic spurs are the externally visible portion of the vestigial remnants of legs found on each side of the vent in primitive snakes, such as boas and pythons. The remnants of a pelvis and femur, which have no connection with the spine, simply "float" in the muscle mass. The femur protrudes from the snake's body and is covered by a horny spur, which resembles a spur or claw. Males' spurs are generally longer and more pointed than females', and are used for clasping and tickling during courtship and mating as well as combat with other males in some species.

Crocodiles

Male and female crocodiles have internal sex organs, which may make it difficult to tell them apart unless you are conducting a close inspection. Both sexes have a "vent," or a slit that houses the sex organs. Unless mating is going on, male and female vents are typically indistinguishable.

Size of animal

Usually, the best indication is size - males grow larger than females in all crocodilian species, and so a very large individual is more likely to be a male. In some species, females may have narrower snouts, and a more slender body, but such traits are highly unreliable indicators of sex. In larger crocodilians, the shape of the vent can provide a guide to the animal's sex. Females tend to have smaller, narrower and flatter vents, whereas males have larger, wider, and more convex vents. This difference is due to the increased elasticity of the vent in males necessary to allow eversion of the penis during copulation.

Eversion of penis in male crocodiles

Crocodiles have a rigid penis (always in *erection)* hidden inside the body that, shot out like a spring to the outside at the time of copulation and is hidden again at the same speed.

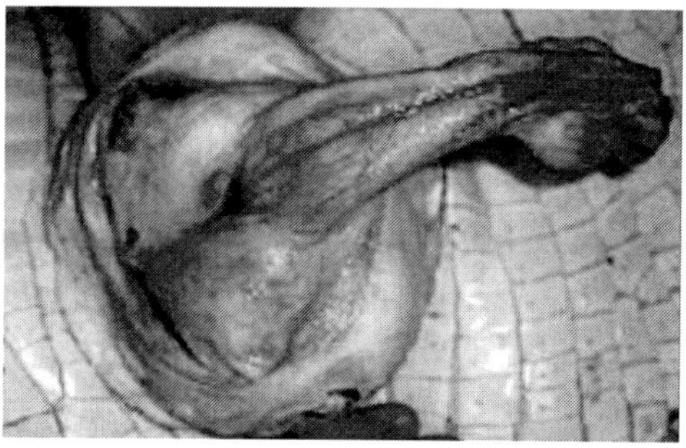

Fig. 3. Rigid penis ie. os penis of crocodile

Fully everted penis of large adult male crocodile, the groove running down the centre conveys semen to the tip, and the two masses at the base are the muscles used to evert the penis during copulation. The male's testes are inside the body cavity. Males have a single penis, not a pair of hemipenes like most other reptiles. It can be confusing because the tip of the male's penis is split into two halves.

Popping of penis (possible only in young hatchlings kept upside down)-

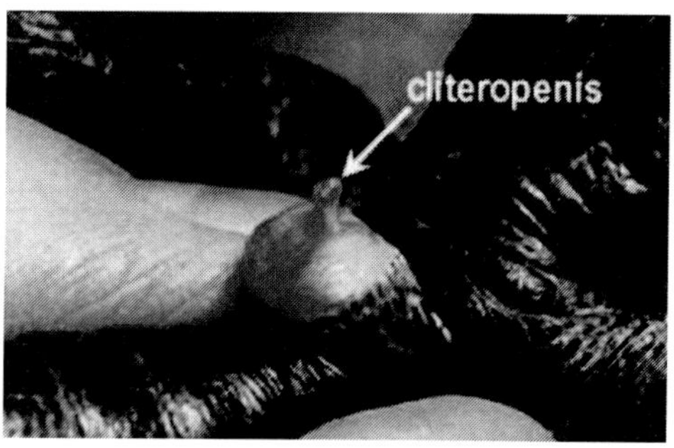

Fig. 4. Cliteropenis of crocodile

Palpation of the ospenis (inside the vent) is required towards the sexing in crocodiles and male crocodiles have ospenis.

Baculum (ospenis) and Radiography based techniques for sexing

The baculum is an extra-skeletal bone (that is, not attached to any other bones of the skeleton) that grows inside the glans (head of the penis) of many mammalian species.

The baculum (also penis bone, penile bone, or *os penis*, or *ospriapi* is a bone found in the penis of many placental mammals. It is absent in the human penis, but present in the penises of other primates, such as the gorilla and chimpanzee. The bone is located above the male urethra, and it aids sexual reproduction by maintaining sufficient stiffness during sexual penetration. The homologue to the baculum in female mammals is known as the baubellum or osclitoridis - a bone in the clitoris.

The baculum (*os penis*) is a bone found within the penis of certain mammals, including many primates, rodents, bats, carnivores, and some insectivores. It is an isolated bone, derived from connective tissue and located at the distal end of the penis, above the urethra. Lower mineral density and reduced stiffness of the baculum compared to skeletal bones may help reduce the risk of fracture under strain during copulation, although breakage can sometimes occur.

More broadly, the stronger the baculum, the longer the intromission is. (Some animals, like the coati - a member of the raccoon family that definitely has a baculum- have an intromission duration as long as one hour.) The data suggest that the physical characteristics of the baculum evolved to help the penis stay in throughout the duration of copulation.

Alligator

Alligators are large reptiles, members of the order Crocodylia. Alligators and crocodiles are, therefore, closely related, and people often confuse one with the other, however, these two reptiles are very different.

The first easy way for sexing is to gauge the length of an adult alligator. If it measures 10 feet or more, it's a male. Females don't grow that long. If it's less than 9 feet in length, it could be either a male or a female.

The second easy way is to see if there are lots of small, newly born alligators around the adult. They will stay by their mother for up to a year and she will protect them. A male gator could eat them, even if he's the father, so the mother usually won't let him anywhere near the babies.

Female alligators also have narrower snouts and bodies than males. Flip the baby alligator upside down and examine the "vent," which is located between the lower legs. Lightly press down on either side of the vent to expose the reproductive organs of the baby alligator. If the alligator is a male, a penis will emerge.

Lizards

Femoral pores (present in both sexes but more obvious in males) on medial aspect hind limbs more obvious in male than female. Some males have head ornamentation .hemipenes can be seen as bulges at base of ventral tail in sexually mature males Note: the green iguana only reaches maturity at 3- 4 years (3-6 foot length) when sexual characteristics will be obvious. Radiography of certain monitor species will reveal the os penis.

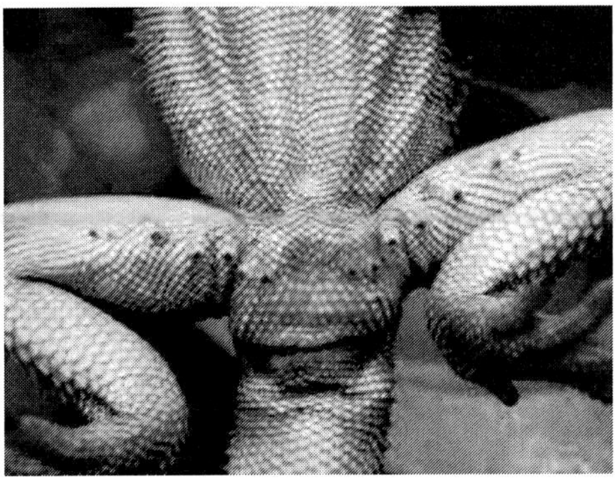

Fig. 5. Femoral pores in lizard

Chelonians

- Males are often very virile and will engage in relentless courtship (shell butting, leg biting). In some cases a female may become traumatized and need separating from an amorous male.
- Male has longer tail than female, or more caudal vent(The male tortoises have a simple penis that is folded in two in the cloaca, inside the tail, reason why the tail of the males is thicker and longer than the females. During the erection, it fills with fluid, deploys and exits, reaching a comparatively larger size).
- Male terrapin has longer forelimb nails than female.
- Male tortoise has concave plastron.

External reproduction in amphibians

Anura is a tail-less amphibian like frogs as an example of external reproduction:The anurans (amphibians without tail, such as frogs) have external reproduction and mating occurs usually in the water. The male, who is smaller than the female, grips the female firmly. This *embrace* is called amplexus.The contractions of the female when expelling the eggs stimulate the male to spray them of sperm in the same moment that they are expelled. The eggs are joined by a gelatinous mass that takes different forms depending on the species.

Internal reproduction in amphibians

1. Urodela is amphibian with tail. eg.salamanders and newts as an example of internal fertilization: Almost all urodela (amphibians with tail, such as salamanders and newts) have internal fertilization. The male is placed in front of the female and releases sperm packages (spermatophores) containing the sperm. The female walks over one of them, collects it with the lips of

the cloaca and places them in the spermatheca, a cavity where the sperm wait for the eggs to pass through the cloaca to make them fertilize. The female lays the fertilized eggs one by one beating them in aquatic plants, except in some species of salamander, in which the female retains them and they are born live larvae **(ovovivivarism).**

2. **Apoda are caecilians which are amphibians as an example of internal insemination:** Apoda (or) caecilians are amphibians without legs with internal fertilization, but unlike in anura, internal insemination occurs. This is possible thanks to a pseudo-phallus **(phallodeum)** that have the males, which they insert in the cloaca of the female for two or three hours.

Endoscopic techniques for sexing: Endoscopy can be used to visualise the gonads.

Molecular techniques for sexing

Determining sex from DNA is the most practical option, or sometimes even the only possibility, in these cases. Molecular sexing is routinely used in mammals, reptiles and birds.

Genotypic sex determination

Species in the genotypic group, like mammals and birds, have sex chromosomes, which in reptiles come in two major types. Many species - such as several species of turtle and lizards, like the green iguana - have X and Y sex chromosomes (again, like mammals), with females being "homogametic," that is, having two identical X chromosomes. Males, on the other hand, are "heterogametic," with one X chromosome and one Y chromosome. Other reptiles governed by GSD have a system, similar to one found in birds, with Z and W sex chromosomes. In this case - which governs all snake species - males are the homogametic sex (ZZ) and females are the heterogametic sex (ZW).

Renal Portal System of Reptiles

Renal Portal System of Reptiles is associated with the passage of venous blood from posterior parts of body i.e. hind quarter regions pass on either to kidney or to liver or both before getting into heart i.e. systemic circulation.

Renal portal system is present in reptiles as well as in aves. Renal portal vein is present in reptiles, below kidneys.

Receipt of blood by Renal - portal vein

- The portal ring (renal portal vein) receives venous blood from the gut and the pelvic region (including the legs) through the external iliac veins, the ischiatic veins, the internal iliac veins, and the caudal mesenteric vein & all these veins are associated with drainage of blood from the dorsal body wall, the cloaca, the sex organs, and the bladder.

- Caudal vein brings venous blood from posterior regions including the tail region.

Outgoing of blood from the portal ring (renal portal vein)

The blood from this Renal-portal vein as well as the caudal vein then passes through the renal parenchyma (mixing with postglomerular efferent arteriolar blood), before returning to the common iliac veins and the caudal vena cava via the renal veins.

Hence, Hind limbs (or hind quarters) injections in reptiles are preferred.

Drugs injected into the caudal half of the body, base of the tail and hindlimbs, may be cleared by the kidneys prior to reaching the systemic circulation (drugs not be injected into the caudal body of reptiles because they will be carried by the renal portal system to the kidneys,where they may be nephrotoxic or rapidly excreted).

Because blood draining the caudal body of reptiles passes through the kidneys before reaching the central circulation, the effect on the pharmacokinetics of a drug injected in that region will vary with its renal extraction rate.

Hence, nephrotoxic drugs become more nephrotoxic to the reptiles if injected into the posterior half of the body i.e.) in hind quarters. Hence, care should be taken when administering nephrotoxic drugs in the hindlimbs, and when possible, anesthetic drugs should be injected in the forelimbs.

21

Clinical Examination of Aves

Birds are extremely vulnerable to handling (even injection related events) stress and hence, chemically immobilize for a detailed clinical examination or intensive sampling procedures).

Commonly reared/owned exotic aves

- Cockatiels
- Budgerigars
- Zebra Finches
- Hyacinth Macaw
- Canary
- Macaws
- Cockatoos
- Love Birds
- Pineapple Conures
- Hahn's Macaw
- African gray parrot

The Respiratory System

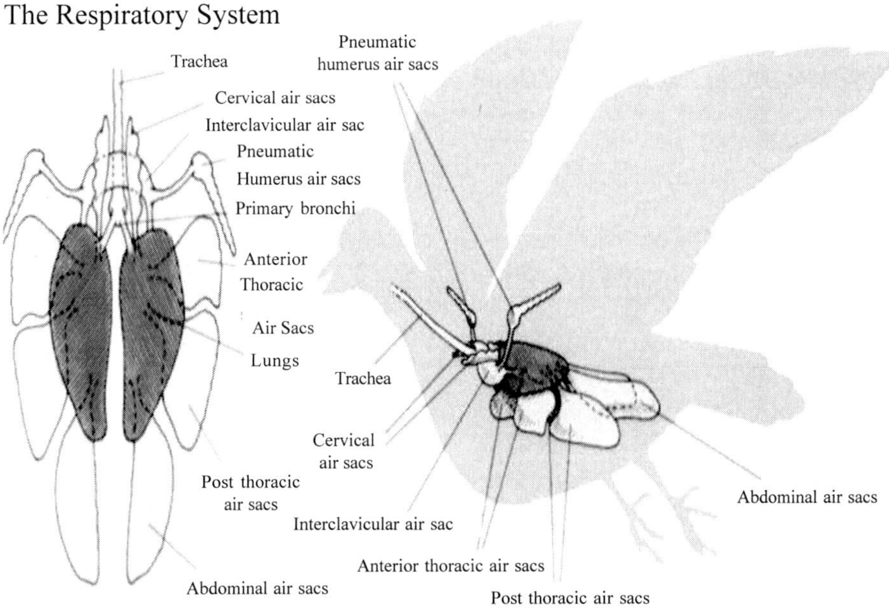

Fig. 1. Air sacs in aves-a speciality

Approximate body weight (in grams) of birds

Birds	Body weight
Macaw	120-160
Quaker parakeet	90-150
Senegal parrot	110-130
Mynah	180-260
Pigeon	240-300
Pionus, Blue-headed	230-260
Cockatoo	220-390
African Grey parrot, Amazon	300-500
Amazon parrot, Orange-Winged	300-450
Electus parrot (only parrot with sexual dimorphism)	388-524
Cockatoo, Moluccan	700-1000
Zebra finch	10-16
Canary	12-30
Budgerigar parakeet	25-35
Parrotlet	30-34
Lovebird	45-70
Conure	60-80
Cockatiel	80-125
Ring-neck parakeet	120-150

Examination of oral cavity in birds

Glottis	Epiglottis
Glottis opens into the airway	Epiglottis forms the superior border of the glottis
Size of the glottis responsible for the voice type.	Size of the epiglottis not responsible for the voice type.
While swallowing glottis moves upward	While swallowing epiglottis moves downwards.

Note

Glottis opens into the windpipe and is responsible for the production of sound. The epiglottis is a cartilaginous flap on top of the glottis that prevents the food from entering into the larynx. The main difference between glottis and epiglottis is their function and the structure.

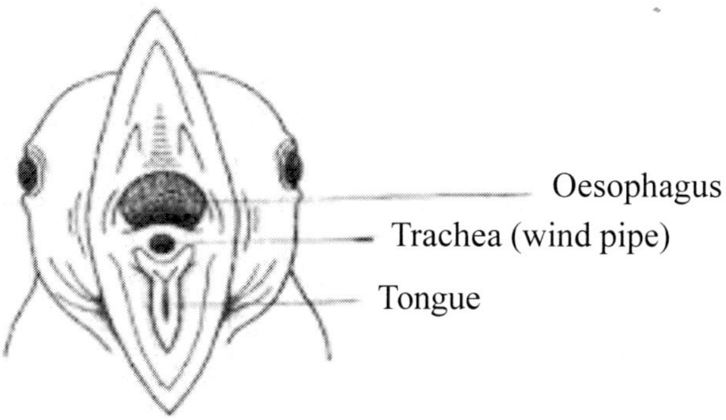

Fig. 2. Oral cavity in aves

The larynx, commonly called the voice box (or) glottis, is the passageway for air between the pharynx above and the trachea below. Glottis has upper epiglottis and lower glottis and glottis is the opening of trahchea at the back of the tongue. The larynx plays an essential role in human speech.

During the sound production, the vocal cords close together and vibrate as air expelled from the lungs passes between them. Larynx does not function in the production of sound as in mammals.

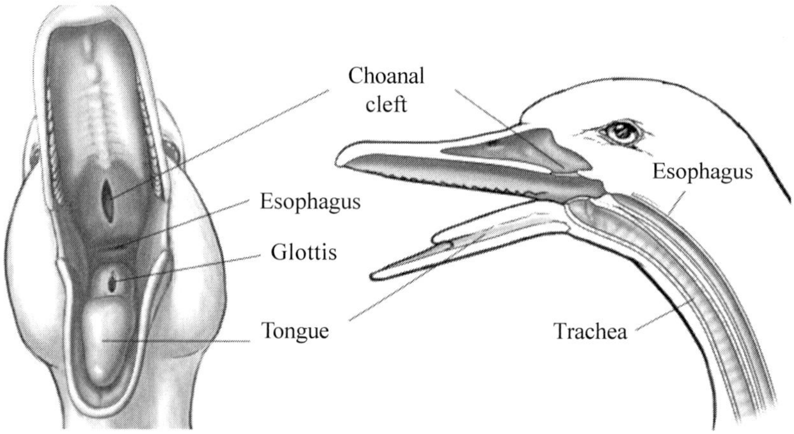

Fig. 3. Oral regions in aquatic birds

Choanae (internal nares) open from the nasal chambers into the roof of mouth.

Oral medication

Population medicine is to be carried out for therapeutic attempts if carried out in group of birds except the high valued and large sized aviary species like flamingo, pelicans etc.

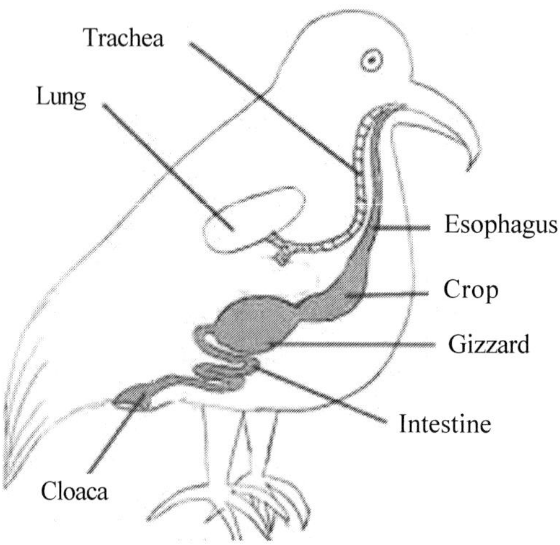

Fig. 4. Digestive organs in birds

Oral delivery of drugs

Avoid wrong delivery of drug into trachea to avoid aspiration pneumonia.

Syringe delivering the drug should be placed on sides inside the mouth of birds.

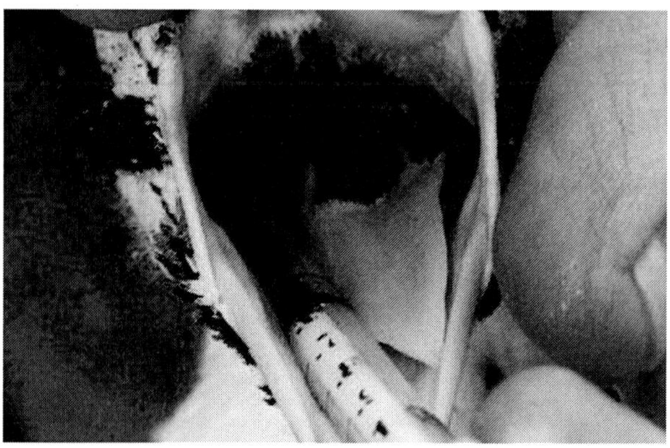

Fig. 5. Oral delivery of drugs in birds

Note on usage of ivermectin in aves

- **Dose rate:** 200μg/Kg b.wt. s/c, oral, pour-on.
- (Also, effective against some coccidia, gapeworms, sternostamatosis etc.)
- But, deaths are documented in finches and budgerigars after inection of ivermectin.
- Ivermectin is toxic in bullfinches and goldfinches when used topically.

COMMON & PROBABLE DISEASES/DISORDERS IN CAPTIVE AVIFAUNA

Commonly encountered clinical problems in captive avifauna

- Helminths / Cestodiasis
- *Plasmodium* spp. & *Hemoproteus* spp.
- External parasites esp.lice
- Gout (visceral and articular gout)
- Bumble foot (esp. in birds that are heavy and long-legged aves).
- Feather-loss (rule out the physiological molting process).
- Egg-drop problem
- Egg-bound syndrome
- Cannibolism /Aggression (rule out the stress factors).
- Breeding related disorders.
- Avian cholera (*by Pasteurella multacida*).
- Ranikhet disease
- Pox
- Ornithosis (zoonotic).
- Rabies (Raptors-in particular.

SIGNIFICANT NOTES ON CHLAMYDIOSIS/PSITTACOSIS

It has zoonotic significance

Etiology: *Chlamydia psittaci*

Susceptibility

All, especially Psittaciformes, Columbiformes and Galliformes.

Clinical signs

Upper respiratory disease, conjunctivitis, weight loss; signs may be variable.

Pathophysiology

Epithelial cell damage affecting respiratory epithelium first, multiple organ systems affected.

Diagnostics

Definitive ante-mortem diagnosis is challenging; culture is a gold standard test.

- Confirmed: bacterial isolation or identification in macrophage, immunofluoroscent antibody (IFA) positive tissue biopsy, fourfold titer increases 2 weeks apart.
- Probable: Single high titer in bird with clinical signs, antigen identified in feces via PCR.
- Suspect: Compatible illness without lab confirmation and existence of single high titer without clinical signs.
- Serology: Complement fixation test (CFT) & elementary body agglutination.
- CBC/chem.: Leukocytosis with heterophilia and monocytosis and increased liver enzymes.

Treatment

Tetracycline therapy for 45-days treatment shall be carried out.(e.g., Doxycycline at dose rate of 150-200 mg/kg of Doxycycline , PO, q 24 hrs or IM with less dose range- in seed, or water for at-least about seven days, as in Amazon Parrots).

Prevention

- Isolation of suspected cases
- Adequate quarantine period is a must.
- Prophylaxis by drugs shall be carried out.

Feather plucking in captive birds & etiological factors

- Molting
- Boredom
- Dietary deficiencies.
- Parasites
- Allergic reactions
- Folliculitis (bacterial).
- Psittacine Beak and Feather disease (PBFD)-virus based.

Use of haloperidol in self - mutilation of pet birds

Haloperidol-the dopamine antagonist currentlybeing used on cockatiels, lovebirds, ring-neck parakeets, African Greys, and several species of cockatoos and Amazon parrots.

Indications: Severe feather plucking/ mutilation of skin and muscle over the back, chest and legs, wing web mutilation/ Amazon foot necrosis syndrome.

Side effects from the use of haloperidol have included depression, depressed appetite, excitability and anorexia. (In most birds, side effects disappeared after discontinuing the drug for several days and then retrying at a lower dose.)

Note

One study reported normal behavior was maintained "by administering haloperidol at approximately 0.4 mg/kg body weight/day (orally) for approximately seven months". (Once or twice a day dosing shall be adapted depending on status).

Treatment of aspergillosis in parrot like birds

- Orally, 4mg itraconazole, using a syringe (as suspension) daily for 6 months.
- Concurrent nebulization with 1% clotrimazole solution (Clotrimazole 1% solution was nebulized at rate of 1ml BID to TID, by placing a pediatric nebulizer mask over the cooperative bird's head), daily for 5-6 months).

Usage of anti-fungal drugs in aviary species

Ketaconazole	10-30 mg/Kg P.O. BID x 21 days
Itraconazole	5-10 mg/Kg P.O. BID x 7-21 days
Fluconazole	5 mg/Kg P.O. SID x 7 days
Nystatin	1 lakh units / 400 gm bird P.O. x 7 days
Amphotericin B	i/v, i/tracheal or 1mg/ml saline nebulized for 15mts BID
Voriconazole(recent)	6-18 mg/Kg P.O. BID x 21 days

Common management methods to prevent flight of brids under captivity

BRAILING: The flexure of one wing,which is held closed by a soft bandage.

PINIONING: Pinioning is associated with the amputation of distal wing of birds to prevent its flight i.e. escape (i.e. Amputation of the distal wing, including the carpal,metacarpal and phalangeal bones).

Procedure

- Under general anesthesia the feathers are plucked from the carpal area and the skin is prepared for surgery.
- A tourniquet(a constricting or compressing device, specifically a bandage used to control venous and arterial circulation to an extremity for a period of time) should be placed in the mid-humoral region, and the large ulnar vein coursing along the caudal edge of the ulna is ligated through the skin just proximal to the carpal joint with chromic gut.

- The skin just dorsal to the carpal joint is incised and reflected proximally to expose the joint.
- Tendons of the lateral and oblique carpal extensors and the joint capsule are incised.
- The distal portion of the wing including the ulnar carpal boneis removed.
- The protuberance of the radial carpal bone is removed with rongeurs to produce a more esthetic surface.
- The skin should be sutured with suitable chromic gut.

Clipping of distal feathers

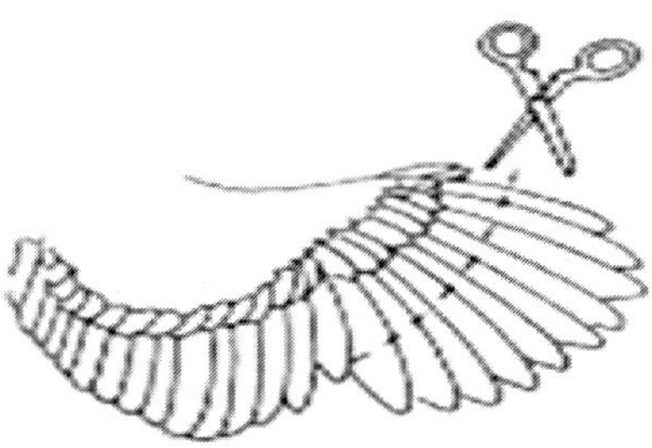

Fig. 6. Clipping of distal feathers in birds

EGG-BOUND STATUS RELATED THERAPEUTIC MANAGEMENT IN AVES

A. Visible egg related therapeutic tips on management of egg-bound status in aviary species

- Use warm water soaking & lubricant
- Remove urates & feces & clean the vent
- If needed, incision on mucosa & then attempt to remove the bound egg
- Pierce the shell tactically, remove contents first and then the shell subsequently.

B. Non visible egg related therapeutic tips on management ofegg-bound status in aviary species

- Use warm water soaking for some time & then place the bird in warm cage & clean the vent.
- IV / Sc Calcium gluconate1% soln (0.01 to 0.02 ml /gm BW for enchanced peristalsis.
- IM Oxytocin 3 to 5 IU/Kg BW.

NOTE: If the egg is not laid in 48 hrs, surgical remedy is required.

Treatment of aspergillosis in aves

- Orally, 4mg itraconazole, using a syringe (as suspension) daily for six months.
- Concurrent nebulization with 1% clotrimazole solution (Clotrimazole 1% solution was nebulized at rate of 1ml BID to TID, by placing a pediatric nebulizer mask over the cooperative bird's head), daily for 5-6 months).

Helminthiasis therapy: Extrapolation of knowledge available in domestic birds shall be utilized with appropriate clinical cautions. Piperezine dose is given below:

For round worms: Chickens: Single dose, 50 mg/bird (<6 weeks old), 100 mg/bird (e"6 weeks old), in the feed at 0.2%–0.4% or in the drinking water at 0.1% - 0.2%.

Turkeys: Single dose 100 mg/bird (<12 weeks old) or 200 mg/bird (≥12 weeks old)

Because only the piperazine moiety is efficacious, doses should be calculated based on mg of active piperazine/bird. Treatment can be repeated after 14 days.

Albendazole usage: Dosage: 5 mg/kg bird weight is reported effective against most roundworm species. A higher dosage of 20 mg/kg is needed to be effective against roundworms and tapeworms.

Fenbendazole and pyrantel pamoate and praziquantel shall be used judiciously in captive birds, depending on the need.

22

Feeding Management in Captive Wild Animals

Management of zoo and exotic animals in zoos are carried out in different ways. In the management of zoo, various cadres of personnel get employed and often, a team-approach is highly required and however, veterinarian is one of the important cadres in the zoo related personnel and veterinary interventions are highly required for management of feeding, housing, breeding and health of various species of wild fauna belonging to multiple taxonomical groups.

In general, the zoo management in a broader sense can be divided in four main categories.

1. Feeding management
2. Housing management and
3. Breeding management
4. Health management

1. FEEDING IN WILD ANIMALS

Feeding in wild animals is different under captive conditions and in free ranging conditions. Feeding is a controlled activity in case of captive wild animal species unlike in case of free ranging wild animal species in which cases, the animal by itself attempt to have some control measures. Differing feed habits are there in case of captive wild animal places that are rich in multiple species of wild animals. Hence, one should have a preliminary knowledge of the feeding related activities in the concerned wild animal species and a basic knowledge of nutrition, proper diets etc. is an essential one. Scientific mode of feeding-strategies forms the basis for the scientific management of wild animal places.

CLASSIFICATION OF WILD ANIMALS BASED ON FEEDING BEHAVIOR

i) Herbivores

They constitute the wide spectrum of different species of wild animals with anatomical adaptations comprising of symbiotic microbial population of bacteria, protozoa etc. The feed resources to these animals have in general low nutritional values but are bulky in nature. Among herbivores, the ones with complex stomach (ruminants) are the most efficient ones and the roughages and forages are most efficiently utilized by the species. Microbial fermentation is the mode of digestion in these species.

Example: Gaur, deer, giraffe, antelopes like blackbuck, wild buffaloes etc.

Pregastric fermenters are also available as wild fauna like kangaroo, wild pig, hippopotamus etc. Similarly, hind gut fermenters like rabbits, guinea pigs, capybara (caecal fermentation) and zebra and wild asses (colon fermentation) also exist under captive conditions. Cecotrophs are the ones that are produced in the morning and are the soft materials that are often consumed directly from the anal region. Animals like rabbit and hares produce these soft fecal pellets that have high protein, fiber and water contents with increased amounts of vitamin B complex. It is noteworthy to note that the bulk eaters like elephants or rhinos have poor digestive efficiency but meet their nutritional requirements by consumption of high levels of feed intake and fast rate of food transit without digesting fiber (as the case with giant panda).

ii) Carnivores

Carnivores are the meat eating animals and require highly digestible and high quality food resources with nearly all the types of nutrients. The various species of this group require most of the times unique type of nutrition. For example, felids need a dietary requirement for amino acid 'taurine' and preformed vitamin A and essential fatty acid 'arachidonic acid'.

iii) Omnivores

Large group of wild animals belong to this in general. Most of the rodents, flying fox, sloth, bears, non-human primates, pigs many species of birds etc. belong to thisgroup. Carbohydrates become the major nutrient received from the plants, while moderate amount of protein and fat are received from meat sources.

SIGNIFICANCE OF BALANCED NUTRITION

1. Longer life span of the animal
2. Maximal reproduction
3. Maximal infant survival rate
4. Appreciable health status
5. Acquiring of good immune mechanisms

GENERAL NUTRIENTS AND FEED STUFF

i) Carbohydrates

This is the chief source of energy in case of wild animals. Ruminants like deer or giraffe or antelope make use of the complex carbohydrates subsequent to the bacterial actions in the rumen and the rumen microflora help the proper digestion of nutrients. Cereals, grains, roots, tubers and fruits have high carbohydrates. Fruits are rich in pentoses and hexoses, whereas the tubers and seeds are rich in glucose.

ii) Proteins

More significance needs to be provided towards the provision of adequate amounts of protein to wild animals especially the carnivores. The proteins comprise the ingredients of internal frame work of cells esp. the interstitial cells like dentine, osteoid tissue, connective tissue etc. Essential amino acids like arginine, methionine, threonine, leucine, lysine etc. are to be given importance during the provision of protein rich diets. It is to be noted that protein deficiency may result in retardation of the growth rate, cessation of lactation in case of nursing animals, impairment of reproduction, decreased body resistance level etc.

iii) Fats

Fats are the important nutrients in case of wild fauna like the domestic animals. They provide the fat soluble vitamins like A, D, E and K. In addition, the fat materials provide some satiety value to the concerned wild animal species in addition to the provisions of the palatability to the feed. Provision of optimal amounts of fat is a must for the wild animal species. Fat provides the most concentrated forms of stored energy and fat reserves in fact help a lot for the provision of energy during the adverse climatic extremes. For example phocine like elephant seal may spend a considerable time in land without any access to food while suckling the pups. In such occasions, fat is the major nutrient factor that helps the survival of the concerned species. Similarly, in case of hibernating animals like bears in cool regions it is the fat that gets accumulated often and is useful as an energy resource in winter months.

iv) Roughages

Tree and shrub leaves, grass and legume silages, straw, fodder, hulls, shells, maize, hay etc. form the roughages. They are bulky in nature but are poor in energy content and are rich in fiber.

v) Concentrates

These are low in fibre but are rich in protein or energy content. Cereal grains, non-cereal seeds like amaranthus green, grain milling by-products like wheat and rice bran, beet pulp, citrus pulp, molasses etc. fall under this category. Fish meal, dried milk products like skin milk powder, sunflower meal, cotton seed meal etc. provide more than twenty per cent crude protein.

vi) Mineral mixtures

Mineral supplements need to be added along with the routine food materials to be offered to the dietary items of captive wild animals. It to be borne in mind that minerals also are supplied by a balanced diets. However, these can be supplied as mixtures including lime stone, dicalcium sulphate, salt, trace mineral mixtures etc. Among minerals, it is the zinc that has effect on the hair growth and calcium with phosphorous are also to be given maximum significance in case of wild animals. Deficiency of minerals like calcium and phosphorus may lead to development of bone disorders like rickets, osteodystrophy etc. Nursing animals need an additional allowance of calcium in their dietary items.

vii) Vitamin supplements

Vitamins like fat soluble ones and water soluble ones are of much helpful in various metabolic functions occurring in the body. Care has to be paid in the provision of adequate amounts of vitamins to the diet of captive wild animals. The vitamins can be supplied along with the main diet as a special mixture to rectify feather loss like conditions. Species like red vented bulbul, frugivours bats, guinea pigs, non-human primates etc. are in need of direct supply of vitamin C because they lack the enzyme L-gluconolactone oxidase required for the synthesis of vitamin C.

viii) Water

Watering in case of wild animals has to be given more significance. Generally wild animals prefer water content and even in the wild, wild animals move to the water holes frequently in every day. However, it is to be understood that certain species may not take water much like blackbucks. The water requirement may be met by water content of food itself or through the oxidation of organic constituents that produces metabolic water. High moisture diets are generally preferred by the wild animals like non-human primates. It is also equally true that high moisture food items are often subjected to the fungal as well as the microbial proliferation. Wild ruminants mostly drink water either in the late evening or early morning. Camels have capacity to take more water at a time. Wild animals like felids require the provision of water *ad-libitum*.

Diets for exotic and zoo animals have been developed through

- Practical experience.
- Food habits in the wild.
- Oral and GI tract morphology.
- Nutritional research on exotic species in the wild and captivity.
- Nutrient requirements established for domestic and laboratory animals and people.
- Anecdotal literature reports (eg, case studies).
- Physiologic status of the animal (eg, young, old, pregnant, etc).
- Body condition.

Feeding strategies in case of wild animals

Otters, badgers, pelicans, penguins, gharials, dolphins, ferrets, pole cats, mink etc. are often fed with fishes. Hence, more care needs to be taken while feeding the fish to the wild animals. Rotten fish or fish with more pungent smell are to be avoided. Gill regions in the fishes need to be examined for the freshness. Avoid the feeding of fishes like carps and herring that contain the enzyme termed thiamenase since this may destroy the thiamine in the diet. Cooked fish or fishes like butter fish and mackerel may be used. Usage of oily fish like herring in fish meal may lead to the oxidation of vitamin A and E in the diet. Wide trays may be used for feeding of species like star tortoises.

SOME EXAMPLES OF FEEDS GIVEN TO WILD ANIMALS ARE

Indian Elephant

1.	Ragi	7 kg
2.	Horse gram	2 kg
3.	Salt	200 gms
4.	Jaggery	250 gms
5.	Grass	200 kgs
6.	Sugarcane	4 nos
7.	Green tree leaves	–
8.	Bamboo / stylo	250 kg
9.	Coconut	500 gms (1 no)

Lion and Tiger

1. Beef (with bone) 10 kg
2. Chicken 1 kg (weekly once)

Bonnet macaque

- Rice 50 gms
- Banana 3 nos
- Orange/Mango ¼ no.(100-150 gm size)
- Guava ¾ no
- Groundnut (WOS) 15 gms
- Bengal gram 15 gms

Jungle cat

- Chopped beef 250 gms
- Bread slice 2 no
- Milk 100 ml

Jackal

- Beef without bone 500 gms
- Liver 100 gms
- Chicken 250 gms weekly once.

Hyena

- Beef 3 kg/day
- Liver 100 gms
- Chicken 500 gms weekly once

Sloth bear

- Ragi (cooked) 250 gms
- Rice gruel + black gram 150 + 50 gms
- Orange / Mango 2 nos
- Guava 4 nos
- Tapioca 100 gms
- Jaggery 200 gms

- Groundnut (WOS) 100 gms
- Honey bi-weekly
- Milk ½ litre
- Radish 100 gms
- Bread slices 2 nos
- Carrot 200 gms

Otter

- Fish 1.5 kg
- Crab (weekly twice) 300 gms
- Sardine 1.5 kg

Porcupine

- Rice 100 gms
- Carrot 100 gms
- Cabbage 100 gms
- Tapioca or sweet potato 100 gms
- Soya bean 20 gms
- Groundnut (WOS) 150 gms

Zebra (adult)

- Wheat bran 2 kgs
- White Bengal gram 100 gms
- Grass and leaves 30 kgs
- Mineral mixture 10 days in a month at regular intervals.
- Lucerne 5 kgs

Panther

- Beef (with bone) 3 kg
- Liver 250 gms
- Chicken 1 kg (weekly once)

Camel

- Wheat bran 2 kg

- White Bengal gram 500 gm
- Grass 30 kg
- Leaves (neem, bamboo,
- Subabul, bauhina) 20 kg
- Salt 50 gm
- Cabbage 2 kg
- Banana 6 no
- Leaves of acacia 5 kg

Indian bison (Gaur)

- Wheat bran 3 kg
- Bengal gram 0.5 kg
- Green leaves/ grass L.S

Barking deer/ Spotted deer/ Sambar deer

- Wheat bran 1 kg
- White Bengal gram 25 gm
- Grass 7 kg
- Green leaves 3 kg
- Salt 10 gm
- Stylo/Lucerne 2 kg

Peach faced love bird, Fisher's love bird, Sky blue mask love bird, Love bird (Split)

- Apple (to all) 1 no
- Banana (to all) 1 no
- Thinai 10 gm
- Paddy 5 gm
- Mixed grain 10 gm
- White Bengal gram 5 gm
- Onion 10 gm
- Greens 10 gm
- Shell grit Q.S.

Parakeet

- Bread slice 1 no
- Apple (L.S) 3 no
- Sathukudi/Mango/Orange ¼ no
- Guava 1 no
- Groundnut (WOS) 20 gm
- Chilly fruit 10 gm
- Garlic 2 gm
- Paddy 10 gm
- Mixed grains 20 gm
- Bengal gram 10 gm
- Sunflower seed 10 gm
- Green gram 10 gm

Indian Peafowl

- Cabbage 25 gm
- Mixed grains 25 gm
- Paddy 25 gm
- White Bengal gram 50 gm
- Greens 100gm
- Garlic 10 gm
- Groundnut (WOS) 50 gm
- Shell grit 25 gm
- Green gram 25 gm

Owl

- Chopped beef or rat 150 gm/2no/day
- (each 100-150 gm size)
- Chicks 10 gm (once in a week)

Budgerigar

- Thinai 10 gm
- Greens 10 gm

- Shell grit 20 gm
- Bengal gram 5 gm
- Green gram 5 gm

Emu

- Green gram 250 gm
- Wheat 250 gm (soaked)
- Broiler finisher grumble diet 250 gm
- Rice 250 gm (cooked)
- Milk 100 ml (boiled)
- Tomato 100 gm
- Green banana 2 no

Marsh crocodile (adult)

- Fish (twice a week) 250 gm
- Bone (vertebral column) 100 gm
- Beef 250 gm

Gharial (adult)

- Fish (twice a week) 1 kg
- Bone (vertebral) 100 gm

Python

- Chicken 1 kg (twice a month)
- Rat 8 no (twice a month) each 150 gm size

Viper

- Chicken 3 no
- Rat 4 no (weekly once) 100-150 gm size

Cobra

- Chicken 3 no
- Rat 4 no (weekly once) 100-150 gm size

Iguana

- Carrot 50 gm (daily)
- Cabbage 50 gm (daily)
- Tomato 50 gm (daily)
- Greens 100 gm (daily)

Star tortoise

- Carrot 30 gm (daily)
- Cabbage 30 gm (daily)
- Tomato 30 gm (daily)
- Greens (L.S) 500 gm (daily)

Feeding habits

- The feeding habit varies from species to species.
- Chewing bones is a preferred activity among lions, tigers and jaguars and the activity is less in panthers.
- These carnivores prefer larger pieces of meat to alleviate hunger more readily than the smaller meat pieces. Lions and tigers carry the beef pieces to one side of the cage before it sits for feeding.
- In lion, tiger and jaguar the posture of consumption was of extending the fore legs and holding the meat while the hind legs are tucked up within the body, where as in panthers all the four legs tucked up within the body.
- Wild dogs eat while they were in standing position in a hurried gulping manner.
- Among the large felines like tiger, lion, panther and jaguar the time taken to consume the meat was from 16.5 minutes to 39 minutes in a very slow manner.
- Tigers soon after feeding they lick the cage wall few times and then drink water, where as in lions they drink water soon after feeding.
- After the weekly starvation in lions and tigers a characteristic restlessness was evinced by the sound and arrival of the food delivery vehicle.
- During the act of drinking the large cats curl tongue backward and then flick it forward, rolling it up slightly into a spoon shape, as they do so and they swallow after every 4 or 5 laps.
- Tigers, Jaguars and Panthers show a preference for chicken meat when offered than beef.

- Almost all species of the carnivores like panther, lion, wild dog and tiger eat quickly in winter than in summer.
- In panther, lion and tiger, smelling and licking of the meat were noticed. Tigers and lions show a greater degree of smelling the licking than the other species.
- Elephants use trunk as prehensile organ and may even pick up grass by using strikes with legs on ground and later, the grass materials may be striked on its own legs to wither away the dirt or sand and then by using the trunk, they may place the feed materials into the mouth. The trunk will not be protruded during eating activities of the elephant.
- Bears have the habit of climbing the trees or rocks in order to remove the bee hives and by using forelimbs, the hives are destroyed and use to suck honey in addition to lapping using tongue.
- Crocodile have the habit of gulping the feed materials.

Sick diets

Most seriously ill-wild animals refuse to eat or just pick at the food. Force feeding often may not be practicable especially in carnivores or herbivores.

1. Soft diet like chicken preferably in cooked form may be attempted as one of the significant diets in wild animal species.
2. Intra-venous fluids like dextrose saline, Ringers lactate etc. may be chosen in wild animals that have totally ceased eating activities.
3. Attempts may be done to provide the most palatable food for the targeted wild animal species.
4. In wild animals especially carnivores with severe gastritis whatever food is offered or ingested, it may be vomited often. In such cases, blend diet may be offered. Egg white may be offered to carnivores with severe vomiting, in addition to administration of 5% dextrose saline solution, in these gastritis affected wild animals.
5. Provide drinking water ad-libitum to all the sick wild animals in general.
6. Provision of bland diet in small quantities spaced in several daily doses may help to minimize the incidences of vomiting or rejection by the concerned wild animal species.

Geriatric captive wild animal feeding

Intellectual geriatric nutrition is the need of the day in many captive wild animal places like zoos, zoological parks and zoological gardens including aviary and various reptilian centres.

Thumb-rules in geriatric captive wild animal feeding

1. Avoid feeding with less-digestible feeds.
2. Avoid full-stomach feeding.
3. Provide adequate quantities of vitamins and minerals.
4. Provide water *ad-libitum.*
5. Maintain hygiene during feeding including watering
6. Avoid long-time stored feeds due to occurrence of aflatoxicosis esp. in case of herbivores with concentrates.

Practical tips on feeding of geriatric captive wild animals

- Feed the aged captive wild carnivores with proteins of high biological value as well as high digestibility. This helps to minimize the protein residue entering the colon where bacteria act on it to produce toxins. Such proteins are more than the quantity given to adult carnivores in general.
- Food is consumed primarily to satisfy energy requirements of captive wild animals. Older wild carnivores generally need fewer calories because they are less active than younger adults. To maintain optimal weight in old animals, caloric intake can decrease to 80 percent of that needed for younger adults. Total caloric intake reductions must take into consideration that requirements for other nutrients may be unchanged or increased. As already noted, dietary protein must increase even if caloric intake remains unchanged. Needs may increase for some vitamins and trace minerals, but that is unproven. Vitamin E is most important to supplement. Aging is associated with many degenerative changes and vitamin E helps prevent damage. Older animals are more likely to be overweight than younger adults.
- The incidence of tumors is lower than expected in animals fed soy protein diets and several soy protein constituents can inhibit tumor growth (They include isoflavones, phytosterols, protease inhibitors, inositol hexaphosphate, and saponins but the soy proteins are also deficient in methionine. Dietary soy protein instead of animal protein is associated with a lower incidence of breast and colon cancer in humans. Hence, attempts may be made to mix such products with meat, thereby reducing animal protein to aged animal to some extent.
- Weight loss and cachexia are important complications of cancer. Cancer affected captive wild animals have to maintain normal weight if their life span is to be increased. It is to be understood that such aged animals may live longer with fewer complications during related treatment-measures. Tumor cells uncouple metabolism which accelerates wasting and poor use

of nutrients and thus the resulting metabolic abnormalities affect utilization of carbohydrates, proteins, and fats. Cancer patients are invariably anorectic but have a basal energy requirement that is twice normal, requiring food intake to be greatly increased. High-caloric density diet are to be fed to increase energy intake and often, up to 50 percent of non-protein calories should be fat; palatability should be enhanced by using animal fat such as chicken fat.

- Antioxidants protect against free radicals which appear as oxygen is used to produce energy and antioxidants are important as protectants and these include naturally occurring nutrients such as vitamin A, Vitamin C, and vitamin E. For example, vitamin E is essential for cell membrane protection against the many chemical reactions generating free radicals and vitamin E is more potent than synthetic antioxidants because it binds cell membranes. When animals are given vitamin E from a young age, the onset slows for some age-related problems such as cataracts, cancer, cardiovascular disease, and decreased immune function. High blood vitamin E levels may lower the risk of some cancers. This effect can be due to vitamin E blocking the formation of carcinogens in the feeds.
- Similar to humans, energy or calorie requirements in felids initially decrease in their senior years but unlike humans, energy requirements start to **increase when aging advances and this is** because, as felids age, they have difficulty in digesting of fats, proteins, and energy.
- In geriatric captive felid species, it may be more important to increase their caloric intake to sustain a normal physique as their body condition and weight naturally declines with advanced age.
- It is important to closely monitor the captive aged-felid's body condition and muscle condition and maintaining healthy body condition and muscle mass, in general reduces the risk for many diseases including cancer, kidney disease, osteoarthritis, and immune-mediated disease. It can slow the progression of age-related changes and increase a captive wild felid's lifespan.
- Water is the single most important nutrient for captive wild animals of any age. Aging, however, interferes with the animal's sensitivity to thirst which is already low, esp. in feline species and predisposes them to dehydration. Chronic dehydration can interfere with normal metabolic function and may speed the progression of subclinical disease.
- Aging, however, interferes with the animal's sensitivity to thirst which is already low, esp. in feline species and predisposes them to dehydration. Chronic dehydration can interfere with normal metabolic function and may speed the progression of subclinical disease.

23

Housing Management of Captive Wild Animals

The aim of any good zoo should be to recreate the habitat from which the animal came as accurately as possible, with enough space to move around and enough stimulation so that they can behave naturally. Monkey cages should have plenty of branches for them to swing from and bird cages should have enough room so that they can fly. Some zoos hide the lion's or tiger's food so that they have to use their senses to explore and find it.

The objectives are

1. To know much about various components of housing like common barriers, standoff barriers, fences, floor, door etc.
2. To reveal information on housing and time budget activity, holding yards and biological needs, feeding and watering facilities, lighting facilities, including the cubicle size etc.

Basics of Animal Housing

The housing of wild animals is one of the important criteria to be observed in case of wild animals in order to have a successful breeding potential and to have a comfortable living conditions under captive conditions maintained in zoos, zoological parks, zoological gardens etc. Any wild animal reared under captive condition needs to be provided the housing arrangement that can ensure a quality of life and longevity to enable the zoo population reared in captive status. The fundamental concept is that the wild animals need to get adequate space for the free type of movements that are generally carried out in the wild conditions to the possible extent.

Components of housing arrangements in wild animals

Each wild animal enclosure needs to be provided with appropriate shelter, perches, withdrawal regions, drinking water facilities, pools or water holes of suitable areas, and other facilities that may facilitate the concerned wild animal species. Such facilities finally should help the targeted wild animal species to display they wide range of their natural behavioural patterns and the housing facilities should also provide adequate protection from the predators to a great extent. Construction of the moat gains more significance in the housing arrangements.

Common barriers

Common six types of barriers that are generally used in case of captive wild animal places are given below:

1. Glass panels
2. Plastic panels
3. Wire-mesh fencing or chain link fences
4. Wet and dry moats of adequate dimension
5. High tensile vertical wires
6. Electrically charged wires
7. Concrete barriers in selected sides

Stand - off barriers

The enclosure barriers are the most and more cautions need to be exercised in order to design these types of barriers especially for the hazardous type of wild animal species like tiger, panther, lion, jaguar etc.

Spread - out railing beyond the barrier

If there is a direct contact between the wild animal species and the visitor, then there are chances for the visitors to get injured by the highly capable animals like lions, tiger etc. Hence, there is an immediate requirement to construct the stand-off barrier like the construction of Spaced-Out railing beyond the barriers which help top revent any accidental contact with the concerned wild animal species.

Security of fences

More care has to be paid in the construction of the fences that has security related features. If not, the visitors as well as the wild animal species may get injured. Particular attention is to be given to protect the children also during the visit to the captive wild animal places.The barriers should not injure the children or anybody.

Natural appearance

The housing arrangements need to merge with the natural surroundings and this avoids the distraction when visitors see the enclosure. Hence, the objectives of visiting of zoos may be achieved. For many wild animal species, housing arrangements should include naturally simulating infrastructures and for example, trees may be placed / grown inside the arboreal species like nilgiri langur. The visible structural elements of the barriers that are in direct line of the vision of visitors and exhibit species should be painted suitably, so as to render those structural elements to appear like those of local soil. The housing arrangements need to merge with the natural surroundings and this avoids the distraction when visitors see the enclosure. Hence, the objectives of visiting of zoos may be achieved. For many wild animal species, housing arrangements should include naturally simulating infrastructures and for example, trees may be placed / grown inside the arboreal species like nilgiri langur. The visible structural elements of the barriers that are in direct line of the vision of visitors and exhibit species should be painted suitably, so as to render those structural elements to appear like those of local soil.

Overhangs are required particularly in case of animals that are capable of jumping to a great height. This helps to give protection to both visitors and wild animal species.

Following wild animal species need the inside-overhangs in general

1. Cheetah
2. Zebra
3. Wild ass
4. Spotted deer
5. Hog deer
6. Sambar deer
7. Mouse deer
8. Musk deer
9. Brow antlered deer
10. Four horned antelope
11. Impala
12. Chinkara
13. Nilgiri tahr

Floor of mammalian enclosures

In case of elephants, the floor arrangements should not be made only by concrete. Natural substrate has to be provided to avoid the foot rot. Similarly, for cervids and antelopes, natural floor is a must. Avoid the presence of any pointed materials during the construction of the housing arrangements. Drainage facilities need to be provided while designing the floor arrangements inside the mammalian or other enclosures. Flooring arrangement needs to be made in order to facilitate an easy cleaning of the premises. Crevices need to be taken care of during the routine management.

Floor of aviaries

Care has to be taken to protect the aviary species from the predators that use the floor or sides, often. Hence, the aviary enclosure or housing arrangement needs to be intellectually established, considering many features required by avi-fauna of multiple species, in general. Rodent control is an important measure for the wild birds that are kept in the confined state. Floors of aviaries should have cement concrete floors in order to prevent the entry of rodents and have to be topped by the layer of about 15 cms earth.

Floor of reptilian houses

The reptilian houses should have land as well as the water-designs that should allow the sufficient space for both bathing and basking. The substrate for the reptile cages should be of pea-sized gravel or sand material depending upon the species of the reptiles.

Doors

The doors of any wild animal species should be constructed considering the following factors in mind:

1. Safety (Secured locking systems must be provided in order to prevent the theft or vandalism and to prevent the unauthorized opening of the cages in which the wild animals have been kept in confined status).
2. Durability.
3. Easy handling nature.
4. Gilletin types of vertical doors are to be avoided and horizontally, sliding doors may be used with proper lock-positions.

Breeding design

The housing arrangement should have facilities to facilitate the breeding related activities whenever required for the concerned wild animal species. For example:

1. You may be required to lower the water in hippo pools to thirty to forty cms when birth of the hippo calf is expected.
2. Hence, the housing arrangements have to be made with all such facilities that can enhance the breeding potential of the wild animal species.
3. Escape route is a must for the male felids during mating with female animal.

Housing for different sexes

Many times, if both sexes are kept in same place, fight may occur and in the process, animal may often gets injured and this will create unwanted problems in the health related management of various wild animal species. Hence, separate housing arrangements have to be constr.ucted for the proper housing of different sexes. Species like tigers, lions etc need separate housing arrangements. Even giraffes may fight with each other many times when the same housing facility is used by both sexes of this exotic-wild animal species.

Anatomy and housing arrangements

1. The entry door of the enclosure has to be constructed in a careful manner in order to avoid the injuries to the wild animal.
2. The opening has to be an adequate one, so that the concerned wild animal species can make entry freely into the enclosure.
3. The entry door of the wild animal species like Giraffe has to be built so high enough to accommodate the long neck of this animal.
4. Elephant should enter into the enclosure freely without any struggles and the housing arrangement has to be done in such a manner that entry related difficulties have to be avoided in general.

Nature of the species and housing

The nature of the concerned wild animal species has to be given more significance whenever a proper housing arrangement is made. Chimpanzees generally are reluctant to approach the water resources except for the drinking purposes. Hence, wet moats are generally preferred ones whenever housing arrangements are made for them. Giraffe do not swim and hence will not have inclination to cross the water moat. Further, the Giraffe are generally reluctant to step over the barriers and also have been very rarely observed to step over the shallow ditch. Similarly, Giraffe can extend the neck to a great extent during the attempting of trying to receive food material if any given by visitor. Hence, during the construction of housing facilities for species like this, all considerations have to be given to such nature of this species. Wet moats with resting platforms appear to be the must in case of housing arrangements for felids like tigers.

Holding yards and biological needs

1. For wild animal species like spotted deer, Sambar deer etc., small holding yards are often used to keep the released cervids (from quarantine places) for some days. This facility in captive wild animal places often helps to keep the wild animals acclimatized with the environment.

2. Snakes need mud-pots for laying of eggs. Similarly, arboreal non-human species like Common langurs need hanging types of wooden rods for climbing activities.
3. Wallowing tank or water source to move freely is to be provided for Elephant, Rhino, Sambar deer etc.
4. Among the felids, emphasis maybe given to provide water filled tank for submerging or sitting in summer periods for tigers, in particular. There should be proper lighting facilities in all wild animal enclosures and this helps to inspect the wild animal even in the night hours also.
5. However, the nocturnal and diurnal activity pattern of the wild animal has to be taken care of while lighting facilities are used in the enclosures.
6. Reptiles like diamond pythons, lizards etc. may require Ultra Violet-B type that has non-visible wavelength and the UV-bulb may be fixed in such a manner that the concerned reptile may get maximum light and it appears better to have the bulb at about 12 inches away from the basking spot.

The place for feeding should be constructed in such a manner that the cleaning of the premises becomes an easy one and the crevices in the feeding trough needs to be attended properly during the maintenance of the feeding trough or place. This helps to avoid the deposition of feed particles in the structures and thereby the chances for contamination of food particles get minimized. Multiple feeding places are the better ones especially for the animals that are exhibited in herds like Spotted deer, Manipuri deer, black bucks etc. The watering facility should be thought of whenever a housing facility is constructed for the concerned wild animal species. The capacity of wild animal species with regard to the watering habits needs to be paid more emphasis. For example, an elephant may require about two hundred and twenty litres of water in a day. Hence, the watering trough should be of adequate size and should have an easy access for the wild animal species to have water whenever it desires. These need to be constructed outside the enclosure and by placing appropriate agents, it becomes possible to prevent or minimize the entry of microbes through the visiting personnel. Place of foot bath should be inspected frequently to avoid the slippery nature of the floor.

Name of the Species	Size of the cubicle in meters (Length, Breadth & Height)		
	Length	**Breadth**	**Height**
Tiger and lions	2.75	1.80	3.00
Panther	2.00	1.50	2.00
Clouded leopard & Snow leopard	2.00	1.50	2.00
Small cats	1.80	1.50	1.50
Elephant	8.00	6.00	5.50

Name of the Species	Size of the cubicle in meters		
	Length	Breadth	Height
One-horned Indian Rhinoceros	5.00	3.00	2.50
Brow antlered deer	3.00	2.00	2.50
Hangul	3.00	2.00	2.50
Swamp deer	3.00	2.00	2.50
Musk deer	2.50	1.50	2.00
Mouse deer	1.50	1.00	1.50
Nilgiri tahr	2.50	1.50	2.00
Chinkara	2.50	1.50	2.00
Four horned antelope	2.50	1.50	2.00
Wild Buffalo	3.00	1.50	2.00
Gaur	3.00	2.00	
Yak	4.00	2.00	2.50
Bharal, goral, Wild sheep and markhor	2.50	1.50	2.00
Wild Ass	4.00	2.00	2.00
All type of Indian bears	2.50	1.80	2.00
Jackal, wolf and Wild dog	2.00	1.50	1.50
Palm civet	2.00	1.00	1.00
Large Indian civet & binturong	2.00	1.50	1.00
Otters all types	2.50	1.50	1.00
Hogbadger	2.50	1.50	1.00
Martens	2.00	1.50	1.00

ENVIRONMENTAL ENRICHMENT MEASURES IN ZOO

- During the meeting out of the physical requirements of various species of wild animals, one has to find ways to stimulate the concerned wild animal species for the purpose of exhibition of more activities in an environment.
- Furnishings of the enclosures in an intellectual manner helps to enhance the activities of the targeted wild animal kept in the confined status.
- Environmental enrichment enhanced the quality of captive animal care by identification and provision of environmental stimuli necessary for the optimal psychological and physiological well-being of the concerned wild animal species in a captive condition.

GOALS OF ENVIRONMENTAL ENRICHMENT

- Followings may be said as the goals of environmental enrichment:
- Enhancement of positive utilization of the environment.
- Finding an increase in range or number of normal behavioral patterns.
- Encountering reduction in the frequencies of abnormal behavior.

- Finding an increase in the behavioural diversity.
- Experiencing an increase in an animal s ability to cope with the challenges in a more natural manner.

ENRICHMENT STRATEGIES

Provision of due enrichment measures varies from species to species. This is because of the variations in the requirements by the concerned wild animal species.

REQUIRED INFRASTRUCTURES

These items may change the stimulus in a favorable manner:

- Toys
- Objects
- Usable surfaces
- Manipulable and movable materials
- Materials for camouflaging
- Increased usable materials
- Facilities that requires probing or analysis by the concerned wild animal species to some extent

Note: Modified feeding patterns (or) places may help the enrichment measures in case of wild mammals.

24

Overall Breeding Management of Captive Wild Animals

Captive breeding programme is generally considered as a process of breeding animals in controlled environments within well-defined settings, such as wildlife reserves, zoos and other commercial/noncommercialconservation facilities.Use of modern reproductive biotechnologies or assisted reproductive techniques (ART) include in general artificial insemination, embryo transfer/sexing, *in vitro* fertilization, gamete/embryo micromanipulation, semen sexing, genome resource banking, and somatic cell nuclear transfer (cloning) in conservation programs for endangered mammalian species.

With captive breeding the ultimate aim should be to release the progeny in the species' natural habitats, for replenishment of wild populations. Young herbivores so released should not be too tame, and their predators have to be curtailed at least initially. Released predators have further problems, as they must be able to hunt effectively, which often involves considerable areas.

SUCCESSFUL BREEDING PROGRAMMES IMPLEMENTED

- Reintroduction of Przewalski's horse was successfully reintroduced in the wild after breeding these equids under captivity and these animals are native to Central Asia.
- Pere David's deer was successfully saved by captive breeding programmes after almost being hunted to extinction in China.
- The Mysore zoo has also been identified as the participating zoo in the conservation breeding of lion-tailed macaques and Nilgiri langur.
- Successful breeding of Nilgirilangur is being carried out at Arignar Anna Zoological Park, Vandalur.

MERITS OF CAPTIVE BREEDING PROGRAMMES

- Recent advances in molecular biology would contribute towards captive breeding of animals that cannot be saved in the wild.

- The low birth and high mortality rate in many wild fauna (as the case with elephants-the mega herbivores) cause the captive population to decline rapidly, thus leading to the necessity for adaptation of successful and well carefully framed captive breeding programmes related to the different species of wild fauna.

DEMERITS OF CAPTIVE BREEDING

- Less expression of natural instincts in captive bred wild fauna
- Fear complex might be absent leading to succumbing to poaching
- Lesser foraging abilities unlike the naturally bred wild animals
- Absence of fully learned natural escape mechanisms unlike the natural ones
- Inbreeding resulting in more heterozygosity / compromised immunity/ diseaseoccurrences
- Re-introduction related field - problems

FACTORS ASSOCIATED WITH BREEDING STRATEGIES

- Environment
- Enrichment in the captive breeding places for the targeted wild fauna.
- Social group-availability.
- Knowledge on biology, anatomy and physiological features of the concerned wild fauna undergoing the captive breeding programmes.
- Assistance from the Animal keepers, mahouts and other care-takers including the authorities.
- Technical assistance from the nearby veterinary institutions.
- Huge funds.

TYPES OF BREEDING STRATEGIES

- Conventional approach of planned breeding
- Modern approaches like cloning of endangered species, establishment of gene banks by cryopreservation of semen, eggs and embryos of endangered species, and resurrection of extinct and endangered species by cloning with the assistance related to the frozen genetic material.

EXCESSIVE POPULATION IN ZOO

In general, there are wide variations in the existence of excessive population of wild animals in a zoological park or zoo or zoological garden. The list of wild animals in excess may vary from zoo to zoo or country to country.

In general, following wild animals may be found in excess numbers in many zoos:

- Spotted deer
- Bonnet macaques
- Rhesus macaques
- Mugger crocodiles
- Black buck
- Lions

POPULATION CONTROL STRATEGIES

- Separation of sexes: This helps in the prevention of the fight between the male-members of same wild animal species. o Separating the sexes is one of the easiest method to be adapted in various zoos and is a widely practiced method of population control strategy in many zoos at present.
- Surgical intervention wherever possible (eg.Vasectomy which is ideal than the castration. This is because of the fact that castration is being associated with the loss of secondary sexual characters like mane in lions.
- Hormonal intervention and others.

Breeding Strategies and Genetic Diversity in Wildlife

S.No.	English Name	Scientific Name	State
1.	Asiatic Lion	*Panthera leo persica*	Gujarat
2.	Barasingha	*Cervous duvauceli*	Madhya Pradesh
3.	Binturong	*Arctictis binturong*	Meghalaya
4.	Blackbuck	*Antilope cervicapra*	Punjab
5.	Clouded Leopard	*Neofelis nebulosa*	Nagaland
6.	Crab eating Macaque	*Macaca fascicularis*	Andaman and Nicobar
7.	Four-horned Antelope	*Tetracerus quadricornis*	Andhra Pradesh
8.	Gour or Indian bison	*Bos gaurus*	Maharashtra
9.	Chinkara	*Gazella dorcus*	Rajasthan
10.	Golden cat	*Catopuma temmincki*	Mizoram
11.	Hanuman Langur	*Semnopithecus entellus*	Delhi
12.	Indian Elephant	*Elephas maximus*	West Bengal
13.	Kashmir Stag	*Cervus elephus hanglu*	Jammu & Kashmir
14.	Leopard	*Panthera pardus*	Uttar Pradesh
15.	Lion-tailed Macaque	*Macaca silenus*	Kerala
16.	Mouse deer	*Moschiola meminna*	Goa
17.	Musk deer	*Moschus chrysogaster*	Himachal Pradesh
18.	Nilgai	*Boselaphus tragocamelus*	Haryana

19.	Nilgiri Tahr	*Hemitragus hylocrius*	Tamil Nadu
20.	One-horned Rhinoceros	*Rhinoceros unicornis*	Assam
21.	Phyre's Leaf Monkey	*Trachypithecus phayrei*	Tripura
22.	Red Panda	*Ailurus fulgens*	Sikkim
23.	Sambar	*Cervus unicolor*	Orissa
24.	Slender Loris	*Loris tardigradus*	Karnataka
25.	Sloth Bear	*Melursus ursinus*	Bihar
26.	Takin	*Budorcus taxicolor*	Arunachal Pradesh
27.	Thamin	*Cervus eldi eldi*	Manipur

To understand the breeding related strategies, the zoo veterinarian should be aware of the biological features related to specific species under cativity

Example:

Biological features related to reproduction in case of elephants:

Body weight: About 5000 kg (Males may weigh more in general and elephants have largest brain among land-animals.

Sexual maturity: At the age of 15-16 years in females & it are at 12 years of age in males and the males have fertile sperms, when they are 18-20 years old.

Oestrus cycle: About 15 to 19 weeks (About 4 months)

Gestation period: 20-22 months (Females can continue to breed to the age of 55-60 years).

Raising of young one: Because males play no part in raising the young and are not needed to protect the mother or baby, their role appears to be purely reproductive.

Longevity of elephant: About 75 years (Captive elephants live longer than the wild due to intense care related measures adapted for rearing of elephants under the captivity).

25

Overall Health Management in Zoos

Veterinarians, biologists, field assistants, hunters, and other individuals who work directly with wildlife have an increased risk of acquiring these diseases directly from animal hosts or their ectoparasites. Plague, tularemia, and leptospirosis have been acquired in the handling and skinning of rodents, rabbits, and carnivores. With regard to disease conditions affecting the captive wild fauna, though many disease conditions have been documented in wild animals reared under captivity at south India, it is also equally true that still there are large number of conditions that may warrant in-depth analysis towards establishing the confirmatory diagnosis in case of captive wild fauna, in various countries.

Management of diseases in captivity is an art to be exercised by the Zoo Veterinarians and often it becomes a team work in which zoo personnel like Director of the zoo or zoological park or zoological garden, Range officers and animal keepers and biologists of the zoos have coordinating roles in the field of wildlife conservation and management.

BACTERIAL DISEASES

Wild life diseases are given more priority in the recent days due to the fact that conservation of any wild fauna cannot be achieved fully, unless due efforts are equally given pertaining to the assessment of health status and the disease management, in the concerned wild animal species.

Bacterial diseases are in plenty in case of wild animals esp. the captive wild animals and they pose problems in the diagnosis as well as the treatment. Hence, one should have a thorough understanding of various bacterial disease conditions that affect commonly the wild animals belonging to multiple taxonomic classes or groups.

SIGNIFICANT BACTERIAL DISEASES

1. Tuberculosis
2. Haemorrhagic septicaemia (Pasteurellosis)
3. Leptospirosis

4. Anthrax
5. Tetanus
6. Enterotoxaemia
7. Salmonellosis
8. *Escherichia coli* infections
9. Wound infections

OTHER BACTERIAL INFECTIONS

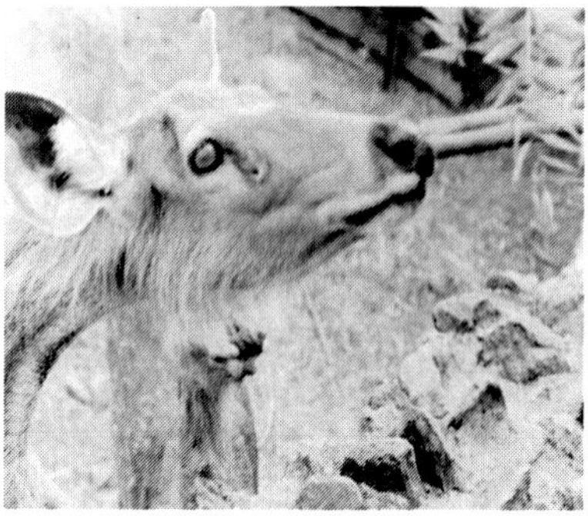

Fig. 1. Feeding of more green leaves

Most of the carnivores get affected by the infections with Streptococcus sp., staphylococcus sp. and Corynebacterium sp. frequently. These organisms may be cultured from animals with neonatal polyarthritis, pneumonia, septicemia and abscesses. Similarly, *corynebacterium pyogenes* is found with abscesses, arthritis, metritis and cystitis. Colic like disorders and corneal opacity like conditions may be encountered in animal like elephant. Corneal opacity, as furnished below is common not only in bacterial infections or parasitic infections like trypanosomosis but also in nutritional deficiencies also.

INFECTIOUS DISEASES

Infectious diseases in wild animals have to be understood well by the veterinarians. These are the significant causal agents for the ongoing morbidity and mortality among various captive and free ranging wild animal species, in various regions of this world. Proper identification of various agents associated with this should be known and their pathogenic potentials for other animals or for man have to be given significance always. PCR plays a major part in effecting the proper diagnosis of the various infectious agents in general. However, conventional techniques also assume significance for the proper understanding of these diseases affecting wild fauna. Significant infectious diseases affecting should be known.

Table: Significant infectious diseases

Disease	Hosts affected
Trypanosomosis	Bovids, equids, canids, felids, equids, suids etc.
Glanders (*Pseudomonas malle*)	Equids like wild ass, zebra etc.
FMD (Aptho virus)	All artiodactylids
Hog cholera (Toga virus)	Suids
Haemorrhagic septicemia	Bovids in particular
Japanese B encephalitis (Flavivirus)	Suids, equids and man.
Louping ill (Flavivirus)	Bovids, shrew, wild sheep, wood mouse and man
Dourine (*Trypanosoma equiperdum*)	Equids
African swine fever	Suids
African horse sickness	Equids and canids
Teschen disease (Enterovirus porcine 1)	Suids
East coast fever (Therileriasis)	Bovids
Rift Valley fever, Bunyavirus	Wild sheep and wild goat

Peste des petits ruminants (Paramyxo viruses)

VIRAL DISEASES

Viral diseases causing problems to the routine performance of the wild animals are caused substantially by many viral agents also. In both the captive and free ranging wildlife regions, the diseases caused by different viral agents are being documented throughout the world. However, the research findings are still to be improved in this regard due to various reasons.

Some common viral diseases among wild animals

1. FMD
2. Rabies
3. Measles (rubeola)
4. Viral hepatitis
5. Kyasanur forest disease (kfd) and others
6. Herpes virus and pox virus infections
7. Feline viral rhinotracheitis
8. Canine distemper

PARASITIC DISEASES

Natural areas in tropical and sub-tropical climates are more likely to enhance development of parasitic loads because of the fact that there are variations in climates of these areas in addition to the variations in the type of vegetation and species of wild fauna. The parasitic diseases have caused serious problems in captive animals and it is to be accepted that some of the diseases bear Zoonotic significance. Hence, treatment and prevention against parasites gain significance always in the wild animal health and disease management.

In non–human primates, Strongyles, *Strongyloides* spp, *Trichuris* spp, *Entamoeba* spp and *Balantidium* spp are noticed which the zoonotically important ones are. The common internal parasites in felids are *Toxocara cati, Ancylostoma* spp, *Taenia* spp, *Dirofilaria immitis*, *Spirocerca lupi* and the common blood protozoa parasites that are often encountered comprise *Trypanasoma evansi, Toxoplasma gondii* and *Hepatozoa* spp. There are numerous nematode parasites in the elephant like liver flukes, ascarids, oxyurids, strongylids, paraphistomes, ancylostomes, syngamids and filarids. Cestodes like *Anoplocephala manubriuta* are also reported. External parasites mange and tick ingestion are also common. Psoroptes spp, Sarcoptes spp and demodex spp are caused mange infestation in wild ruminants. In case of reptiles like snakes, tick infestation is more common. The common ticks are *Aponomma* spp, *Amblyomma* spp, and *Hyalomma* spp. Internal parasites like *Capillaria* spp, *Rhabdius* spp. *Ophidascaris* spp, *Isospora* spp, *Eimeria* spp, *Kalicephalus* spp, *Polydephis* spp are similarly encountered in various species of wild fauna.

METABOLIC AND NUTRITIONAL DISEASES IN WILD ANIMALS

Metabolic diseases mean the diseases that occur due to the "imbalance between the rate of input" of dietary nutrients and the "output" of products (product like new born, milk for young one etc.) and lead to the occurrence of metabolic derangements in the affected wild animal species.

Metabolic diseases usually result from a disturbance in the normal balance of the physiological mechanisms that maintain stability (or) homeostasis. Captive wild ruminants are prone for occurrence of many metabolic diseases as the case with the domestic ruminants.

Examples of metabolic diseases include overproduction or underproduction of hormones, which control specific body processes; nutritional deficiencies; poisoning from such agents as insecticides, fungicides, herbicides, fluorine, and poisonous plants; and inherited deficiencies in the ability to synthesize active forms of specific enzymes, which are the proteins that control the rates of chemical reactions in the body.

Trillions of bacteria live in the primate gut, contributing to metabolism, immune system development, and pathogen resistance. Perturbations to these bacteria are associated with metabolic and autoimmune human diseases that are prevalent in the current societies. It has been documented that the captivity and loss of dietary fiber in nonhuman primates are associated with loss of native gut microbiota and convergence toward the modern human microbiome, suggesting that parallel processes may be driving recent loss of core microbial biodiversity in many specis including non-human primates.

Some common metabolic diseases of wildlife are

1. Parturitient paresis (milk fever) in wild ruminants
2. Lactation tetany in wild equids
3. Ketosis (acetonemia) in wild ruminants
4. Fatty liver in mammals and birds
5. Diabetes mellitus in mammals and birds
6. Rickets and osteoporosis
7. Osteomalacia and fibrous osteodystrophy
8. Haemochromatosis and amyloidosis in captive birds

WOUNDS, ABSCESSES AND INJURIES

These are very common among wild animal species esp. the captive ones. In-fighting is the common cause often.

1. Abscesses may occur if immediate treatment is not done due to multifaceted causes.
2. Long time persisting wounds are common among elephants in particular and routine treatment protocol needs to be adapted in all these cases.
3. In many captive animals, wounds may get further complicated by affections with maggots.

Treatment of chronic wounds

Chronic Wound infections in animals not responding to conventional treatment modality are the important cause of morbidity. Infection is responsible for delayed wound healing.

- Removal of hair particles on and around the wounds, removal of tissuedebris, slushing with isotonic saline solution followed by application of hydrogen peroxide solution with proper cleaning within minutes are the primary steps required in the chronic-wound management.
- **Citric acid** treatment was found most effective and economical approach for the successful treatment of chronic infected wounds in animals not responding to conventional antibiotic treatment and local wound care. Citric acid (3% to 5%) treatment (7 to 20 applications externally over the cleaned wounds) treatment is most effective and also bears economical approach

for the successful treatment of chronic infected wounds in animals not responding to conventional antibiotic treatment and local wound care.

- **BIPP** (Bismuth-lodoform-Paraffin-Paste) ointment – application (A paste of composition lodoform 40% w/w, Bismuth Subnitrate 20% w/w and Paraffin Liquid 40% w/w) for daily or once in 2 days application is required for months over the wounds (The paste is to be evenly spread onto a suitable length of sterile gauze and packed into the wound-cavity).
- **Triple sulpha powder** (Each gram powder contains: Sulfadimidine sodium 110 mg, Sulfadiazine sodium 110 mg and Sulfamerazine sodium 110 mg. Indications: Triple Sulfa is indicated for use in case of infections (esp. respiratory and intestinal infections) caused by micro-organisms sensitive to sulphonamides) shall be packed (in gauze) in the wound cavities.
- The animal studies revealed that treatment with **topical insulin** (spray & cream) lead to faster wound contraction and re-epithelialization. The total dose of 0.25 units of **long-acting insulin-zinc suspension** may be injected directly into the wound every other day for few days and generally, the serum glucose which gets decreased will come to normal after few (three hours, mostly) hours.
- **Chitin and chitosan** with beneficial intrinsic properties and high potential for wound healing are attractive biopolymers for wound management.

26

Physical Restraint of Wild Animals

In the wildlife conservation and management, restraint and handling of wild/zoo and exotic animals play a prominent role. Zoo veterinarian has to deal with animal handling on a regular basis for various purposes like routine health check-up, research purpose (assisted reproductive techniques, blood collection for genetic health analysis, radio-collaring), or for conservation and management purposes (capture of problematic animals, translocation. introduction and reintroduction) and for the marking of animals. So, proper management called for good restraint in wildlife.

Types of Restraint

1. Physical / Manual restraint
2. Chemical restraint

1. Physical / manual restraint

Simple procedures such as brief examination, injection or venipuncture can be carried out using physical restraint alone for captive animals. Most of the zoos has squeeze cages where animal is allowed to feed and restrained its movements for veterinary care.

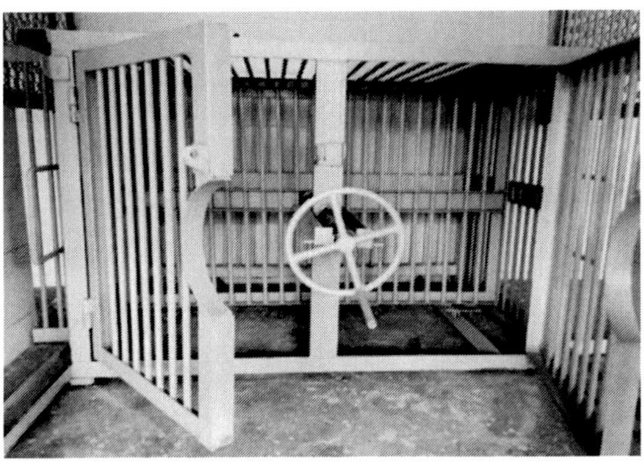

Fig. 1. Squeeze cage at LaCONES Animal Holding Facility for Physical Restraint of Wild Felid: Leopard at LaCONES-CCMB

SQUEEZE CAGES AND CHAIN LINK FENCES

- The squeeze cages need to be adequate size for the concerned wild animal under target. The squeeze cages are in-built ones in case of felid enclosures.
- These cages are mainly used for an efficient control of captive felids like lion, tiger, panther, bears, hyena, jackals, wild dogs, fox etc.
- Hydraulic squeeze cages are available for an efficient control of even the large sized mega herbivores like elephants.
- Well padded squeeze cages are available for the control of cervid species like spotted deer, sambar deer etc.
- Chain link fences are used to restrain many species of wild animals including non-human primates like Bonnet macaques in an efficient manner.

Other devices of physical restraint are

TRAPS: Traps are routinely used to capture mass population of wild animals that are laid at places where the animals frequently visit such as water holes. The traps are laid in a funnel shape where the animals are driven from large area leading it into the trap. Sometimes, food or live bait (e.g. goat for carnivore sp. or large felids) is kept near traps to attract animals for capture. Even the opposite sex animal can also be used to attract the counterpart. In case of animals in zoos, the traps are used in their feeding cell or night shelter.

SNARES: Snares can also be used to capture problematic animal but the snares needs to be monitored for long hours so that as soon as the animal is trapped in snares, it has to be relieved immediately from the snares to prevent strangulation. These physical (manual) restraint methods have several limitations. For instance, physical restraint needs long term planning and it is very expensive to perform physical capture in the wild such as hiring of helicopters and other vehicles for driving/chasing animals. Individual subject animal (such as aggressive animal) from a group of animals cannot be tracked and anaesthetized independently using physical restraint. Also, physical method cannot be applied in captive animals especially while dealing examining and offering veterinary care to the sick and injured animals. It leads to serious stress in the animals kept in captivity and sometimes, it may prove fatal. Thus, in such instances, chemical capture and handling would be an ideal capture method for immobilizing zoo captive animals.

BALES OF STRAW MATERIALS

The bales of straw materials are more easy to use due to it's availability and cost.

However, it can be used mainly in case of deer related restraint strategies especially to restraint the deer inside the fenced area

USE OF BLANKETS FOR RESTRAINT

- Blanket materials are particularly useful in controlling the semi-conscious cervids and more useful during the control of primates falling from top.
- Blanket materials are particularly useful in controlling the semi-conscious cervids and more useful during the control of primates falling from top.

USE OF PLYWOOD BOARDS FOR RESTRAINT

These are the large pieces of plywood with handles fixed in one side, so as to have a better grip of the board whenever the captive wild animal is approached for various purposes.

USE OF NET GUNS & KRALLS FOR RESTRAINT

- The net guns are always used for the physical restraint with capture of free ranging aviary species. However, the cost factor of this has to be taken care of. Krall is used mainly to restrain the elephants in free ranging regions

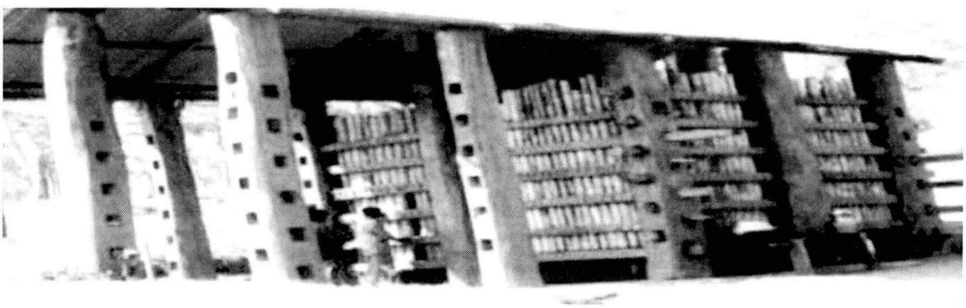

Fig. 2. (Krall for elephant-restraint)

KETCH-ALL POLE & ELECTRIC RODS

The ketch-all-Pole gadgets may be used for control the highly aggressive wild carnivores of smaller size. Snares are used to control the species like wild boars, camels etc.

Electric rods are currently used as a means of defensive action. In case of highly aggressive animal, this may be used for an effective control whenever required.

GADGETS BASED ON SIGHT AND SOUND

The **puppets** are mainly used to capture the freely swimming birds in a lake etc.

NETS: Variety of nets such as mist net, drive net, projection (or) cannon net (or) net can be used to capture aggressive (or) injured animals and nets with extension of arms is a preferred one esp. for captive birds.

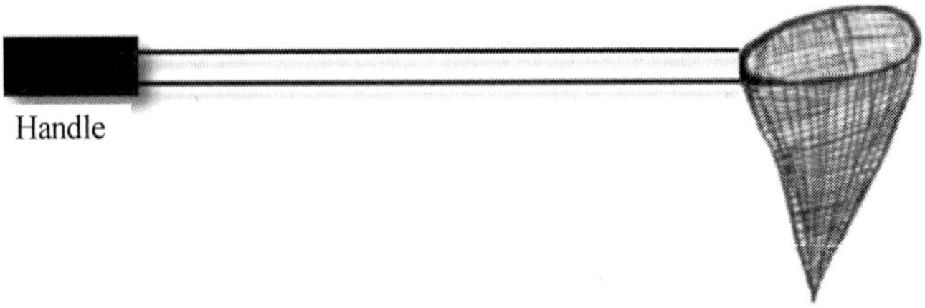

Fig. 3. Net with handle

Mist nets are of fine ones and can be spotted out only out of serious observations. These are used mainly for the restraint of cervids like spotted deer, antelopes like blackbuck. However, they need to be placed with suitable height.

The **visual barriers** directing the wild animals in one direction with facilities for the placement of obstacles may be used for the proper restraint of cervids.

The **spot lights** are used with adequate illuminative power, in the night periods. The eyes of the wild animals will glow often in this targeted spot light. The animals may be restrained subsequently.

The **carbondioxide fire extinguisher** based gadgets are simply used to have control over the wild animal by means of developing some foam or noise in front of the concerned wild animal especially in case of some emergency conditions.

The **hoods** made of clothes are used for the control of the big sized birds like ostriches, emus, cassowary etc.

RESTRAINT USING "SENSES"

Cooling: The cooling related reflex can be used to control the wild animals like serpentines.

Vision

- Vision related reflex can be used to control the wild animals and such types of restraints are often used to control the vision based stress reactions also in case of wild animals.
- It is to be remembered that the blind folded wild animals may not show much excitement unlike the wild animal which has not been blind folded.
- Complete coverage but with the proper ventilation using *thick cloth like tarpaulin* may be of useful in quitening the concerned wild animal. This feature is to be taken care of during the calming down of the free ranging wild animal like leopard etc.
- It is to be remembered that the nocturnal wild animals may be less active in broad day light and similarly, the diurnal wild animals may be less active in night time.

Psychological tool: Voice may be helpful to some extent for the pro per restraint of the wild animal. However, it may not be taken as a more reliable tool for the restraint of the wild animal.

Smell: Sometimes, the presence of excreta from same animal or the same species may have some degree of calming effects.

Snake hook & elephant hook: Please note that the snake hook needs to have an adequately lengthy handle to provide safety to the operator or restraining personnel associated. Transparent plastic tubes may be used for the proper restaint of serpentines.

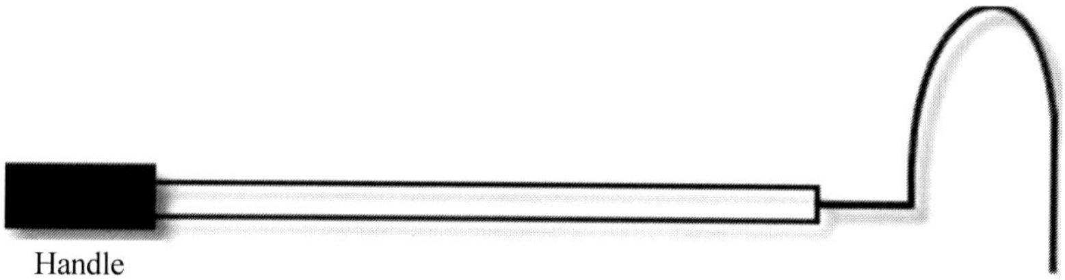

Fig. 4. Restraining hook for elephant

Fig. 5. Ankush for elephant

FOOT HOLD TRAPS AND DROP NETS

These foot hold traps are mainly useful to restrain the carnivores in the free ranging regions like the wolf, hyena, jackals etc.

- Drop nets are used to capture the non-human primates, cervids, antelopes etc. but more caution is needed to use these gadgets for the restraint purpose.
- Nets made of nylon or cotton with sufficient durability may be used for an efficient restraint of the wild animal.

PRESSURE FORCE, CUSHION AND MATTRESSES

- The pressure force to be exerted by fingers help to exercise more control in the birds captured. However, some experience is required for it s efficient usage.
- Cushion may be used to give specific support in selected spots during the restraining operations of cervids in trucks or fenced chambers.
- Mattresses can be used safely but with cautions in cervids, antelopes etc. and these gadgets are of useful as barriers mainly.

MISCELLANEOUS GADGETS

Mouth gags may be useful for small sized wild mammals like jungle cats, foxes, jackals etc. However, needs a clear assessment. Snares also may be used to restrian the wild animals at a distance.

Adjustable partitions are used in between the animals like carnivores. The enclosures for lions or panthers often have the partitions that can be operated from outside in a more safe manner.

The drop gates with pulley system can be used to capture and restraint of non-human primates, wild pigs etc.

27

Chemical Immobilization of Wild Animals

Chemical restraint is a form of animal restraint technique in which a drug or a chemical is used to restrict the movement (walking, running, aggression) of an animal or sometimes just to sedate or to calm down the animal. Chemical restraint is a safe and effective capture method when applied correctly and with due precaution.

PURPOSES OF CHEMICAL RESTRAINT

- Disease diagnostic purpose
- Therapeutic purpose
- Vaccination purpose
- Examination of highly excitable species
- Biological research purposes
- Veterinary research purposes
- Translocation
- Transfer
- Transport
- Wild animal conflicts related events (herbivore and carnivore and omnivore may get associated with these conflicts)
- Random health assessment in free ranging areas
- Rescue purposes
- Management purposes

Chemical restraint is advantageous over physical capture because it allows examining and treating sick and injured animals or animals caught in snares or traps in the wild by poachers. It enables restraint of selected aggressive animals within a group of animals, and the equipment required for chemical restraint is easy to transport from one place to another in the field. However, chemical capture may have disadvantages such as occasional failure of the equipment on site, undesirable side effects of drug in unknown excited or diseased animal, improper darting of an animal due to occasional operator's mistakes. Further, chemical capture method cannot be applied for mass capture of animals within a group. Nonetheless, chemical restraint has become a valuable tool in wildlife health, research and management since it facilitates the handling of animals as and when required for medical procedures and experimentation. However, the state of chemical restraint may vary from immobilization (restricting animal movements), to tranquilization (calmness), to complete anaesthesia (complete loss of consciousness). Various modern capture methods require a high degree of expertise and experience, as well as knowledge of physiology and behaviour of an animal to be captured.

However, one of the biggest challenges facing Wildlife Veterinarians in India is the lack of expertise and experience in wildlife handling and also knowledge of basic physiology of various species. Therefore, wildlife veterinarians need to be fully conversant with a wide array of environmental and biological variables while using chemical restraint on wild animals. In order to minimize risks of anaesthesia to subject animals, Veterinarians also need to be able to react appropriately using the correct equipment with sufficient skill to deal with anything that may go wrong during the capture.

ANAESTHESIA EQUIPMENT

Anaesthetic drugs are generally administered by remote darting systems by means of a wide range of equipment such as aluminum or plastic syringes called "Darts". The darts are fired from a distance by a variety of dart guns or blow pipe for administering immobilizing and tranquillizing drugs intramuscularly into wild animals from a reasonable distance. Pole-syringes are used to inject animals that are in close proximity, such as animals in squeeze cages, crates or crush passageways. The drugs can also be injected with ordinary syringes after the animals have been captured in nets or by other mechanical means.

VARIOUS ROUTES OF DRUG ADMINISTRATION

1. Oral-drugs can be mixed in water and food
2. Hand-held syringes-Regular syringe, jab-stick
3. Remotely projected syringes or darts-Blow-pipe, blow-gun, gun, pistol

1. **Oral route:** The immobilizing drugs can be mixed in the food or water as bait. However, it has limitations especially in free-ranging animals that the bait may be consumed by the non-targeted animals, or aggressive animal may consume more than the desired dose or if the drug gives undesirable

smell, animal may reject the bait or regurgitate the food. This drug delivery will be applicable in captive or trapped animals.

2. **Hand-held syringes:** When the animal is held in the trap cage or in squeeze cage, regular or ordinary syringes made of any metal/aluminium, plastic or glass with dart needle having sleeve can be used for delivering the drug.

   a) Jab-stick is a modified syringe that allows operator to keep away from animal while injecting the drug. The stick will be attached with a syringe and attached needle. The drug will be administered using a pressure. Different types of jab-sticks, made of aluminum, plastic or fibre glass are available.

   b) An extendable jab-stick of 4.5 m is preferred for delivering anaesthetics in captive animals or partially anaesthetized animals. Even the repeated injections of desired doses can be injected using modern jab-sticks.

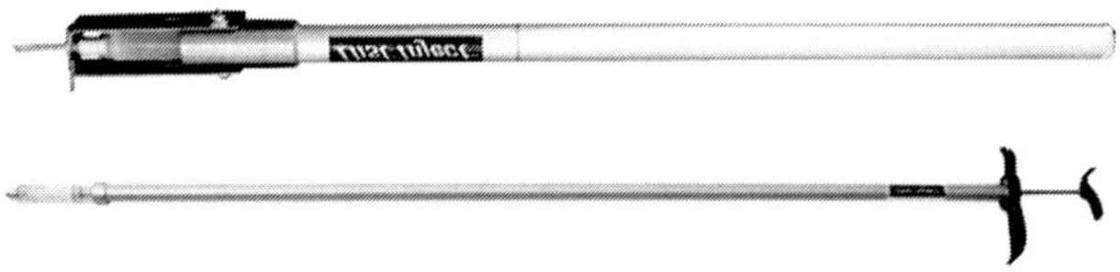

Fig. 1. Pole syringe & Jab-stick for immobilization of captive animals

Projectile Dart Syringes: Most of the chemical immobilization procedures in wild animals are performed using dart syringes which are injected using either blow-pipe or dart gun or pistol. The dart has three components-needle with sleeve, barrel of syringe/dart for drug and rear side stabilizer which provides direction while darting.

The preparation of dart is very important and needs much practice and experience. For filling a dart with a drug, first push the rubber plunger of the dart barrel back and fill the dart with the drug from the anterior opening. Then cover the needle hole with a rubber sleeve and fix the needle on the syringe hub. The dart is then pressurized by filling the gas from the rear end of dart and finally the loaded dart is put in the blow-pipe ready for darting. Dart syringes of varying capacity (1 ml to 5 ml) are to be darted via blow-pipe

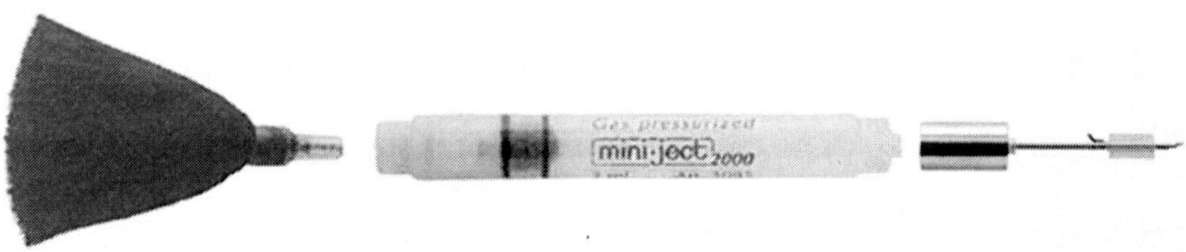

Fig. 2. Dart syringe: Photo credit: Dist-Inject

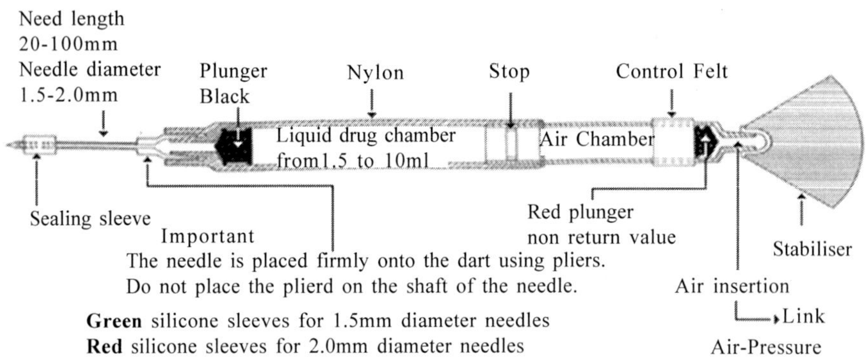

Fig. 3. Cross section of dart syringe showing different pa rt:Photo credit: Dist-Inject

Collared needle

These provide a better grip.

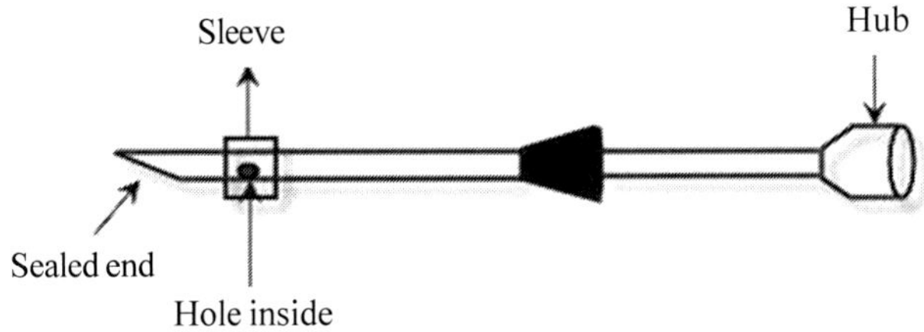

Fig. 4. Collared needle

Barbed needle:

These offer a best grip but skin-injury may occur during removal.

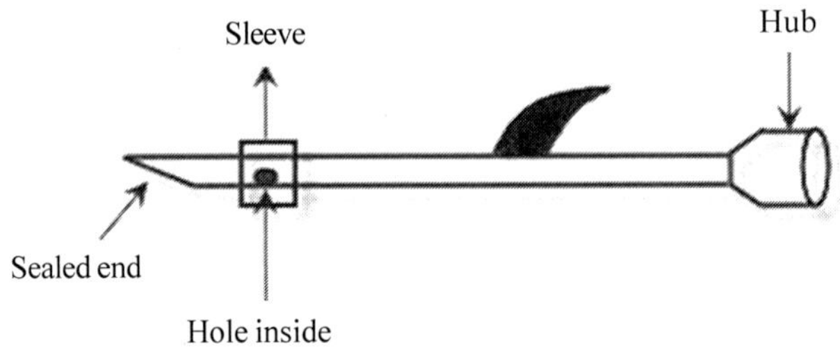

Fig. 5. Barbed needle

a) **Blow-pipe**: Blow-pipe is the commonest dart projector made of PVC or aluminum for darting. The length of blow-pipe tube is generally 1-2 meters. It can propel a plastic dart of maximum of 5 ml capacity to over a short distance of 10 meters.

b) It is mainly used for wild felids and ungulates in captivity. The physiological results of immobilization drugs delivered by dart depend on dosages, the site of darting, success of dart placement and drug delivery in the muscle, as well as the physiological state of the animals prior to and during anaesthetic induction. The key to success in anaesthesia and analgesia in wildlife is being flexible and adapting to changes.

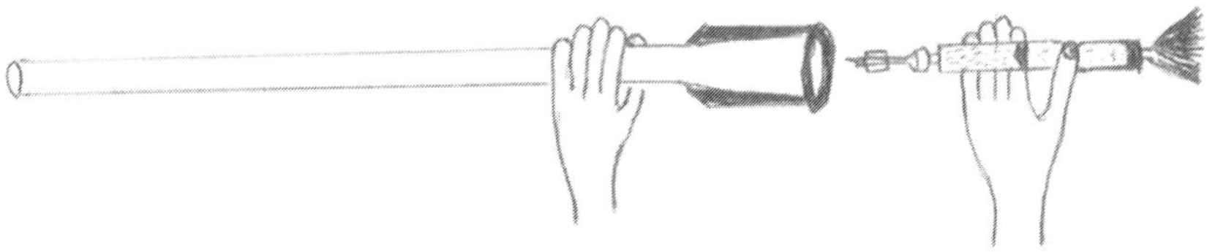

Loading of dart into the blow pipe

Fig. 6. Preparation of blow pipe

c) **Air pressure dart Gun:** It is commercially available as Tel-inject. The dart is similar to a blow-pipe but bigger in size. Some dart guns have interchangeable barrels and depending on the barrel diameter used, darts of 2 ml, 3 ml and 5 ml capacity can be used. There are four models with some variations of the Tel-Inject dart gun available:

   i) **Pistol:** It is the simplest of all the models. Pressure to fire the dart is built up by using either a foot pump or a carbon dioxide cartridge. The pistol has an effective range of 20 to 25 meters, but it does not have an accurate sight. It is recommended for darting animals in pens and at close range.

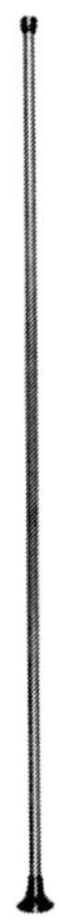

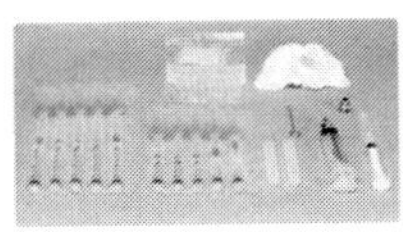

Fig.7. (Blow pipe used for darting and size varies from 1 to 2 meters)

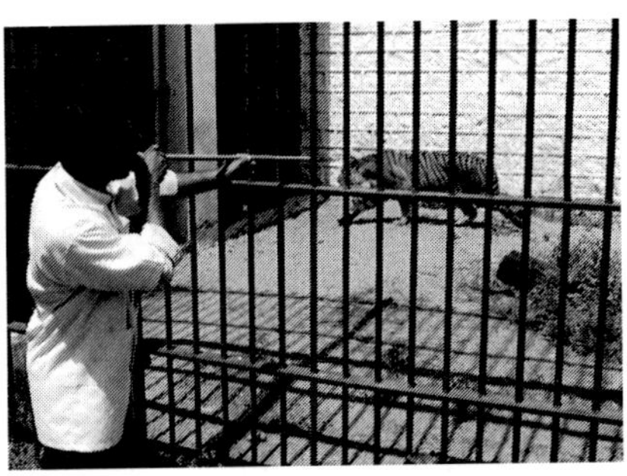

Fig. 8. Darting of a captive Tiger using a blow pipe that covers a range of approximately 5meters: Pic courtesy: CZA

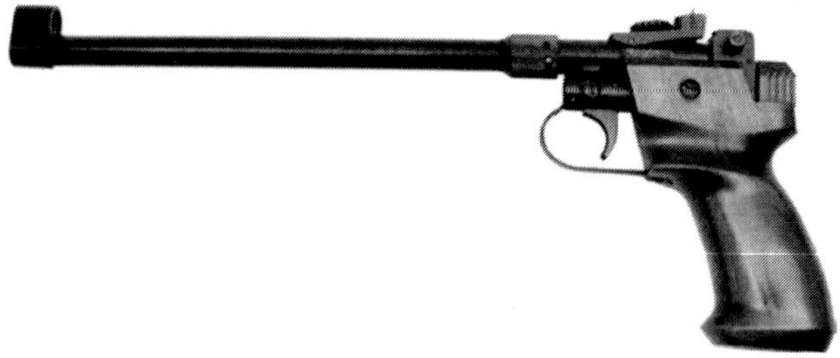

Fig. 9. Pistol for immobilization of wild animal: Photo: Dist-Inject

Cross bow

The cross bow is not much used now a day. Further, it is to be taken note of that the cross bow is not suitable for species under hundred Kg. This may be due to the high impact capacity that may be developed by the projected one.

Types of Projectors

Palmer Cap-Chur equipments or Dist-inject or DAN-inject equipments (or) Teleinject equipments are commonly used to effect the immobilization of multiple species of wild animals, in general.

ii) **Rifle:** This model has a sight with two possible settings for accurate aiming up to 30 meters. Pressure is supplied either by a foot pump or a carbon dioxide cartridge. Another Rifle model is a powerful dart gun having effective range for firing darts over chamber by a 20 ml syringe fitted with a special adapter. The pressure in the rear air chamber is regulated by a blue valve. The pressure can be checked by gently probing the back of the valve with a blunt piece of thin wire that fits into the opening. The needles may be smooth or collared and have a solid, hard tip and two small holes on the sides above the tip. These holes are closed by a plastic cover that slips back when the needle penetrates the skin and muscles of the animal. In this way, the pressurized immobilizing drug is released. The firing mechanism used in Rifle is compressed air or carbon dioxide instead of a powder charge and is therefore silent. The advantage of this silence is that when an animal in a herd is darted, the others are not disturbed by the sound of the shot. The darted animal also does not become panic-stricken and run off because the impact of the dart is not associated with a loud noise. The darts are light and therefore do not damage the muscle tissue and injure the animal. The equipment is accurate at both close and long ranges when suitable allowances are made for wind velocity and direction. With special needles, elephants and rhinoceroses can also be darted. Special needles are available for animals of different sizes.

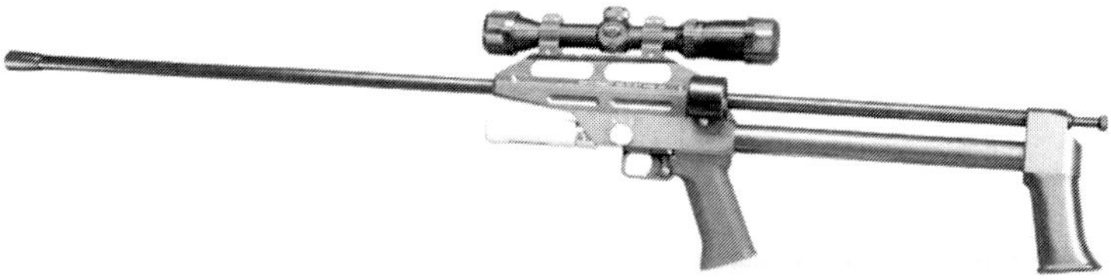

Fig. 10. Rifle for immobilization of wild animals:Photo: Dan-Inject

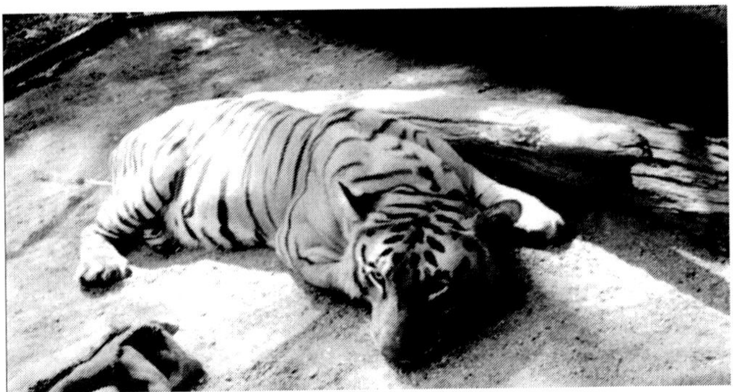

Fig. 11. Captive Tiger was anaesthetized with a combination of ketamine-xylazineusing a dart syringe projected via a Blow-pipe:Photo:Govindaraj Giridharan

Darting Sites: The preferred sites of darting are shoulder and hindquarter. The muscles of the shoulder, the biceps and triceps, are among the best places for remote injection in ungulates. It is better to avoid the upper part of the shoulder because the dart needle may become embedded in the cartilage or scapula.

In skinny and emaciated animals, the hindquarters maybe a preferable site of dartin as the darts may strike the spine of the scapula and result in fracture, hemorrhage or dart blockage. Darting on the shoulder region gives shorter induction in comparision to the darting on the hind quarter. Large herbivores such as elephant, rhinoceros or hippopotamus, have well developed muscles in the withers or hump, which provides a suitable darting site.

In Giraffe or buffalo, the brisket (pectoral area) can be a suitable dart site when no alternative sites are available, but fat portion interferes with the absorption of drug thereby delaying the induction. The well-muscled area is a commonly selected dart site. It is possible to dart most ungulates from any angle into the hind leg but the dart must hit perpendicular to the surface to prevent deflection and to ensure deep IM injection.

The mid-lateral part of the hind leg should be avoided due to the proximity of the femur (and a large bony protuberance, notably in Rhino). Placement of a dart high up on the hind leg from behind and to the side should be avoided as the bony prominences of the pelvis may deflect the dart.

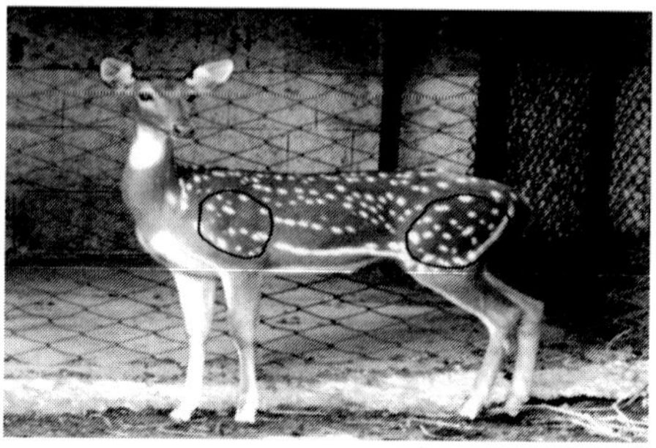

Fig. 12. Preferred areas that are markded on the Axis deer for IM injection by darting ie. the preferred areas are the large muscular region on the hindquarters and shoulder: Photo: Sadanand Sontakke

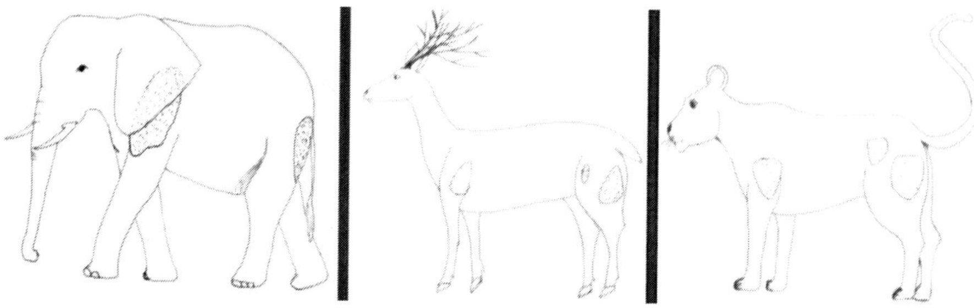

Darting sites in Elephant   Darting sites in Cervid   Darting sites in Felids

Fig. 13. Sites for darting

Table 1: Recommended sizes of dart needles for use in wild animals

Species	**Needle Size (diameter x length in mm)**
Lion, Leopard, Tiger, Cheetah and wild dog	1.5 x 35
Axis deer, Sambar, Nilgai, Eld's deer and barasingha	1.5 x 35
Blackbuck, Chousinga, Chinkara and Barking deer	1.5 x 25
Elephant, rhinoceros and giraffe	3 x 60

Avoid using needles with a narrow bore. Needles with smaller diameters have thinner walls and tend to bend more easily on impact; the pressure within the dart chamber will be greater and the force of injection will be more likely to result in the dart being forced back. The dart contents sprayed into the air may be dangerous to humans so be cautious. Needles fitted with a bulb or a barb on the shaft can be used to prevent the dart from being forced backwards and out of the animal as the drug is injected. Using a barbed needle will help to retain the dart on the animal body for some time but these needles can cause excessive soft-tissue damage as the needle moves up and down in the tissue when the animal is being chased.

Animal immobilization form

Date _______________ Animal Number ___________________________

Name____________ of ___________ Investigator(s) _________________
Species _____________________ Sex: M/F/UN (Tick) ______________
Age _____________ Month ________ Yr ________ (Estimated or Actual)
______________________ Weight ____________kg (Estimated or Actual)
_______________ Purpose/Experiment ___________ of _____________
Capture ________________ Location of Capture ___________________

Ambient Temperature __________ F°/C° Weather Conditions ____________
___________________________ Time _________ Drug Dose (mg or ml)
____________ Method _____________ Location ____________________

Time ________________ Animal ________________________________
Immobilized ________________________Time_______________________

Animal Recovered ____

Vital Signs ____

Time ______________________ Temperature ______________________

Pulse ___________________ Respiration _________________________
Condition of Animal Indicate ____________________ Excellent ________
Good __________ Fair ________ Poor ______ Injuries ________________
or _______ Abnormalities _______________ Noted __________________

____

Samples Taken ____________________________________ Time ________
Type (Indicate Blood, Tissue, Tooth, Etc.) __________________________
Radio Colar Frequency _________________________________ Radio Signal
Checked _______________ Transponder Number ____________________

Transponder Checked _______________________________ Ear ________
Tag _______ Number(s) ________________ and Colour (S) _____________
____________________________ Other Measurement ________________
________________ Body Length ____________________________________
_______________________ CM Tail Length _________________________
____________ CM Shoulder Height ____________ CM ______________

Girth ______________________ CM__________________________________

Comments ____

Signature of Veterinarian

(Adapted from Kreeger *et al*., 2002)

____

28

Chemical Immobilization of Elephants Wild Felids and Ungulates

CHEMICAL IMMOBILIZATION OF ELEPHANTS

Chemical immobilization of elephants needs an understanding of it's special features as a priority. Lungs are adhered to the chest wall by fibrous tissue and there is no pleural space. This fact must be taken into consideration when the elephant is cast or put into positions that may inhibit respiration.The trunk of the elephant is a vital organ. An injured or paralyzed trunk is a serious problem; if it cannot be corrected, the elephant will starve.

Seventy percent of the airflow into the lungs is via the nares in the trunk. At the approximate location where the nares enter the bony skull, there is a sigmoid flexure and a sphincter arrangement that allows the elephant to pull water and dirt up into the nares but prevents inhalation into the lungs. Elephants have highly vascularized ears, which are the major organ of heat regulation. An elephant customarily stands flapping its ears on a warm day. During immobilization the elephant is incapable of moving its ears, and hyperthermia may develop with prolonged restraint when the ambient temperature is high.

Table 1: Sedative and Chemical restraint agents used in elephants

Agent	Asian Elephant			
	Sedation		Immobilization	
	Total dose	mg/kg	Total dose	mg/kg
Acepromazine	10-30	0.004-0.005		
Carfentanil			5-12	0.002-0.004
Etrophine			6-20	0.002-0.004
Xylazine	180-360	0.04-0.08		0.15-0.20
Xylazine/Ketamine				0.12/0.33
Acepromazine	10-30	0.004-0.005		
Butorphanol	25-55	0.01 +/- 0.003		
Carfentanil			3-12	0.002
Etrophine			4-20	0.0015-0.0030
Xylazine	100-640	0.08-0.1		0.15-0.20
Xylazine/Ketamine				0.14/1.14

NOTE

- Free ranging elephants may require a higher dose than a docile captive animal and Asian elephants may require more than comparably sized Africans.
- No inexperienced person should attempt to sedate or immobilize an elephant without prior consultation with experienced veterinarians.
- In a zoo the procedure for immobilizing an elephant should include draining of any pools in the enclosure and chaining the elephant so it does not fall into a moat or empty pool.
- Etorphine hydrochloride (M99) is valuable when it is necessary to obtain complete control of an elephant. It is a marvel of biology that 5mg of a drug given to an elephant weighing 5,000 kg can immobilize it within 15-30 minutes. The dose is 0.0022 mg/kg for the Asian elephant and 0.0017 mg/kg for the African. The dose expressed in different terms would be 1 mg/450 kg in the Asian and 1 mg/600 kg in the African.
- Effects of etorphine will be observed within 10-15 minutes. The trunk hangs limp or loses some of its investigativeness. The animal will start to sway back and forth. Keepers or handlers must stay away from the animal from this point on because the elephant may fall suddenly. Recumbency occurs within 20-30 minutes.
- At the conclusion of the necessary period of immobilization the antidote, diprenorphine (M50-50), is administered intravenously in an ear vein. The dosage is double that of the etorphine. The elephant will begin to investigate with its trunk within 1 - 2 minutes.

CHEMICAL IMMOBILIZATION OF WILD FELIDS & UNGULATES

Immobilization of wild felids is challenging and requires experience and expertise while approaching a wild cat. Wild felids either in captivity or in the wild need to be immobilized for various reasons- for veterinary medication, surgical procedures, blood collection, sterilization, for carrying out assisted reproductive procedures or even capture and translocation of injured animal or man-eater from the wild. Nowadays, due to human-animal conflict, wild leopards are straying in the human premises in search of food thereby creating havoc in the public. Such situations need to be quickly attended by capture of strayed animal using the available anaesthetics.

RECOVERY OF CHEMICAL IMMOBILIZATION IN WILD FELIDS

Uncontrollable recoveries because of prolonged sedation are a serious concern in wildlife research since the sedated free-ranging animals could be easily preyed upon. A few deaths have also been recorded in tigers because of profound respiratory depression following ketamine–xylazine anaesthesia. It is therefore very important to determine a suitable antagonist for the speedy recovery of anaesthetized endangered wild felids. Alpha-two adrenergic antagonists such as yohimbine, tolazoline and atipamezole have been used effectively in ungulates for antagonizing the anaesthetic effects of ketamine–xylazine. Although common in ungulates, there are hardly any reports on reversal of anaesthetic effects by administering suitable antagonists. It has been observed, that yohimbine is an effective reversal of ketamine-xylazine anaesthesia that hastens the recovery of anaesthesia within 5-10 minutes of IV administration of yohimbine.

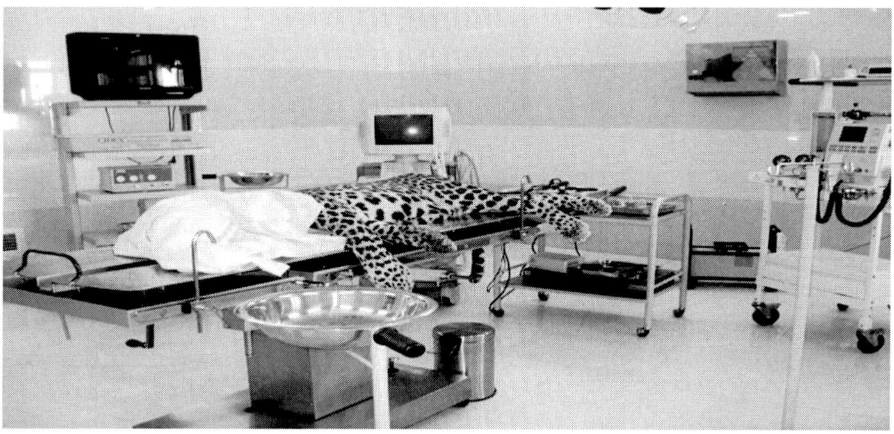

Fig. 1. A State-of-art Operation Theatre at LaCONES equipped with modern instruments required for anaesthesia monitoring in wild animals. An anaesthetized Leopard is seen on the operation table before performing electro-ejaculation procedure

CHEMICAL IMMOBILIZATION OF WILD UNGULATES

Wild ungulates are very nervous and temperamental animals and therefore, chemical immobilization in wild ungulates may be associated with a high percentage of complications and fatalities. Several drugs, such as ketamine hydrochloride, xylazine hydrochloride, tiletamine, zolazepam,and medetomidine, have been routinely used to immobilize a number of wild animals. Of these, ketamine and xylazine are the most commonly used drugs that are readily available in India.

Reversal of anaesthesia in wild ungulates

Wild ungulates are very sensitive and are easily prone to fatalities due to capture shock. Identifying a suitable antagonist for immediate recovery from the effects of chemical immobilization is equally important in wild ungulates so as to avoid hazards of regurgitation, aspiratory pneumonia, and distention of rumen in ungulates. Moreover, it is also important in free-ranging animals to avoid predation in the wild. For more than a decade, the authors from Laboratory for the Conservation of Endangered Species (LaCONES)-CCMB, Hyderabad, have been working on Spotted deer (*Axis axis*) and Blackbuck (*Antelope cervicapra*) as models for critically endangered deer species and antelopes in India to develop various assisted reproductive technologies such as semen collection, ultrasonography for monitoring ovarian follicular response to oestrus synchronization regimes, they have optimized anaesthetic combinations as well as reversals in these species for easy handling and speedy recovery to avoid any distress and effect on their research experiments.

CHEMICAL IMMOBILIZATION OF OTHER LARGE HERBIVORES

Immobilization in Large herbivores such as Elephant (*Elephas maximus*), Rhinoceros (*Rhinoceros unicornis*), Wildbuffalo (*Bubalus arnee*) and Giraffe (*Giraffa camelopardalis*) etc. requires wide experience of handling these animals before undertaking any of these procedures.

Table 2. Chemical Immobilization of large herbivores such as Elephant, Rhinoceros, Giraffe etc. in captivity or in free-ranging conditions.

Species	Drugs	Total Content (mg)	Total volume (ml)	Reference
Elephant Male	Etorphine+Acepromazine	8 - 8.932-35	3.25-3.50	Sale *et al.* (1981) WII Manual
Elephant Female	Etorphine+Acepromazine	8.3-8.08.333-32	3.0-3.25	Sale *et al.* (1981) WII Manual
Rhinoceros	Etorphine+Acepromazine	2.45-4.90*10-20	1.0-2.0	Sale *et al.*(1986) WII Manual
Rhinoceros	Etorphine	1.5-2.5	1.5-2.5	Seal 1976
Wild buffalo	Etorphine+Acepromazine	510	51	Seal 1976
Gaur	Etorphine+Acepromazine	8.0-10.010.0-25.0	8.0-10. 01.0-2.5	Seal 1976
Giraffe	Etorphine	11	11	Snyder *et al.* 1992

DOSE OF CHEMICALLY IMMOBILIZING DRUGS IN HERBIVORES AND CARNIVORES (in mg/kg)

HERBIVORES

Spotted deer (*Cervus axis*)

- Xylazine and ketamine: 6 and 1.2, IM
- Meditomidine and ketamine: 0.05-1.0, IM and 0.8-3.2, IM

Hog deer (*Cervus porcinus*)

- Xylazine and ketamine: 6 and 1.2, IM
- Meditomidine and ketamine: 0.05-1.0, IM and 0.8-3.2 IM

Swamp deer (*Cervus duvaucelli*)

- Etorpine and xylazine: 0.003 and 5-8 mg/animal, IM
- Ketamine and medetomidine: 2 and 0.25, IM

Blackbuck (Antil ope cervicapra)

- Xylazine: 20 mg/ animal, IM

Nilgai (*Boselaphus tragocamelus*)

- Etorpine, acepromazine and xylazine: 0.03, 0.12 and 0.16- 0.23, IM

Barking deer (*Muntiacus muntjac*)

- Xylazine and ketamine: 3 and 2, IM

CARNIVORES

Wolf (*Canis lupus*)

- Xylazine and ketamine: 10 and 2, IM

Himalayan black bear (*Ursus thibetanus*)

- Tiletamine/ zolazepam and medetomidine: 0.5 and 0.01, IM

Sloth bear (*Ursus ursinus*)

- Ketamine and xylazine: 7.5 and 2, IM
- Ketamine and meditomidine: 3 and 0.05, IM

Red panda (*Ailurus fulgens*)

- Ketamine and meditomidine: 5 and 0.1, IM

Civet and binturong

- Ketamine and xylazine: 10 and 1-2, IM

Lion (*Panthera leo persica*)

- Ketamine and xylazine: 04.5 and 1, IM

Tiger *(Panthera tigris)*

- Ketamine and xylazine: 5 and 1, respectively IM

Snow leopard (*Panthera unicia*)

- Ketamine and meditomidine: 2.5-3.0 and 0.06-0.08, IM

Leopard *(Panthera pardus)*

- Ketamine and medltomidine: 3 and 0.07, IM

Small felids (cats)

- Ketamine: 5-10, IM
- Ketamine and xylazine: 3-5 and 0.06-0.08, IM

OTHERS

Macaques and langurs/Leaf monkeys:

- Ketamine and medetomidine: 5-10 and 0.05, IM

  NOTE: The combination of Xylazine and ketamine or even ketamine alone shall be used.

29

Handling of Chemically Immobilized Animals

Once the animal is darted, immobilized animal should be under the expert care of an experienced wildlife veterinarian. The veterinarian needs to monitor the complete immobilization process and should know what to do if something goes wrong. Keep the darted animal in sight and allow the drug to act completely which may generally take 5- 25 minutes depending on the species, sex, drug used, and body condition of animal. Any noise or excitement may cause immobilized animal to wake up or take flight which may make animal search difficult.

Following lateral recumbency, check the animal for pedal and tail reflexes by prodding it lightly with a bamboo stick from the rear. Once confirmed of complete anaesthesia, approach the animal. The dart should be carefully removed from the site of injection, and intra-mammary preparations of antibiotics used for the treatment of mastitis, which can be squeezed into the dart wound to counter infection and the possible formation of an abscess at the dart site. Animal body should also be thoroughly checked for any wound or abrasions that may have occurred during capture procedure and such wounds should be cleaned with antiseptic solution (e.g. povidone solution) and an antibiotic ointment should be applied.

Ruminants (ungulates) always suffer from bloat when immobilized for a long time. Therefore, they must always be rested on their sternum, with their limbs folded under their bodies and their head and neck held higher than their chest to avoid bloat. The head of the animal must be held upright and usually one person is needed just for this task. The mouth must be lower than the rest of the head with tongue kept out of mouth so that any excess saliva can drain away, because the animal cannot swallow when immobilized. Immobilized animals should never be left in the sun for too long. When it is hot, shade should be provided or the animal must be carried to a shady tree. Large animals should be carried on a stretcher.

In cold weather,blankets (or) sacks should be used to cover the body of the animal to prevent it from losing too much heat. Although animals should never be captured in hot weather, this sometimes happens in emergencies. This involves the danger that the immobilized animal may overheat. In such situation, the animal can be sprayed lightly with water to cause evaporation and cooling. Some animals do not close their eyes and cannot blink when they are immobilized. An eye ointment should be applied in the eyes to lubricate them and prevent them from drying out. A dark, soft blindfoldover the eyes must be tied to prevent damage from dust and also the damage to the cornea. Ears shall also be plugged with big cotton rolls to avoid the auditory stimuli. When an immobilized animal is transported over dusty roads, the eyes must also be protected by a blindfold. It is advisable not to make much noise near the immobilized animal as the animals can hear well while they are [immobilized.

As a precautionary measure against secondary bacterial infection, a dose of long-acting (LA) antibiotic such as Teramycin LA or Penicilin LA should be injected subcutaneously or intramuscularly after capture.

PHYSIOLOGICAL MONITORING OF IMMOBILIZED ANIMALS

Monitoring of immobilized animal is essential to determine changes in the physiological variables so as to correct irreversible injury, ensure adequate anesthetic depth, and assess the effectiveness of supportive care, if required. Anesthetic monitoring requires solid understanding of normal and comparative physiology and anatomy, as well as the effects of immobilization and anaesthetic drugs. The techniques used in humans and domestic animals can also be applied to wildlife species. However, more research is necessary to validate the accuracy, sensitivity, and reliability of monitoring equipment in nondomestic species.

The portable monitoring systems (e.g., pulse oximeter, blood gas and electrolyte analyzers) and technology to measure physiological variables offer opportunities to improve monitoring procedures in wild animals. Each anaesthetic event for individual animal should have a permanent record. Minimally, it includes examination and history findings, recent or estimated body weight, drugs used, start and finish of anaesthesia, endotracheal tube size, and problems encountered.

Ideally, the anaesthetic record includes systematic recording of physiological variables throughout the anaesthetic procedure. The frequency of measurement or assessment is determined by the variable. For example, heart rate is assessed around every 5 minutes.

ANAESTHETIC DEPTH

Depth is determined by the drugs, dosage, species, and physiological status. The presence of adequate muscle relaxation does not necessarily imply unconsciousness or analgesia (e.g., muscle relaxants). Corneal reflex and anal tone are usually present at surgical anaesthetic levels. In mammals, eye position often changes with anaesthetic level. This change can be validated as anaesthesia is deepened and lightened. A fixed dilated pupil, unresponsive to light and with no corneal reflex is an indication of excessive anaesthetic depth or brainstem ischemia.

BODY TEMPERATURE

Measurement of body temperature using rectal thermometers is a standard procedure during all anaesthetic episodes. Thermometers made of glass should be avoided as it poses risk of breakage and rectal injury to animal. Digital thermometers are useful if they have a short measurement time. Thermometers should be able to read over a wide temperature range. Hypothermia is common in small animals because of the large surface area-to-volume ratio. Some of the drugs may suppress normal thermoregulatory mechanisms thereby causing hypothermia. On the other hand, hyperthermia is also common immediately after immobilization of both captive and free-living mammals because of excitement and struggling while darting.

DEHYDRATION

Determination of relative hydration is difficult to interpret in wild animals because of the wide range of skin types and pattern in variety of wildlife species. Gently grasping a fold of skin and rolling it between fingers is a more reliable technique. Normally a hydrated skin moves easily, whereas in dehydrated animals, a "sticky" feeling exists. Dehydration also produces dry mucous membranes, sunken eyes, and decreased tear production. In dehydrated animals, the urine production usually decreases and specific gravity of urine is increased.

RESPIRATION

Auscultation of lungs for evaluation of the respiratory system requires a good-quality stethoscope with appropriate head and length of tubing. Usually during anaesthesia, respiratory rates lower down, although it depends on the anaesthetic used.

CARDIAC FUNCTION

The main function of the cardiovascular system is oxygen and nutrient delivery to tissues, and the removal of carbon dioxide and waste (e.g., lactate). Adequate cardiovascular function implies sufficient capillary flow to fulfil these functions. Unfortunately, no reliable, accurate, and effective way to measure capillary flow exists. Although cardiac output can be measured, it is not feasible for routine monitoring in Veterinary practice. Heart rate is an important determinant of cardiac output. Bradycardia and tachycardia needs to be monitored in a systematic manner in the chemically immobilized wild animals of different species.

NOTE: Marked tachycardias, bradycardias, and arrhythmias can decrease blood flow.

PULSE OXIMETRY

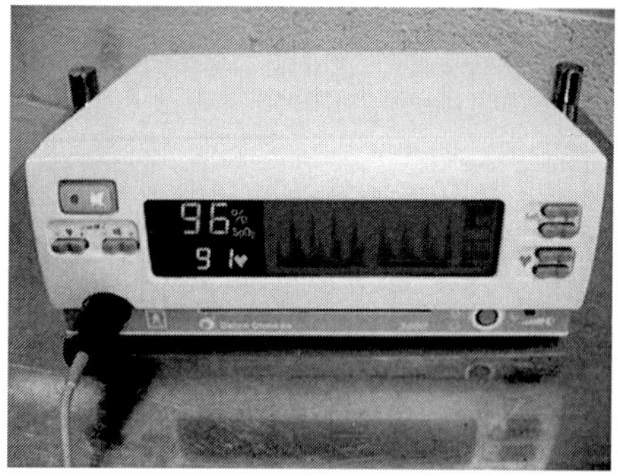

Fig. 1. Pulse oximeter displaying oxygen saturation (SpO_2) in the blood & the pulse rate

Pulse oximetry is indicated for monitoring oxygen saturation (SpO_2) in the blood and for controlling external oxygen administration (Fig. 12). The latter allows for administration of the lowest concentration of inspired oxygen compatible with safe levels of arterial oxygenation. Commercial pulse oximeters also measure pulse rate. Pulse oximeters estimate arterial haemoglobin oxygen saturation by measuring pulsatile signals across (transmission) or by reflectance (reflection) from per fused tissue. Potential sites for placement of transmission pulse oximeter sensors include the ear, tongue, buccal mucosa, paw, vulva and tail. The oxygen saturation range is measured between 0 to 100 % and level below 80 % in the blood in considered as alarming. Accordingly the external oxygen needs to be supplied. Pulse oximeters require adequate plethysmographic pulsations to allow them to distinguish arterial light absorption; therefore, they are inaccurate in the presence of decreased blood pressure, decreased pulse pressure, and vasoconstriction. The presence or absence of a pulse is quickly detected, but the presence of a pulse does not ensure adequate blood flow.

ELECTROCARDIOGRAPHY (ECG) MONITORING

ECG is indicated for routine monitoring of cardiac function and whenever an abnormal pulse or arrhythmia is detected. The ECG monitor for human medicine can also be used for wildlife species. The ECG should have a multichannel oscilloscope with non fade tracing and freeze capabilities. Also, it must be able to record at speeds of 100 mm/s and amplify the signal to at least 1 mV equal to 1 cm. The ECG of mammals resemble each other in general form, with clearly defined P,QRS, and T components. Standard lead positions described in cats and dogs can also be applied for wild animals. To improve signal detection, stainless steel suture is passed through the skin and attached to the electrodes.

SAFETY PRECAUTIONS DURING IMMOBILIZATION

There is always an inherent risk to the animal as well as to the Veterinarian and associates during capture and handling of wild animals. Knowledge on safety and how to deal with accidents is an important part of animal capture. Following precautionary measures need to be taken to prevent drug accidents:

1. Ensure that you are thoroughly trained in the use of capture drugs.
2. Know basic first-aid techniques, including cardiopulmonary resuscitation.
3. Before a capture operation, check your communications and transport infrastructure to ensure that you can respond quickly in an emergency.
4. Use capture drugs only in the presence of a second person who is trained in their use and in the management of accidents.
5. Respect the potency of these drugs-never take chances and never underestimate a potentially dangerous situation.
6. Always concentrate on what you are doing, and work in an orderly fashion.
7. Never eat, drink, smoke, or rub your eyes when working with capture drugs.
8. If you have cuts or abrasions on your hands, put a plaster on the affected area or wear gloves.
9. Be careful never to inhale drugs that are in powder or aerosol form.
10. Never work with opioid drugs in a moving vehicle; exercise extreme care in a helicopter.
11. Never work with opioid drugs without having the human antidote at hand in the first-aid kit or emergency kit.
12. Take extreme care with loaded darts. Carry them in a container. Darts that work with compressed air or gas, or with a spring, should only be armed immediately before use.
13. Always keep basic notes on capture drugs and emergency treatment, as well as emergency telephone numbers, in your drug box, first-aid kit and emergency kit.
14. Sufficient quantities of water should always be available to wash off spilt or splashed drugs.

CAPTURE MYOPATHY

Capture Myopathy is one of the important pathological changes that occur in case of wild animals due to the stress factors during the restraint operation. This condition may affect different species of wild animals that may endanger the life of the wild fauna. Hence, the attending veterinarian needs to understand base line information about the various features pertaining to the capture myopathy.

Clinical signs of capture myopathy

- Stiffness
- Torticollis
- Tremor
- Lameness
- Emaciation
- Hemoglobinuria
- Myoglobinuria
- Cramping of muscles in strange or unnatural positions may be seen in the affected wild animals.
- Death may occur finally if not attended in a proper manner.

Treatment of capture myopathy

- Depending on the clinical status, corticosteroids may be given to combat the inflammatory responses.
- The animals have to be attended with vitamin E injection and Selenium-vitamin E combinations.
- Sodium bicarbonate may be given by means of intra-venous route at rate of fourto six mEq per kg body weight.
- Parenteral B complex vitamins may be provided along with balanced nutrition.
- Corrective measures against the hyperkalemia and the thermo-regulatory derangements.
- Respiratory problems need to be corrected if any.
- The affected wild animal needs to be kept in a place with cool environment.

CONCLUSION

In Zoos, handling of the wild animals is done on a daily basis for performing the various routine health check-up, research purpose for conservation and for the marking of animals for which the safety of the handler/veterinarians and also the prevention of stress to the wild animals during handling is of utmost importance. Therefore, proper management calls for good restraint in wildlife.

30

Visit to Zoo (Zoo Management)

Visiting the zoo should be understood in terms of conservation by all and it is to be remembered that the zoo is a captive wild animal place wherein the public and particularly the children have ample opportunities to see the various species of wild fauna which includes not only the native species of wild mammals, reptiles, aves, amphibians, butterflies etc. but the exotic speciess of wild animals also in general. Similarly, visiting sanctuary i.e. free ranging area helps understanding about the free-ranging wild fauna of the protected wildlife areas.

VISIT TO ZOO

Zoo is the collection of number of wild animals in captivity and is an organized non-profit and stationary institution setup by state governments in majority, local administrations, trustee bodies and registered scientific societies, that own and maintain captive wild animals under the direction of professional staff and provide appropriate care for the purpose of conservation and breeding of different wild animal species especially in endangered wild animals.

In terms of administration, generally the captive wild animal places like zoos or zoological parks or zoological gardens or reptilian centres including the snake parks and the crocodile banks or avian centres are currently managed in India by Director/Curator, Deputy/Assistant Director, Range officer, Forester, Guards and Animal Keepers. Duties of these personnel vary depending on the cadres and the 'Zoo-Director' is overall in-charge of any captive wild animal places, in general.

HISTORY OF ZOOS

The earliest recorded zoological collections associate with cheetah that is currently extinct in India. Emperor Ashoka in third century B.C. respected the ashrams of saints that always had deer and birds. Manageries were the places meant for the collection of animals in earlier periods. Documentations are available about the fight between the lions or tiger and man in a captive state. Even mythical five headed cobra was mentioned in earlier records. Hunting of lions and cheetah and tigers was carried out in large numbers once upon a time.

The earliest recorded zoological collections associate with cheetah that are currently extinct in India. Emperor Ashoka in third century B.C. respected the ashrams of saints that always had deer and birds.

Manageries were the places meant for the collection of animals in earlier periods.

Place and year of starting of Zoo

Vienna zoo	-	1752 (first inception of zoo in the world)
Paris zoo	-	1793
London zoo	-	1826
Philadelphia zoo	-	1874
Calcutta zoo	-	1854 (first inception of zoo in India)
Trivandrum zoo	-	1857

ZOO AND ITS FUNCTION

Zoo is a place where the collection and breeding of wild animals including birds are carried out in a systematic manner under captivity with the permission of appropriate authorities with the functions that are associated with education, captive breeding, basic and applied research, conservation, protection, health care, management and displaying in addition to the recreation.

STAFF PATTERN IN A ZOO-SETUP

- Large zoos have in general more departments and more employees in addition to more number of wild animals and wild animal species, unlike the small or min zoos.
- Administrative set up should be understood well by the zoo veterinarian in order to have the successful implementation of various duties allotted in the captive wild animal places.

ROLE OF DIRECTOR

- Director (or Curator) of the zoo is the executive and a chief person in any zoo. Min job is to expose the activity to everyone, the public, the zoo society and to the government level.
- Management plan is prepared actively by the zoo director about various issues prevailing in the zoos. Master plan is also prepared in a detailed manner.

- Various groups of personnel like range officer, forester, animal keepers, veterinarians, administrative staffs etc. are closely associated with the provision of required inputs for the up keeping of zoo and it becomes a team work with a director as a chief person.
- Deputy Director helps directly the Director of the zoo in the routine management of zoo and Assistant Director assists the Deputy director in this regard.
- Generally both the Deputy Director and Assistant Director are responsible for the public affair and maintenance of the zoo in particular. They assume much of the burden for the day-to-day function of the Director.

ROLE OF RANGE OFFICER

- Range officers look after the wild animals in their range under control. They actively associate with any activities pertaining to the care of wild animals falling in their range.
- Range officers apprise to the higher officials about the welfare measures required for the up keeping of the health status in the wild animals. Administrative activities are being assisted in a systematic manner.

ROLE OF ANIMAL KEEPER

- The animal keepers are entrusted with the cleanliness of cages, enclosures, animal houses, moats, their surroundings including removal of excreta, removing of weeds and bushes.
- They are involved with discouraging of teasing activities by the visiting persons or public. Tigers, lion tailed macaques, hippos, crocodiles, chimpanzees etc. are the frequently teased wild animal species.
- Security of the cages or enclosures are given more priority by these group of personnel and they need to offer assistance during the treatment of wild animals by the zoo veterinarian and it is an accepted one that animal keepers are familiar with the habits and vices of the wild animals that are under direct care in the cages or enclosures.
- They offer information associated with birth, death, abnormality if any like intensive vomiting, diarrhoea etc.
- Reports on any damage to the structure of enclosure or cage are immediately made by these persons to the concerned range officers or other officials when they are visiting the enclosures, cages etc.

- Reports about anorectic wild animals or finding of wound on the wild animals body or any kind of visible sickness condition is immediately reported to the veterinarian in particular.
- They generally ensure that no materials remain in the animals vicinity that are likely to hurt the wild animal maintained under captive conditions like wire bits, mesh, ropes, plastic materials, sharp pieces, nails etc.

CLASSIFICATION OF ZOOS IN GENERAL

Zoos are classified into 4 types

Category	Large zoo	Medium zoo	Small zoo	Mini zoo
Area in Hectares	>75	50-75	20-50	<20
No.of animals exhibited	>750	500-750	200-499	200
No. of species exhibited	>75	50-75	20-49	20
No.of endangered species exhibited	>15	10-15	5-9	>5

OBJECTIVES OF MODERN ZOOS

Zoo has got multiple functions that basically associate with the health care and management of the captive wild animals.

Significant ones are given below:

1. Education
2. Captive breeding
3. Research
4. Recreation

1. Education

The purposes of education are linked to the followings-

i) Knowledge dissemination of wild animals and their conservation to persons visiting the zoos or zoological parks or zoological gardens.

ii) Acting as a central area for the purpose of dissemination of the biological information and evolving of educational programme for visitors, school/biology teachers and students in order to create awareness for the wildlife conservation. The common persons who visit the zoos start asking many questions subsequent to the sighting of the concerned wild animal species.

2. Captive Breeding

Imbalance in eco-system occurs due to the following reasons:

i) Poaching and hunting.

ii) Death due to diseases.

iii) Death due to poisoning.

iv) Death due to natural hazards like earth quakes.

v) Habitat destruction due to multiple reasons (natural and man-made)

Hence, the wild animal species may become extinct in the course of time and it is a fact that many species of wild animals are in the stage of extinction if the management does not have a scientific type of management features. Hence, captive breeding becomes one of the important objectives in case of zoos. It is often becoming a mandatory one for the captive wild animal places like zoos to have both male and female wild animals of the particular wild animal species under threat. Such a type of management under *ex-situ* conditions helps for the prevention of number of wild animals of particular species in an area.

Conservation efforts are directed mostly in that direction to protect the wild animals that belong to various species. Hence, zoos, zoological parks and zoological gardens become the better places for the captive breeding of the selected species of wild animals for which the available infrastructures are being utilized.

3. Research

Both the basic and applied research features are required for an effective conservation of wild animals. Research areas comprise microbiology, pathology, physiology, clinical sectors, nutrition, ethology, genetics, biotechnology, reproduction, meat hygiene, anatomy etc.

Such research features may be of more helpful in the health and disease management of wild animals in both captive and free ranging regions. Awareness is being created among the common public about the conservation and the value of wildlife protection and value of individual wild animal species.

4. Recreation

Aged persons, children, common man, disabled persons and others visiting the zoos get attracted to the sighting of various species of wild fauna in one place. Wild animals in the zoos often comprise both the exotic and natural wild animal species. Particularly visiting the zoo is a full day recreational activity to the younger group of people and children in particular.

CENTRAL ZOO AUTHORITY OF INDIA (CZA)

Seeing the mushroom growth of many unplanned zoos in India, in order to have a better control and assessment of the conditions suitable for the living of the confined wild animals, all the zoos were brought accordingly under the purview of the WILDLIFE PROTECTION ACT, 1972, the Central Zoo Authority of India was set up, later and it helps in overseeing the management of zoos in India. Central Zoo Authority of India came into existence in February, 1992.

This organization grants recognition to various zoos maintained in the country, keeping due regards to the norms and standards codified time to time and it often associated with the setting up of minimum standard for the upkeep and the management of zoos.

ROLE OF VETERINARIAN IN THE ZOO

The role of the veterinarian in the zoo is of utmost importance as the veterinarian's plays a major role in the health and disease management of the wild animals in the zoo. Technical suggestions need to be offered with regard to the management of health and diseases in case of the captive wild animals belonging to various species. Veterinarians in the zoos have multitasks in general.

HEALTHCARE OF NEWLY ARRIVED WILD ANIMALS

The newly arrived wild animals has to be properly taken care of by taking the wild animal in a safe manner to the quarantine unit and the related health care measures may be carried out in a planned manner. Clinical observation, sampling etc. may be carried out depending on the wild animal species under investigation.

PROPHYLAXIS, THERAPY AND POSTMORTEM

Prevention is given much emphasis in addition to the treatment of the sick wild animals.

For prophylaxis the following measures are undertaken in a zoo periodically-

1. Vaccination of wild animals.
2. Periodical examination of wild animals has to be carried out in a systematic manner in order to find out any disease in the beginning stage itself.
3. Surgeries have to be performed whenever required as the case with infighting incidences or breeding programmes.
4. Subsequent to the diagnosis of the case, suitable therapy is to be carried out in a systematic manner.
5. Regular deworming of the animals.

6. When animals die due to diseases or other reasons, post-mortem has to be carried out in a systematic manner. Post mortem is one of the important components that is to be taken with more care and cautions. Veterinarians involving post mortem of wild animals should take care of the features related to the Zoonotic diseases in particular like anthrax or salmonellosis.
7. Meat inspection:Spoiled feeds if found may be discarded. The meat received needs to be inspected in a systematic manner and the diseased ones if any have to be discarded.

Any nodular growths or worms affected regions may be discarded. Fish also needs to be inspected for the healthy status. Rotten fish if any has to be immediately discarded.

TRANSLOCATION AND TECHNICAL ASSISTANCE TO THE ZOO PERSONNEL:

- If any animal is to be translocated, immobilization is to be carried out and safety of the wild animal under immobilization has to be ensured always to the possible extent.
- Whenever any technical assistance is required, it has to be offered in a systematic manner with regard to the translocation.
- Care has to be taken to avoid any type of wound or injury to the wild animal under transport during the translocation and similarly safety measures have to be carried out with regard to the immobilization.

STUD BOOK IN ZOO

The stud book for the significant species needs to be maintained in zoos.

For example, the stud book for Asiatic lion should contain the following details:

1. Name of the enclosure
2. House name and number
3. National Stud book number
4. International Stud book number
5. Sex
6. Sire (National Stud book number)
7. Dam (National Stud book number)
8. Date of birth
9. Since when Date of death

10. Any other mode of disposal
11. Remarks if any (Details, if rescued or transferred).

DISPLAY OF WILD ANIMALS IN ZOOS

Wild animals are displayed (Fig. 1) in an informative manner to the visiting persons or public and followings are undertaken in general for the display of wild animals in zoo set up:

1. Taxonomic arrangement (Non-human primates as first unit).
2. Zoo geographical arrangement (wild animals of India and Australia or other country).
3. Ethological arrangement (Common langurs and Chital in a group).
4. Mixed species-exhibits (eg. Spotted deer and black bucks).
5. Ecological arrangement (Common animals of desert system).
6. Miscellaneous arrangement.

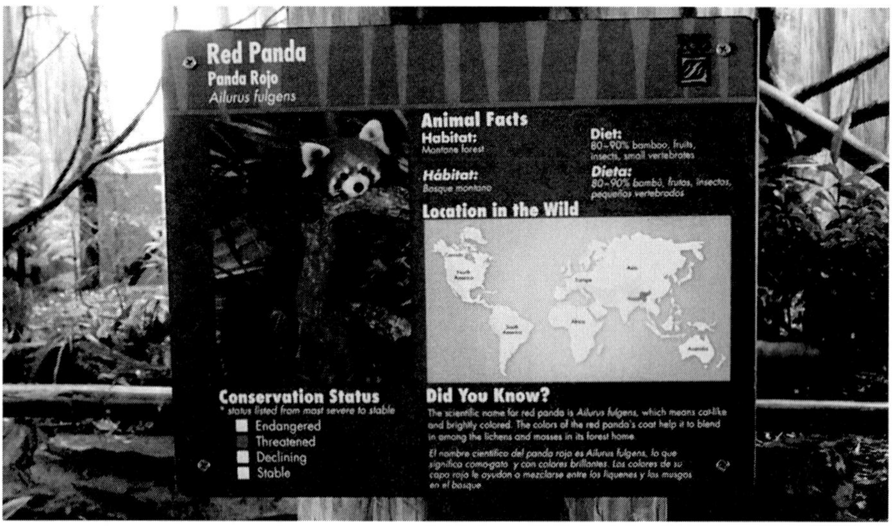

Fig. 1. Display board in a zoo enclosure

COMMON WILD ANIMALS IN INDIAN ZOOS

1. *Commonly held carnivores*: Lion, tiger, panther, jungle cat, hyena, jackals, wild dog, otter, fox, wolf, jaguar etc.
2. *Other wild animals*: Gaur, wild pig, nilgai, spotted deer, sambar deer, porcupine, sloth bear, giant squirrels, zebra, Indian pangolin, hog badger, kangaroo, rhinoceros, giraffe etc.

3. *Reptiles*: Cobra, king cobra, Russels Viper, rat snake, green snake, krait, reticulated python, rock python, monitor lizard, Indian soft shelled turtle, mugger, gharial, salt water crocodile, alligators, caimans etc.
4. *Aviary species*: Peacocks, cockatoo, cockatiel, African grey parrot, grey horn bills, rosy pelicans, painted storks, budgerigars, love birds, swan, sarus crane, egrets, born owls, vultures, kites, shikara etc.

ZOO VETERINARY HOSPITAL

Central zoo authority of India has prescribed number of veterinarians required for various types of zoos and the type of zoo helps to determine the number of veterinarians in this case. However, it is understood that health and disease management in the zoological park is most significant one to be maintained successfully for the welfare of the confined wild animals in the zoos.

Basic requisites of zoo veterinary hospital

1. Squeeze cages
2. Trap cages
3. Immobilization related gadgets
4. Drugs (All types including immobilization and treatment related ones including the prophylactic ones)
5. Clinical laboratory
6. Post-mortem room
7. X-ray unit
8. Modern Diagnostic equipments
9. Antivenin
10. Antiseptics and disinfectants
11. Coveralls, gloves, specimen-containers, sample-containers etc.

VETERINARY MEDICAL RECORD SYSTEM IN ZOOS

The different diseases occurring in various wild animals belonging to multiple species are to be documented in a proper form.

1. Post mortem records should be maintained in a proper manner. Similar is the case with treatment register.
2. Reference books that are required in the routine day to day therapy of wild animals should be available in the zoo.

3. Different terms for males, females and young ones of various wild fauna need to be well known to veterinarians working in various zoological parks, zoos and zoological gardens.

QUARANTINE UNIT

Procedure in which the newly arrived animals into the zoo are kept in confinement in a separate place for a specified length of time-

1. Each zoo should have the housing and isolation capabilities separately in order to truly quarantine the animals. It is better that the place of quarantine should be away from the zoological park or zoological garden or the zoo.
2. The quarantine period may be extended depending on the clinical assessment by the attending veterinarian if there is a requirement for that, technically.

IMPORTANCE OF QUARANTINE

1. To prevent the entry of the disease-causing pathogens into the zoo.
2. Detection of disease causing pathogens
3. Introduction of Zoonotic diseases in particular is highly avoided or minimized

QUARANTINE PERIOD

The quarantine period may be a varying one depending on the concerned wild animal species. In general a minimum of 30 days period is required for the quarantine of various species of mammals.

However, if any new member of same species is added in this period, from that day of addition, again a period of 30 days may be counted. Similar protocols may be adapted for reptiles, amphibians and fish also.

ACCESS TO QUARANTINE UNIT

Following persons are the only personnel to enter the quarantine unit:

1. Veterinarians of the zoo.
2. Staff members responsible for the animals in the quarantine unit.
3. Other persons who are specified to enter the quarantine unit by the authorities.

STRESS AND THE QUARANTINE ACTIVITIES

Stress is a major factor in case of wild animals in general. It is to be understood that isolation of a social animal from all co specifics for the purpose of quarantine may be a psychologically stressful event. Hence, the stress causing factors need to be minimized to a greater extent. Vaccination may be considered whenever required.

ISOLATION UNIT

This unit is meant for the confinement of wild animals that are found to be affected by any infectious diseases that may affect other co-exhibits or nearby wild animals of the same group or the wild animals of another species in a zoological park-environment. This actually helps to contain the disease and hence, the possible spread of the disease is highly prevented to a greater extent. Subsequent to the isolation, the wild animals kept in the isolation unit have to be treated appropriately and the health condition has to be ensured.

31

Visit to Wildlife Sanctuary (Management in Free Ranging Wildlife Region)

WILDLIFE SANCTUARY

Wildlife Sanctuary is a natural habitat, owned by the government or private agency, that safeguards particular species of birds and animals to make sure that viable population of the wildlife and their habitats are maintained.

Conservation methodologies, to be meaningful can associate the following two forms:

1. *In-situ* conservation: in forests (mainly the National Park and Wildlife Sanctuary)
2. *Ex-situ* conservation: in captive wild animal places (zoo, zoological park zoologicalgarden, captive reptilian centres, captive aviary centres etc.)

IN-SITU CONSERVATION

This type of conservation includes conservation of plant and animals in their native ecosystem or in man made ecosystem where they naturally occur. This type of conservation is applied only to wild flora and fauna and not to the domesticated animals and plants, because conservation is achieved by the protection of population in nature. It mainly aims at preservation of lend races with wild relatives in which genetic diversity exists and/or in which the weedy/ wild forms present hybrids with related cultivars. In-situ conservation includes a system of protected areas of different categories e.g., National park, Sanctuaries, Biosphere Reserves, cultural landscapes, National monument. The *in-situ* conservation of habitats has received high priority in the world conservation strategy programmes. Launched since 1980. Institutional arrangements, especially in countries of the developing world, have been emphasized.

NATIONAL PARKS

A national park is an area, whether within a sanctuary or not, by reason of its ecological, faunal, floral, geomorphological, or zoological association or importance, needed to for the purpose of protecting & propagating or developing wildlife therein or its environment and where no human activity is permitted.

At present, as quoted in the web-site of Ministry of Environment and Forests in India, currently, India has a network of 700 Protected Areas (103 National Parks, 528 Wildlife Sanctuaries, 65 Conservation Reserves and 4 Community Reserves).

Table 1: Difference between National Park and Wildlife Sanctuary

Basis for comparison	Wildlife sanctuary	National park
Meaning	Wildlife Sanctuary is a natural habitat, owned by the government or private agency that safeguards particular species of birds and animals.	National park is the protected areas, which are established by the government, to conserve wildlife and also develop them.
Preserves	Animals, birds, insects, reptiles, etc.	Flora, fauna, landscape, historic objects, etc.
Objective	To make sure that viable population of the wildlife and their habitats are maintained.	To protect the natural and historic objects and wildlife of an area.
Restriction	Restrictions are less and it is open to public.	Highly restricted, random access to people is not allowed.
Official Permission	Not required	Required
Boundaries	Not fixed	Fixed by legislation
Human activity	Allowed but up to a certain extent.	Not allowed at all

NATURAL RESERVES

Various natural reserves existing in the wildlife regions provide the complete protection for the wild animals belonging to the different species.Many times, human interventions are made for positive purposes in order to give more protection to the wild fauna and flora. It is to be understood that various natural reserves hardly comprise one percent of the earth s land areas.

Most of the other areas are used for production of food, timber, pulpwood or other raw materials. Hence, in all these areas, wildlife conservation related measures need to be strengthened and if necessary, human intervention (Broader land use strategy) may be made in order to enrich the protective measures for the welfare of wild fauna and flora.

BIOMES AND ECOLOGICAL EQUIVALENTS

Major global units of flora and fauna are termed as biomes.With regard to the ecological equivalents, the wild animals in one region may differ from their taxonomic classification but taps particular environmental resources within the ecosystem.

WETLAND HABITATS AND THE AVIARY SPECIES

Wetlands have the concerned wetland aviary species that have specialized legs and the legs are equipped with webs that help or facilitating for the better movement on mud or water logged surfaces. The beaks vary in size and shape, so as to catch the prey species (mostly the fish) from water.

BIOSPHERE RESERVES

Biosphere Reserves is undisturbed natural area, is dedicated to conservation of biological diversity and genetic integrity of plants, animals and microorganism in their totality as well as scientific study. A protected area that can be declared as a biosphere should satisfy the following essential criteria:

1. Should provide a network of protected terrestrial and coastal environments which form a coherent system on a world scale.
2. Should occur in each of the 193 biogeographical provinces of the world distinguished in the classification of Udvardy (1975), so as to exhibit the maximum genetic diversity.
3. Should show a complete range of the different types of human interference, from ecosystems untouched to those which have been degraded by humans.
4. Structure and size should ensure the efficient conservation of the desired ecosystems.
5. Should have sufficient resources available for ecological education, training and research to be carried on in respect to conservation of nature.
6. If possible, should have geographical continuity with other types of protected areas.
7. Should have adequate long-term legal protection.

SPECIFIC WILD ANIMALS (LOCATION)

- Slender loris (Tamilnadu)
- Slow loris (North-eastern India)
- Red Panda and Binturong (Eastern regions)

- *Hyalobates hoolock* (Arunachal Pradesh and Assam)
- Pig tailed macaque and Assam macaque and Leaf monkey (or) capped langur (Assam).

Globally Habitat is classified as followings:

1. Polar region
2. Deciduous forest
3. Coniferous forest
4. Evergreen forest
5. Grassland
6. Mediterranean scrub
7. Desert
8. Tropical rain forest
9. Mountains
10. Oceans

Table 2: Biographical classification of India

	Regions	Percentage
1.	Trans-Himalaya	5.6
2.	Himalaya	6.4
3.	Desert	6.6
4.	Semiarid	16.6
5.	Western Ghats	4.0
6.	Deccan Peninsula	42.0
7.	Gangetic Plain	10.8
8.	Coasts	2.5
9.	North East	5.2
10.	Islands	0.3

COMPONENTS OF WILDLIFE HABITAT

The components of wildlife habitat may be multiple. However, for the purpose of understanding, major zones are given below:

- Food
- Cover
- Water
- Space

Role of wildlife veterinarians in disease management at wildlife sanctuary, national park, and other forest regions

Ring vaccination: Domestic animals around protected wildlife regions (within 5 kms from border of forests) need to be protected by vaccination against FMD, HS, Anthrax etc.

Selective removal of diseased animals: Immobilize esp. high valued animals like lion, tiger, elephant etc. and treat them and release in wild later

Selective removal of carcases: Diseased wild animals if found dead are to be isolated and dead animals need to be removed for scientific disposal of the carcases and have to be probed for the existence of disease0-causing pathogens.

Reduction in population density: As per the policy changes of forest department, reduction of population shall be carried out. Higher the density, more favourable is the condition for the disease to take epizootic form.

Immunization of wild animals: High conservation-valued animals need to be taken care of during disease-outbreak.In many countries, by helicopter, immunizations are carried out against infectious diseases like anthrax etc. by remote drug-delivery equipments.

Control of vectors in disease outbreaks, as with fasciolosis: Bush control, removal of vector populations like snails etc. shall be carried out if need arises. Mosquitoe proof measures shall be thought of in cases of severe outbreaks of malaria in and around the forest regions.

Transporting of the wild animals: Any wild animal kept for a long time under captivity due to disease or disorders shall be sent to zoos nearby by engaging transport techniques.

Restraint of problematical animals (public problems related ones): Capture of rogue elephants or wild animals associated with the human-wildlife conflicts shall be captured by either physical or chemical restraint measures.

Eliminating the causal agent: Place barriers against the infected water source and discourage other wild animals to approach the infected water source eg) Botulism cases. Population approach shall be carried out for treatment of diseases. If the disease becomes alarming one, baits shall be used for mixing with appropriate drugs like dewormers and orient toward the targeted wild animal species of that region.

Immobilization for sending of wild animals to zoological parks as founder population: Subsequent to the request by forest department, selected wild animal species shall be immobilized and may be transported to the zoological parks or zoos or zoological gardens as per the demand and requirements for establishment of founder populations in captivity.

Animal dispersal methods: Animals need to be dispersed from the infected regions or areas or ponds or lakes by using firecrackers, smoke-generating machines, gunshot sounds, human voice amplified by a public address sound system etc.

Assistance in research: Scientists associated with research in specific wildlife species need to be assisted subsequent to the permission from the concerned state forest department by either physical or chemical immobilization of wild animals eg) Capture of elephant or tiger for radio-collaring purposes etc.

Periodical sampling of wild animals: To assess health status, random examination of wild animal species need to be carried out like assessment of important prey animal species like wild pigs, non-human primates etc. in tiger regesrve areas and this will help in enhancement of wildlife healh esp. for the predators like tigers.

Random examination of wild animals like elephants shall be undertaken to have technical information on health and disease management measures needed for those species.

Post-mortem examinations: When kills are encountered or when immobilizations are carried out for administrative or technical purposes, samples need to be taken with documentations to throw more light on diseases and disease-causing pathogens in free-ranging wildlife regions.

Engagement in awareness-creating measures: Tourists or public visiting wildlife regions or children in and around forest regions in particular need to be provided awareness related programmes to understand about the wild animals and the importance of conserving wild fauna of the designated regions.

PERMISSIONS REQUIRED FOR INTERNATIONAL TRANSPORT OF ANIMALS

India is a signatory to the Convention on International Trade in Endangered Species (CITES), and any international transport of wild animals is governed by this convention. The Director-Wildlife Preservation, Government of India, is the nodal officer for CITES permits, and the country is divided into four regions: The Northern Region consists of the states of Uttar Pradesh, Punjab, Haryana, Himachal Pradesh, Jammu & Kashmir and Rajasthan and the union territory of Delhi and Chandigarh; the Eastern Region consists of the states of Bengal, Bihar, Assam, Arunachal Pradesh, Sikkim, Mizoram, Nagaland, Orissa, Tripura, Meghalaya and Manipur; the Southern Region consists of the states of Tamil Nadu,Andhra Pradesh,Kerala and Karnataka and the union territories of the Andaman & Nicobar Islands, the Lakshadweep Islands and Pondicherry; and the Western Region consists of the states of Gujarat, Madhya Pradesh,

Chattisgarh and Goa and the union territories of Daman & Diu and Dadra & Nagar Haveli.

The Regional Deputy Director (Wildlife Preservation) can be contacted for obtaining the mandatory CITES permits for international transport of wild animals. Once a CITES permit has been obtained, permission may be obtained from the Director General of Foreign Trade for international transport of wild animals.

CRATE-SIZES FOR DIFFERENT SPECIES OF WILD ANIMALS (Length, Breadth and width of crates).

Tiger/lion: 195 x 75 X 105cm

Bear: LBW: 180 X 75 X 100 cm

Leopard and Jaguar: 120 X 60 X 90 cm

Crocodile/ alligator/ gharial: 195 X 60 X 40 cm (Small sizes are preferred).

Python: 75 X 90 X 45 cm (Handles on both sides to carry the crate)

Cobra (or) other snakes: 60 X 75 X 30 cm (Handles on both sides to carry the crate)

Munia/ budgerigar: 75 X 75 X 22.5 cm (Sufficient for 2-25 munias); wire mesh size 150 mm x 600 mm

Kite/ Shikra: 60 X 45 X 45 cm (For one bird; perch at 50 mm, should have enough space to turn around); wire mesh size: 150 mm x 600 mm

Pheasants: 60 X 45 X 60 (For one bird; if the tail is long, the length may be increased accordingly. Wire mesh size 100 mm x 600 mm)

Emu and cassowary: 75 X 60 X 150 cm

Small birds: 75 X 75 X 25 cm (Sufficient for 10 parrots)

SIGNIFICANT SPECIES-SPECIFIC CONSIDERATIONS FOR TRANSPORT

A. Deer species

- The maximum number of animals that may be transported at a time is four or five.
- With smaller species, two females may be transported in a crate; with larger species, only one female may be transported in each crate. However, it is preferable to transport only one animal in a crate.
- As per the need both the sexes can be transported in separate crates.

B. Carnivores

- Preferably only one animal should be transported in each crate/ container. When more than one animal must be transported in a crate, it is preferable to have animals from the same enclosure or those that have lived together.
- Males need to be transported separately in individual crates.

C. Primates

- Up to four animals may be transported together at a time.
- With larger primates, only one animal may be transported in a crate.

D. Birds

- Storks, cranes, ratites and raptors should be transported individually.
- Parakeets may be transported in pairs in boxes.
- Ducks, teals, geese, pigeons, bulbuls, galliforms (females), corvids, sparrows and other finches may be transported in groups.

E. Reptiles

- Crocodiles should always be transported singly.
- Turtles and tortoises: Large animals should be transported singly; smallones may be transported in groups.
- King cobras, cobras, pythons and other cannibalistic snakes must always be transported individually in crates/boxes with locks and signage marked "danger/handle with care - venomous snake".
- When reptiles suchas crocodiles,chelonians,snakes and lizards are to be transported/released, check for evidence of any injury, metabolic bone disease, ecto-parasites, stomatitis, scale-rot, dysecdysis, bloat, retained eye caps, swollen eyes or abnormal discharges from the eyes, nostrils, mouth, etc.

In the case of crocodiles, the teeth should be clean and white, not brittle or translucent. Similary, any accumulation of algae on teeth may often reflect lack of feeding in crocodiles. Fasting prior to physical capture appears to be desirable in reptiles. Transport boxes or container should be of adequate width and depth to prevent chelonians from climbing and damaging their shells.

Snake bags need to be tied firmly to prevent escapes. Boxes should be locked. Reptiles are very susceptible to dehydration during transportation and require to be provided water.

Moist gunny bags have proven to be useful when transporting large numbers of young crocodiles (total body length less than 1.5 m) over short distances (200-250 km or 5-6 hours).

32

Drug Delivery in Zoo and Wild Animals

The ability to inject a drug into a free ranging animal using a remote injection system is a main stay of zoo and wild life medicine and the accepted and routine procedures of today for anesthetizing free ranging, dangerous, or hyper excitable animals are to be well understood for the proper preventive medical procedures, medical treatment, surgery, or scientific study. However, all these were earlier existing only as a dream, until remote injection-based gadgets like darts, blow pipes and distant drug-delivery gadgets like pistol and rifle were duly developed, in conjunction with safer injectable anesthetics. Such developments in addition to the laser or sensor aided technologies in the distant drug-delivery gadgets have further greatly facilitated the systematic medical care of zoo and free-ranging wild animals and has provided investigators with access to many different free-ranging species for field studies.

DRUG DELIVERY SYSTEMS

Drugs can be delivered or administered by different routes:

1. Oral

Baiting of animals can be resorted to in certain conditions. Prebaiting to remove the bait-shyness is important. Strong smell, colour and, taste of the chemical may mar successful baiting.

2. Parenteral

a) Remote Injection and Drug Immobilisation: Parenteral administration of drugs using a hypodermic needle is an old practice. Giving an I/M injection, let alone i/v route, is a problem faced by veterinarians who are dealing with fractious domestic animals and still worse with wild animals in their free ranging conditions.

b) Pole Syringe (Jab Stick): This is a device that comes in handy for animals in cage or animals that can be approached in close quarters without any risk, like deer. This is a modified syringe with the piston that is extended with a rod. This rod can be held in the hand and jabbed on to a muscular region, the barrel of the syringe is housed in a tube with a window to see the volume of the drug present and push out the air if, present. The handle that acts as an extension of the piston helps to push in the drug when jabbed or prodded.

c) Projectors

i) Blowpipe: Usually this is a plastic tube with smoothened inside. A mouthpiece may be attached to one end for the ease of blowing. Plastic syringes up to a capacity of 3-5 ml can be darted to a distance of 3-5 meters ordinarily.

ii) Blowgun: Blowgun with an extension to blowpipe is used for long ranges. A foot pump with a pressure gauge is used. Because of the unwieldy size it is not very popular.

iii) Crossbow: This is more of a sports weapon than a professional gadget. However a quantity of 3 ml can be injected by the inertia developed by the arrow shaft. Attachments to cross bows with explosive capsule syringes are available. The weapon is very powerful and should be used with caution in small animals. Crossbow is very inconvenient in the field with heavy under growth and cannot easily be concealed from the target animal.

iv) Shotguns/Rifles/Pistols: Depending on the range to which the syringe is to be projected, it could be a simple air gun with a break open principle. Carbon dioxide cylinders or $N0_2$ is used. Maximum range can be attained by using blank powder cartridges. However an effective range more than 60 metres is difficult to achieve. Even this is done by a parabolic trajectory.

Depending upon the power of the blanks (0.22) it is called as "very low", "low", "medium", and "high". Some manufacturers prefer to designate by the colour of the charge as red, black, orange and yellow.

Some rifles have an adjustable rear sight to enable to get an accurate trajectory. Certain models use the same powder cartridge but increasing or decreasing the explosive chamber by turning a knurled knob regulates power.

v) Projectiles (Darts or Syringes): Once the dart syringe hits the animal the needle penetrates. The injection of the drug is effected by pressurizing the rear side by the air, butane, LPG or by generation of carbon dioxide (citric acid + soda bicarb with water). A quick injection is achieved by using a cartridge that will explode when the dart syringe hits the animal. This is the most commonly used technique and is very convenient in the field conditions, especially for large animals. The syringe after the impact must deliver the drug intramuscularly. The plunger activation can also be achieved by a pressurized chamber behind the piston or by an impact detonating mechanism otherwise called as the explosive capsule. The plunger can be pushed forward by (a) compressed air pumped from behind the plunger, (b) generation of carbon dioxide by mixing an acid with an alkali or (c) a spring held in compression. For these types of plunger activation, the tip of the needle is closed and holes drilled on the side.

A sleeve is put and this slides back when the needle penetrates the muscle making the hole patent facilitating the injection of the drug. The needles are provided with collars or barbs to ensure attachment to the animal that assists in following it prior to its falling down. The needle to be used on elephants and rhinos are to be reinforced to avoid the breakage on impact and provided with holes on the sides. In general the pressurized syringe mechanisms are more suitable for small and thin-skinned animals, while the explosive types are used for thick skinned large animals.

IDEAL DRUG DELIVERY

Characteristics of an ideal drug delivery system are listed below:

1. Capable of delivering large quantities of the drug.
2. Effective over a wide range.
3. Accurate.
4. Simple in design, easy to handle and reliable for field use.
5. Safe.
6. Minimum damage for the animal.
7. Re-usable syringe and darts.
8. Sterilizable.
9. Inexpensive.

CLASSIFICATION OF DRUGS USED

1. Peripherally acting drugs.

a) Paralysing agent e.g., Nicotine.

b) Muscle relaxants e.g., Curare, Gallamine, Succinyl choline.

2. Centrally acting drugs

a) Opiates e.g., Morphine, Etorphine, Fentanyl, Carfentanyl, Surlentanyl.

b) Sedatives.

- Phenothiazines e.g., Acepromazine.
- Butyrophenones e.g., Azaperone, Haloperidol, Droperidol.
- Benzodiazepine e.g., Diazepam, Midazolam.

c) Dissociative anaesthetics

- Cyclohexamines e.g., Ketamine, Tiletamine (used with zolazepam), Phencyclidine (now discontinued).
- Xylazine.
- Meditomidine, Ditomidine.

3. Adjunct drugs

a) Hyaluronidase.

b) Atropine sulphate.

4. Reversing drugs

a) Alpha blockers: Yohimbine, Tolazoline, Phentolamine, Atipamezole.

b) Opium antagonists: Diprenorphine, Levallorphan, Nalaoxone, Naltrexone, Nalmefene.

5. Supportive drugs

a) Eye ointments

b) Antibiotics

c) Steroids

d) Fluids

e) Stimulants

f) Vitamins.

Paralysing agent

Nicotine is an alkaloid only of historical importance in present day wildlife haracterized. However, several tamed Asian elephants, which became uncontrollable due to musth were haracterized with nicotine. The initial stimulation, which is noticed in other animals, is not observed in elephants. Quick onset and predictable results in spite of external disturbance are the important advantages of this alkaloid when elephant haracterized in a festival crowd is required. Easy availability and low cost make it a drug of choice for stray dog control. However poor margin of safety, lack of antidote and individual idiosyncrasy prevent its use in regular wild animal immobilization.

Muscle Relaxants

There are two groups of muscle relaxants, reversible and non-reversible. Succinyl choline chloride, which is a non-reversible drug, has been in use for deer immobilization. However, the assessment of accurate body weight and lack of antidote have reduced its extensive use.

Both curare and gallamine are reversible type of muscle relaxants and their use in domestic animals has given good results. High solubility of gallamine helps its use in large animals like elephants. In elephant it has given satisfactory results but the animal that has been reversed with neostigmine may again became paralytic. Atropine will have to be incorporated with these drugs to avoid excessive vagal depression on heart when neostigmine is used to reverse the drug action. The reversal is dramatic with neostigmine. The animal is fully conscious and experiences pain. Hence it is not recommended.

Centrally Acting Drugs

1. **Opiates:** The original opiate, morphine has been given only a limited trial. The later compounds like etorphine, fentanyl and carfentanyl have been approved as the most useful immobilizing agents. They are very compatible with other chemicals and their action can be reversed. These can be combined with tranquillizers of phenothiazine group, butyrophenones and xylazine.
2. Sedatives:
   i) **Phenothiazines:** Amongst the phenothiazines, acepromazine is the most extensively used drug. As a sedative its drawback is it produces relaxation of penis and this may be a problem in transportation of male elephants on foot under sedation for long distances. In India only chlorpromazine and triflupromazines are available which are very less potent.

   ii) **Butyrophenones:** Among butyrophenones only haloperidol and droperidol are available in India. Haloperidol being long acting is not used much for animal immobilization. Haloperidol gives satisfactory sedation in elephants, Haloperidol can be used to haracteriz recently captured animals. Azaperone and droperidol are commonly used for haracterized.

   iii) **Benzodiazepine:** All compounds of benzodiazepins like chlordiazepoxide, diazepam, and nitrazepam are available in India, they are very mild and can be used for transport, acclimatization and taming. A new, compound midazolam can be used as a synergist along with drug immobilization.

3. Dissociative Anaesthetics

   i) **Cyclohexamine** Among the cyclohexamines, Ketamine is the most commonly used chemical. Phencyclidine once extensively used is not manufactured now. Tiletamine, a butyrophenon, in combination with zolazepam is used. Ketamine provides very interesting catatonia. Glassy eyes in monkeys are characteristic. Ketamine can be combined with acepromazine or xylazine or diazepam.

   ii) **Xylazine** is a non-narcotic, sedative analgesic and muscle relaxant. Animals appear to be sleeping and produce snoring. In elephants and bulls it causes relaxation of penis. A seemingly sedated animal may rouse explosively. Disturbance during the induction period may delay or even nullify the effect. The elephants may stand and sleep with xylazine. Once an apparently sedated elephant when approached by the crowd ran for a distance of two haracteri and then became immobilized. Xylazine with Acepromazine or ketamine in elephants can produce haracterizedtion if the animal is exposed to solar radiation.

4. Adjunct Drugs:

   i) **Hyaluronidase:** This is an enzyme mixed with immobilizing drugs to increase the rate of absorption from the injection site. The enzyme breaks down connective tissue, and thus, speeds absorption. The drug is marketed in India as Hylase. Generally 150 to 300 IU is added to each haracterize dose. It has been used with succinyl choline chloride, etorphine and fentanyl with apparent decrease in the latent period.

   ii) **Atropine sulphate:** This drug is used primarily to decrease salivation that is often seen with phencyclidine and ketamine. Atropine blocks the parasympathetic nervous system to decrease salivation. It decreases sweating, gut motility, bladder tone, gastric and respiratory secretions. Since there is dilatation of pupil, eyes must be protected from sunlight. Atropine may be mixed with the immobilizing drug, but is often given after the animal is down. Ideal way is to atropinise before Immobilizing drugs are given.

5. Reversing Drugs: This class of drugs is used to reverse the effect of another drug and is often called as antagonists. They are used to negate the effects of an immobilizing drug so as to enable the animal to be on its feet and on its own.

a) Cyprenorphine (M 285) this was the original antagonist used for etorphine, but has generally been replaced by diprenorphine (M 5050).

b) Diprenorphine (M 50 50 or Revivon): This is the antagonist primarily used to reverse the effects of etorphine. It is marketed as M 50 50 (2 mg diprenorphine per ml in a 20 ml vial) and Revivon (3 mg diprenorphine per ml).

c) Nalorphine hydrobromide or hydrochloride these drugs have a structure similar to morphine and compete with morphine at the receptor sites to act as a reversing drug. They are used mainly against fentanyl and carfentanyl. The drugs are marketed as Lethidrone NC and Nalline.

d) Naloxone hydrochloride: This drug has similar action as nalorphine, but does not produce the agonistic effects similar to those of morphine. Naloxone is preferred to nalorphine for reversing the effects of fentanyl.

Supportive Drugs

This class of drugs is used in association with chemical immobilization. An immobilized wild animal may show indications for use of many other drugs as supportive therapy. In all instances these drugs are to be used after the animal is immobilized and examined.

a) Eye ointments: These may be used in preventing infections into the eye and drying of the cornea, when the animal is immobilized in the field. It is suitable with ketamine since the eyes are kept open by the immobilized animal.

b) Systemic antibiotics: These are generally given if the animal has evidence of infection or has potential for infection through injury or dart wound. Since the animal is to be released in the wild, a long acting antibiotic is preferred.

c) Steroids: May be used for supportive therapy in animals under stress.

d) Intravenous fluids: May be used in animals that are severely affected by dehydration or suffering from acidosis.

e) Respiratory and cardiac stimulants: These drugs may be indicated but should be used with extreme caution under veterinary supervision.

f) Injectable vitamins: May be given as a boost for severely debilitated animals.

Capture myopathy, shock, hypothermia, respiratory failure, cardiac failure, bloat, pneumonia, miscellaneous injuries and secondary infections are some of the problems that require immediate attention and appropriate treatment. Hence it is a necessity that some trained personnel are present to handle these situations during captures operations.

Other modes of drug deliveries

Drug delivery by means of oral administration in wild animals:

- Tasteless drugs are easy to administer in case of elephants. Flavoured human drugs are generally palatable in case of elephants.
- Drugs need to be mixed with palatable feeds (eg. Honey for bears, Liver of herbivores for wild felids, bread-loaves with sugar cane for elephants etc.)
- Tubing (except elephants and crocodiles) can be done in many wild animals, provided the animal is duly restrained and specially designed mouth gag is placed in between the molars. However, entry of tube into trachea is to be taken care of always.

Drug delivery by Intramuscular injections in wild animals:

This is to be done at muscular areas only.

- Use one and half inch needle in the large triceps area.
- Long needles may be necessary for the I/M injections into the hind quarters of elephants and dose of even up to 30-50 ml may be given in one site. However, it may produce swelling. Hence, monitor the elephant frequently. Darts may be used for I/M injection in case of free ranging pachyderms.
- Nuchal crest shall be used for IM injection in rhinos.
- Forelimb-regions shall be chosen in reptiles because of the presence of renal portal system.

Drug delivery by sub-cutaneous injections in wild animals:

- Not much desirable as the I/M route in general.
- Use it only when specifically recommended.
- Shoulder-skin area (or) anal fold area if present as in case of elephants may be used.

Drug delivery by intra-venous injections in wild animals:

- Use the bllood vessels at the posterior aspects of ears that are easily accessible for I/V injections in case of elephants, rhinos, wild pigs etc.
- In elephants, large veins on the proximal foreleg and disto-medial rear leg can also be used for this purpose but be careful with the safety measures and in young elephants, the large superficial vein running up the medial aspect of the hind leg is a good site for I/V injection.

- In bears, camels, giraffe etc. jugular vein shall be used as in most of the wild animal species; in camels, upper quadrant of jugular vein shall be used for drug-delivery, unlike giraffe.

Drug delivery by rectal route in wild animals:

- Use a well lubricated sleeved arm / finger and insert into the rectum
- Insert as for as possible
- Take a lubricated hose
- Pass the hose into the rectum aiming the hose antero-dorsally.
- Pass the hose till you encounter the resistance
- Now administer the enema solution (liquid paraffin or soap-water may be used as enema).
- By using 10 ml or 20 ml or 50 ml syringe, drugs shall be administered in multiple species of wild animals.
- Racking may be done with manual removal of dung material as in elephants during the occurrence of constipation based colic conditions.
- Rectal route is highly useful for administration of enema and drugs.

Drug delivery in exotic aviary species

Administration of medicines by intra-nasal route

- Intra-nasal route may be of useful in birds but bulk volume of drugs may be difficult to administer during usage of this route.
- This route is used for nasal flushing also as done in case of infra orbital sinus infection in which cases 1-3 ml of chosen drug is used in budgerigars and up to 10-15 ml is used for cockatoo or larger macaw and may be even up to 40 ml in case of falcons.

Administration of medicines by I/M route and Sub-cutaneous route-

- Body weight of the birds should be well understood by the clinician

Table.1. Body weight of important avian species

Name to the Species	Range of Body weight (grams)
Zebra finch	10-16
Canary	12-30
Budgerigars	25-35
Parrotlet	30-34
Love birds	45-70
Conure	60-80
Macaw	120-160
Quaker parakeet	90-150
Senegal parrot	110-130
Mynah	180-260
Pigeon	240-300
Pionus, Blue-headed	230-260
Cockatoo	220-390
African Grey parrot, Amazon	300-500
Amazon parrot, Orange-Winged	300-450
Eclectus parrot	388-524
Cockatoo, Moluccan	700-1000

In general, preferably the pectoral muscles (or) quadriceps muscle areas are used for the depositing of drugs in case of intra-muscular injections. Sub-cutaneous route is chosen at the axillary region or loose skin in shoulder.

Table. 2. Volume of drugs for injection by IM route

Birds	Volume of drug (I/M)
Budgerigars, canaries, finches etc.	0.1 ml
African gray parrot or Amazon parrot	0.5 ml
Cockatiel, small conure etc.	0.2 ml
Brids weighing more than 1.5 Kg	Volume upto 1.5 ml per site can be given

Administration of medicines by I/V

- This route is mainly used in case of emergency or in case of larger sized birds like cranes, storks etc.
- Take care of the hematoma development or bleeding that may often occur.
- This is very important esp. in case of smaller sized aviary species.
- Wing wein is used for blood collection or IV administration but in large sized or long necked bird, jugular vein also shall be used with more care.

Administration of medicines by intra-osseous route

- This is useful when I/V route or S/C route is not possible to be used due to smaller size of the birds etc.
- Intra-osseous cannula is used to administer blood, fluids, colloids etc.

Site

- Proximal tibia for short-term therapy
- Distal ulna in medium –sized to large birds that requires days of therapy.

Merits

- Reduced patient-resistance is observed during the adaptation of this route of administration of drugs.
- Less stress is experienced when compared to the repeated venipunctures.
- In birds in which the venin cannot be traced as in case of highly sick birds or in smaller sized birds, this route may be of tremendously useful for drug administration.

Transport

Transportation of wild animals of different taxa requires great amount of experience and expertise. Snakes can be transported in small carry bags whereas elephants are transported in big trucks under sedation. Often captive elephants are transported long distances on foot. Care should be taken while transporting carnivores. They can reach out through the bars and maul the attendants.

Transport cages should show the details of the dispatcher, place, date and time of dispatch, short note on the background of the animal and medications done if any. Transporting personnel should also carry a detailed note on the source of the animal, purpose of transport, receiver's address, telephone number and other details that are required to contact in case of emergency. Details of the transponder, if implanted, should also be available. International transport of wild animals needs official permit from the governments concerned, health certificates and details of preventive vaccinations and de-worming schedules followed from a qualified veterinarian. Animals that are endangered require CITES permit and preferably a transponder implant.

If the transportation enclosures are heavy, they must have a provision to be loaded using a forklift or for hoisting using a crane, especially when the transport is of a multi-modal nature. There must be provision for providing food and water depending upon the distance to be transported. During transportation the cages may be covered to avoid the external stimuli as well as to prevent excitement and stress. Depending on the distance of travel, sedatives, preferably long acting ones, can be given. However, heavy sedation for long periods can cause bloat in ruminants.

Aquatic and wallowing animals have to be sprinkled periodically with water during transport to prevent drying of the skin. Transportation of animals in general must be done during the cooler hours of the day and preferably at night when the animal is less active. Provision for rest for the animal as well as for the crew has to be considered especially during long distance transportation. Presence of leftover fodder or even dung of the same animal or the same species in the cage will have a relieving effect on the transporting animal. Prey species like deer may hesitate to get inside a cage in which a predator species like tiger was transported, due to the smell, especially when the cages are not cleaned properly., Even when the prey species is forced inside the cage it may cause stress to the animal.

33

Blood Collection in Different Species of Wild Animals

Guinea pigs: Saphenous vein / Jugular vein / Cranial vena cava Cardiac puncture.

Rat and Mice: Orbital sinus / Jugular vein.

Rabbits / hares: Jugular vein / Ear vein shall be preferred, in general.

Amounts up to 5 ml of blood can be safely drawn from the auricular marginal vein, using a 23- to 25-gauge needle (or) a 23-gauge butterfly attached to a syringe or tube. The jugular vein should be avoided for blood collection if the rabbit suffers from a respiratory problem or shows respiratory distress. It may become cyanotic during the procedure. Alternate sites for blood collection are the cephalic and the lateral saphenous veins. (Their locations are the same as in dogs and cats. These veins are fragile, and a hematoma is easily formed).

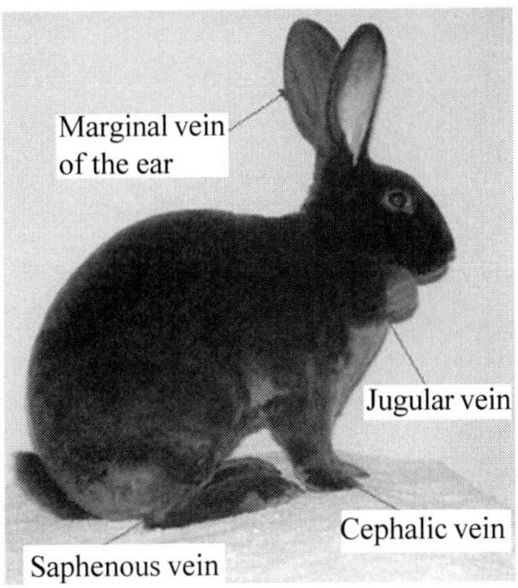

Fig. 1. Loacation of veins in rabbit

Blood collection in canids

- Chemically restrain the wild canid species carefully and place the animal in the harac recumbency.

- Extend the foreleg and occlude the vein with the thumb positioned near the elbow of the canid species
- If needed, clip hair around the sampling site with small clippers.
- Sterilize the area (skin or hair) by using a swab soaked in 70% alcohol / surgical spirit
- Raise the cephalic vein with one thumb by holding pressure across the proximal end of the foreleg.
- Grab the leg and place a thumb adjacent to the vein to pull the skin and stabilize the vein. Position the needle with bevel facing upwards parallel to the skin overlying the cephalic vein.
- Insert the needle through skin and into the vein at a 25° angle up to 0.5-0.75 cm and when blood appears in the syringe hub retract the syringe plunger to let blood fill the syringe. Do not apply too much suction as this may collapse the vein disrupting the blood flow into syringe.

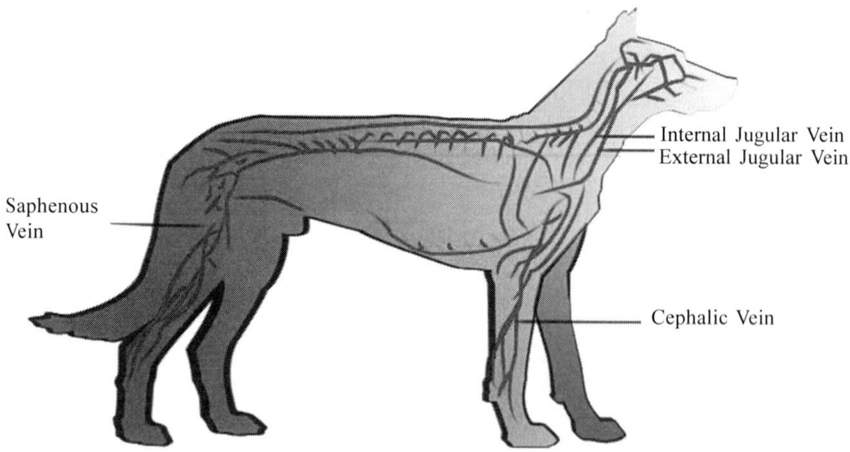

Fig. 2. Loacation of veins in canids

Blood collection in felids

Femoral vein in chemically restrained felid is one of the better route for collection of blood. However, in larger felids like lion, tiger, jaguar and panther, the lateral coccygeal vein is the better choice for the collection of blood.

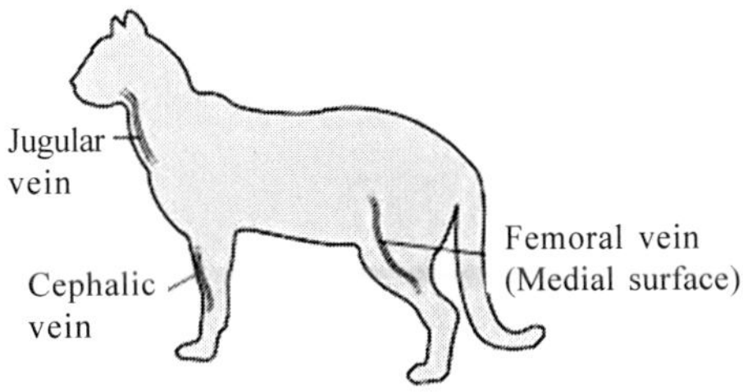

Fig. 3. Loacation of veins in felids

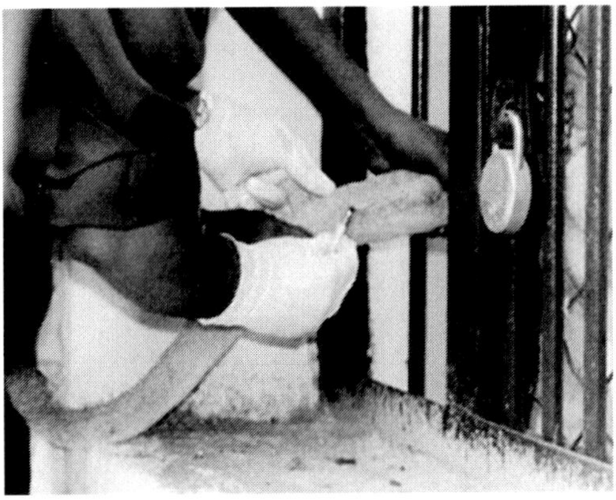

Fig. 4. Loacation of tail-vein in large felid

Blood collection in elephant

External ear vein based collection:

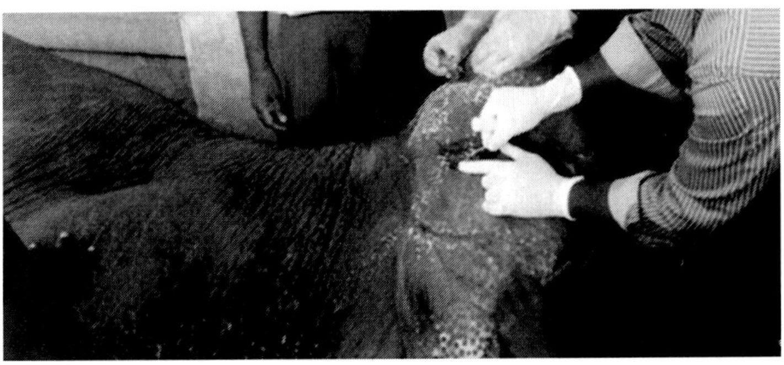

Fig. 5. Loacation of external-ear vein in elephant

Blood collection in wild pigs

External ear vein is commonly used for the collection of blood sample in wild pigs subsequent to the proper restraining methods. Anterior vena cava shall also be used for the successful collection of blood in wild pigs.

Tail bleeding

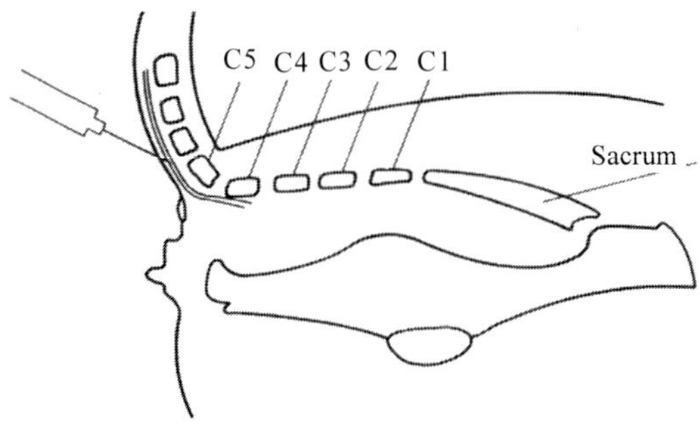

Fig. 6. Loacation of tail-vein

Cross section of the 5th coccygeal vertebra:

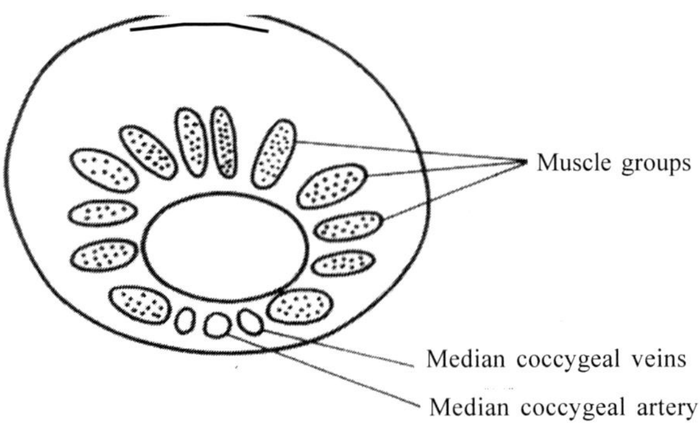

Fig. 7. Loacation of median coccygeal artery & vein

Blood collection in Bonnet macaque

Cephalic vein based collection:

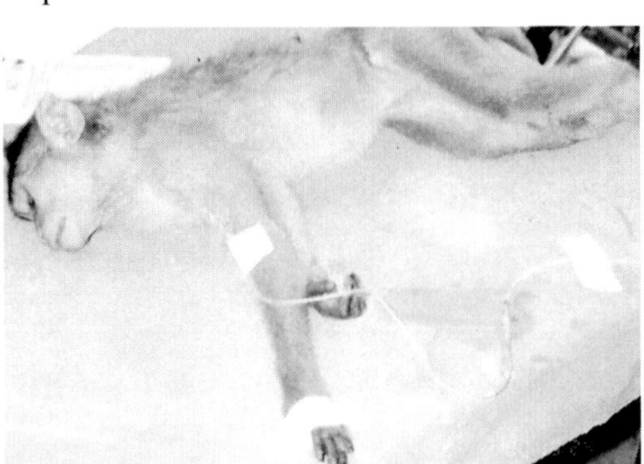

Fig. 8. Loacation of cephalic vein in Bonnet macaque

Blood collection in marmoset

Femoral vein based collection:

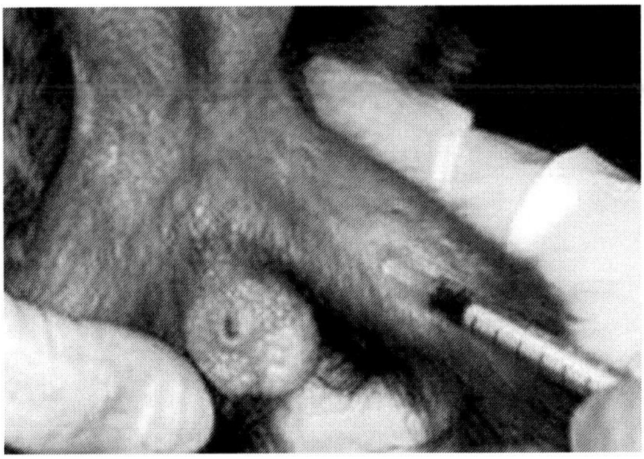

Fig. 9. Loacation of femoral vein in NH primate

Blood collection in rhinos

Small volumes of blood shall be collected readily from the auricular vein noticed on the outside of the rhinoceros's pinna, from the tail or coccygeal vein or from the radial vein and it is to be understood that it may be easy to collect the blood in standing position placed in a chute with carrying out of feeding activity preferably with the palatable feed items for diversion of the rhino from the pain factor dur to needle pricking.

Blood collection in serpentines & lizards

Ventral coccygeal vein is often used towards collection of blood samples from various species of reptiles, as revealed below:

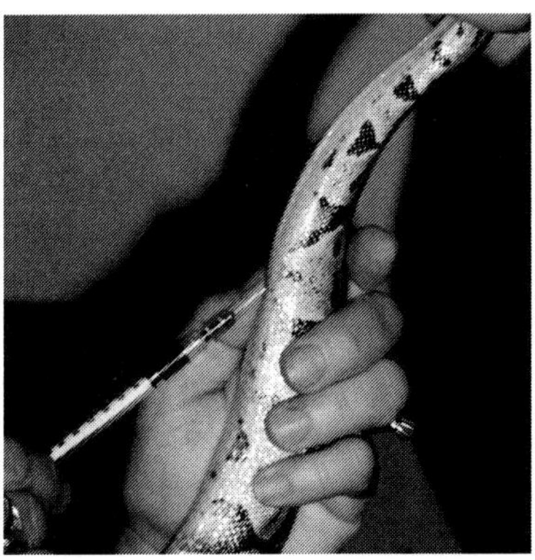

Fig. 10. Loacation of tail-vein: posteriror area to cloaca in snake

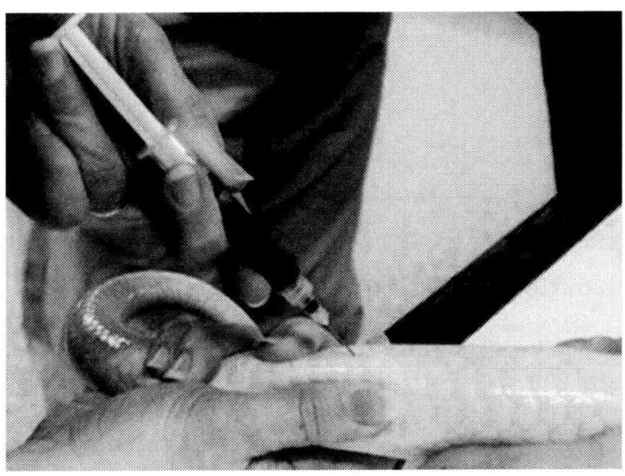

Fig. 11. Loacation of tail-vein for collection of blood

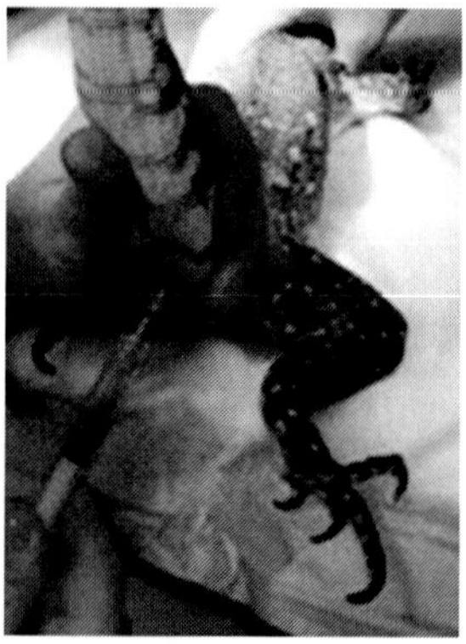

Fig. 12. Loacation of tail-vein in lizard

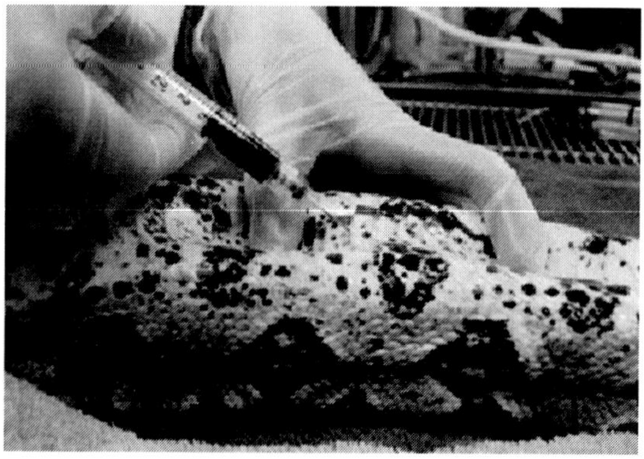

Fig. 13. Intra-cardial blood collection from snake

Intra-cardial route shall be used for collection of blood sample from reptiles, as revealed below in dorsal recumbency:

Blood collection based on the supra-occipital plexus technique in crocodiles:

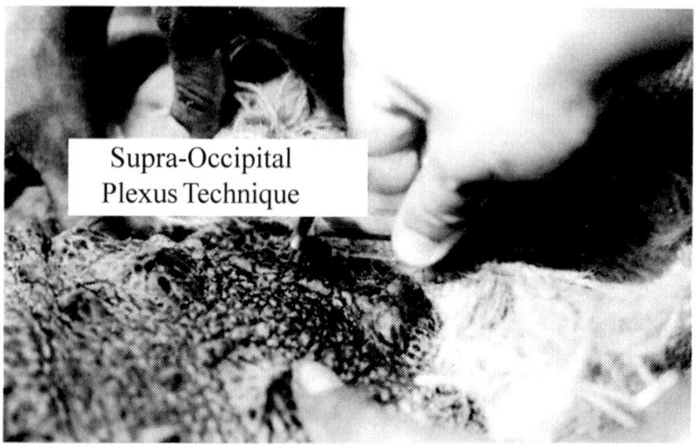

Fig. 14. Blood collection in crocodile using supra-occipital sinus technique

Blood collection using ventral coccygeal vein in crocodiles

Blood collection in chelonians using "Subcarapacial" (subvertebral) venous sinus/vein (if the jugular venipuncture is unsuccessful): This sinus is located on the midline of the cranial aspect of the carapace, in the region where the cervical vertebrae join the shell (Several vessels form a venous sinus at this location, including the common vessels and the caudal cervical branch of the external jugular veins). An increased risk of lymph contamination exists at this sampling site.

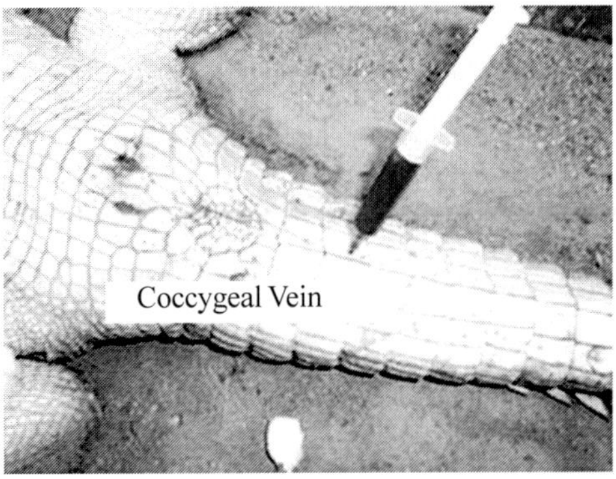

Fig. 15. Site of ventral-coccygeal vein in crocodile

For collection of blood, always position the chelonian in the ventral recumbency, preferably at the edge of a table & forelimbs are restrained. Person performing the venipuncture either extends the head and bends the neck ventrally (or) pushes the head back into the shell.

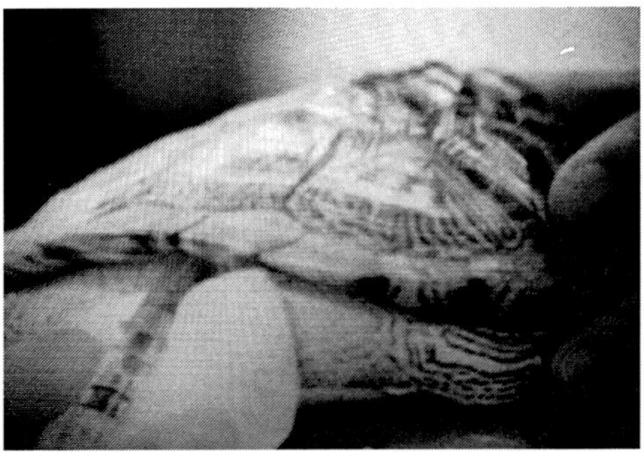

Fig. 16. Sub-vertebral sinus based blood-collection from chelonian

Blood collection in aves

In aviary species, wing vein is often used for the collection of blood samples:

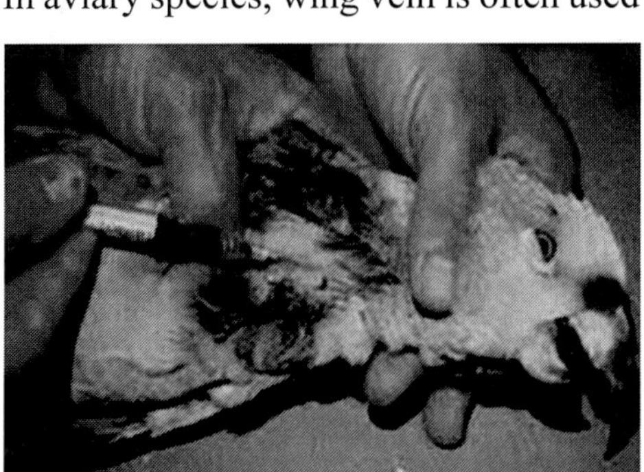

Fig. 17. Jugular vein based blood-collection

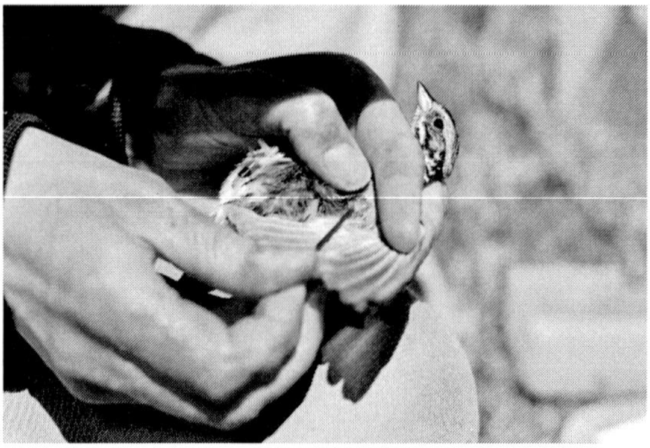

Fig. 18. Wing vein & capillary tube based blood-collectioin

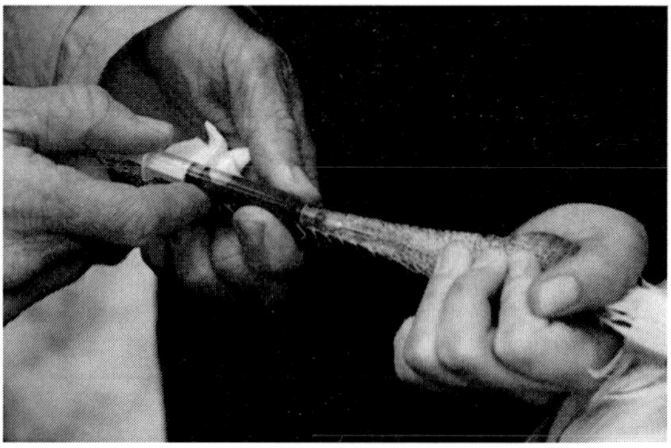

Fig. 19. Blood collection from blood vessel in leg

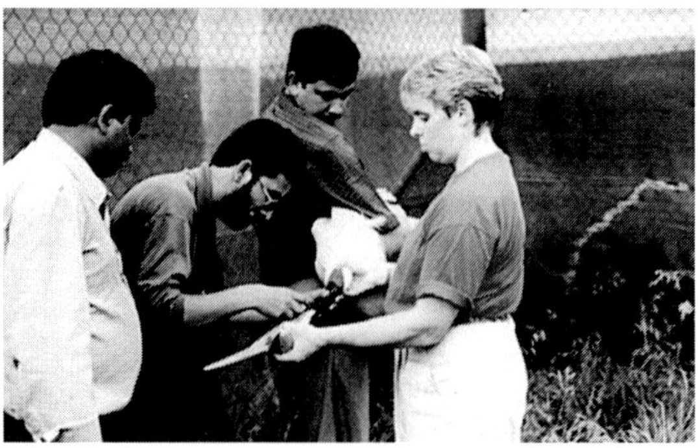

Fig. 20. Blood collection using jugular vein in long-necked bird

34

Examination of Vetero-legal Cases

RULES FOR POST MORTEM EXAMINATION OF VETEROLEGAL CASES

- A veterolegal post mortem examination should be done by written order from the Police or the District Magistrate.
- Before examination carefully read the police report.
- The examination should be in daylight.
- The post-mortem examination should be thorough and complete.
- All the details observed by the Veterinary officer should be carefully noted in the post mortem report on the spot of the post-mortem examination.
- The notes and report to be sent to the court must tally with each other
- A veterinarian should have a fair knowledge of the normal pathological appearance of the viscera.
- Time and date of arrival of carcass should be noted.
- There should be no unnecessary delay in holding mortem examination.
- No unauthorizd person should be allowed to be present at the time of post-mortem examination.

PROCEDURE FOR POST-MORTEM EXAMINATION

A. External examination

The following steps should be followed for the external examination:

- Note the general condition of the carcass.
- Note the species, age, breed and sex of the animal.
- Examine the body surface for injuries, burns, swellings etc.
- Look for the discharge from the natural orifices.
- Examine the visible mucous membranes.
- Examine the external genitalia.

- All the bones should be carefully examined for presence of fracture and joints fordislocation.

B. Internal examination

For the internal examination of carcass the following procedure should be adopted.

i) Necropsy procedure for equines:
   - Place the horse on the right side down.
   - Make an incision through the skin in the ventral neck in line from chin to anus dorso-laterally around the mammary glands or penis.
   - Skin of the left side of the neck, thorax, and the abdomen is reflected back as much as possible without making further incisions into the hide.
   - The left fore and hind limbs are severed by cutting all muscles and attachments.
   - Finish skinning the thorax and abdomen to the tops of the spinous processes of the vertebrae.
   - Incite through the midline from the xiphoid cartilage to pubis and from pubis to thelumbar region through the abdominal wall.
   - Pull upward and forward the large flap of abdominal wall and cut the diaphragm dorso-ventrally close to its attachments.
   - The abdominal viscera are removed in the following order: great colon and caecum, left kidney, left adrenal, the small colon, the small intestines, liver, right kidney, right adrenal, and the stomach.
   - The thoracic cavity is opened by cutting the ribs along their ventral ends from the thoracic inlet to the last rib.
   - Remove thoracic organs by severing the oesophagus, trachea and other attachments, then lifting the heart and lungs out while cutting the remaining attachments.
   - Cut the symphysis of pubis. Saw through the shaft of the ileum above the coxofemoral joint. Examine the internal genital organs, rectum and urinary bladder.

ii) Necropsy procedure for bovines, ovines and caprines:
   - The bovine carcass should be placed on the left side down in order to keep the rumen out of the way.
   - The right fore and hind limbs are severed by cutting all muscles and attachments. It is better to disarticulate the right hind limb.

- An incision is made through the skin on the midline from between the jaws to the perineal region. Incise around the mammary glands or penis.
- The skin of the right side is reflected back as much as possible.
- The abdominal wall is removed by making incision along its periphery.
- The rumen, reticulum, omasum and abomasums are opened *in situ*. Remove the contents and examine.
- The thoracic cavity is exposed in the same manner as in the case of equines.
- The lungs and heart are removed with trachea and oesophagus.
- The urogenital organs are removed in the same manner as that of horses.

iii) Necropsy procedure for swines:

- Place the carcass on its back on the table or site selected for the necropsy.
- Incisions are made so as to drop the limbs to the horizontal position.
- Remove a strip of the ventral body wall from chin to the pubic region, thereby exposing the trachea, oesophagus, thoracic and abdominal cavities.
- At the sternum, make the incisions passing through the costal cartilages.
- The anterior end of the sternum is raised with the left hand so the heart is not.
- The portion of the ventral abdominal wall is incised to' wards the pubis to expose the abdominal organs.
- The ventral abdominal wall is left attached to the pubis so that it can be used to cover the abdominal cavity after necropsy.
- The thoracic cavity is opened by breaking the ribs.
- The, thoracic organs are removed while attached to the oesophagus and trachea.
- First remove the spleen and omentum.
- Push the small intestines to the left side in order to examine rectum.
- Cut the oesophagus posterior to the diaphragm.
- The liver, stomach, and intestines are removed together.
- Remove the adrenal glands before the kidneys are removed.
- The kidneys are removed by tearing its peritoneal covering.

- In the female, the uterus is severed as far posteriorly as possible.
- Examine the seminal vesicles and other accessory organs in boar.

iv) Necropsy procedure of canids and gelids:

- Place the animal with its dorsum upon table.
- The head is extended and the neck is straightened.
- Make an incision from the point of symphysis of mandibles to the ischial arch.
- The mammae are examined at this time.
- Separate the skin from the underlying tissues.
- The legs are pulled to the sides
- Cut the coxofemoral joints and separate the hind limbs.
- Make an incision from the xiphoid cartilage to the pubis.
- Make transverse incisions from the midline to the dorsal extent of the body cavity.
- The abdominal cavity is exposed by removing the flaps.
- To expose the thoracic cavity, cut the harac cartilage or ribs.
- Examine all organs in situ without severing the attachment.
- Lift the organs up and incise for closer examination and return them to body cavities afterwards.

The organs should be examined in the following order:

a) Mouth cavity, tonsils, pharynx, larynx, and salivary glands.

b) Cervical oesophagus and trachea, Lungs, heart and thoracic oesophagus.

d) Liver, spleen, adrenals, kidneys, meters, urinary bladder, genitalia, pancreas, stomach, duodenum, and intestine.

e) Central nervous system.

VETEROLEGAL WOUND

Wound: A wound may be defined as a solution of continuity of the skin. The vetero-legal wounds may be classified as follows:

Incised wound: Incised wound is produced by sharp cutting weapon, such as razors, knives of various kinds, swords, axes, choppers, etc. The edges of the wound are smooth, even, clean, cut and well defined. Incised wounds are characterized by gaping from retraction of the divided skin and tissues. The wound is due to the splitting of the skin and compression against the underlying bone.

Lacerated Wounds: Lacerated wounds are caused by tearing of the tissues. In this type of wounds the edges are torn and irregular; these wounds are generally caused by barbed wires and the claws, teeth or horns of animals. These are common in street vehicle accidents, from either impact or fall.

Punctured Wounds: Punctured wound is also called as penetrating wound and is caused by pointed bodies such as knives, daggers and spears or by more or less pointed instruments. In this type of wound, the external opening is small but the object may penetrate deep into tissues or may enter body cavity like abdomen.

Gunshot Wounds: Firearm Wounds, the gunshot wound is produced by various kinds of firearms. The appearance of these wounds depends upon the following conditions of the individual case under examination.

a) The kind of the weapon employed.

b) The nature of the projectile.

c) The velocity of the projectile.

d) The nature of the powder used.

e) The range at which the weapon was fired.

f) The part of the body struck.

g) The direction of tire.

Table 1. Distinction between ante-mortem and post-mortem wounds.

Ante-mortem wounds	Post-mortem wounds
Copious arterial haemorrhage	No haemorrhages sometimes slight venous.
Presence of inflammation & reparative process	Absence of inflammation or reparative process
There will be gaping of the edges owing to the normal stretched condition of the skin.	No gaping of the edges
Blood is clotted	Blood is not clotted
Spouting of blood from arteries	No spouting of blood

Causes of death from wounds: The causes of death from wounds may be divided into direct and indirect.

Direct causes: Direct causes of death from wounds are as follows:

Haemorrhages: It may be external or internal injury to a vital organ: Severe injury to a vital organ such as the lungs or heart.

Shock: Death may occur from shock without any visible injury as in the case of a severe blow on the heart region or the abdomen.

Indirect causes: The indirect causes of death from the injury are as follows:

- Inflammation of internal organs.
- Septicaemia or pyaemia.
- Necrosis of internal organs.
- Infective diseases: Tetanus, which may develop through the entrance of the causal organism through wounds.

Fractures: Fracture is a solution of the continuity of a bone. Fractures of bones comprise a considerable proportion of the injuries met with in vetero-legal practice. Although simple fractures of bones are not dangerous to the life of the animal.

Classification of Fractures: Fractures are classified according to the degree of injury and the structures involved. Fractures may be classified either as complete or incomplete.

Complete fractures: Fractures in which the bone is broken through its thickness come in this category. Complete fractures are again subdivided into simple, compound and complicated.

- Simple fracture is one in which the bone is broken but there is no breach of continuity of the skin.
- Compound fracture is one in which there is an external wound leading to the break of the bone.
- Complicated fracture is one which involves structures other than the bone. Large vessels may be severed, muscles frequently lacerated, nerves cut or otherwise injured, lungs may be punctured by a broken rib, and the brain may be lacerated by a bone of the fractured cranium.

Incomplete fractures: Fractures in which a part of the thickness of the bone is broken come in this category. These fractures are further subdivided as follows.

- Greenstick fractures are those fractures in which one side, of the bone is broken and other side is bent. This type of fracture is commonly seen in puppies and other young animals, frequently in the radius and ulna of greyhound.
- Splintered fractures are haracterized by separation of particles or splinters of bone as a result of direct violence. This is sometimes seen w hen a horse receives a kick from the heel of the shoe of another horse on the inner aspect of the tibia.
- Fissured fractures are haracterized by the presence of cracks in a bone, without any displacement.
- A Star fracture is one from which in course of time fragments and spicules of necrosed bone become detached.

The Causes of Fracture: Fractures maybe caused either by direct causes (exciting causes) or indirect causes (predisposing causes) Fractures in animals are caused by blows from sticks, kicks and collisions, vehicle accidents, falls from heights and jumping over walls. Fractures may also be caused by unopposed or in coordinated action.

BURNS: Burns may be defined as the destruction of tissues caused by the application of heat, or of chemical substances to the external or internal surfaces of the body Burns include all lesions whether produce by fire, water or chemical action. A scald may be defined as a lesion which results from the application of liquid at or near boiling point or from steam.

Etiology

- Exposure to flame or radiant heat.
- Contact with hot objects.
- Scalding with hot liquid.
- Lightning stroke and electrocution.
- Corrosive chemicals, such as, acids, phenols and strong alkalies.

Symptoms

- Erythema of the skin.
- Diffuse oedema of the skin and subcutaneous tissues.
- Formation of small vesicle; rarely and sloughing of the skin.
- A circular patch of hairs, together with the superficial layers of skin, suddenly falls away, leaving a red wound which soon begins to suppurate.
- Charring of tissue in severe burns and oozing of plasma.
- Animals with severe burn; are reluctant to move and resent handling.
- Shock and toxaemia in very severe cases of burns or scalds.

SCARS

Scar is formed as a result of the healing process of a wound, scar tissue is usually devoid of hair and sweat glands, the presence or absence of known scars from injury operation is of importance in the identification of the living and dead animals. Incised wounds may cause long tape like scars, more or less depressed below the surface of the skin. Broad and irregular scars are caused by lacerated wounds, Scars from lacerated wounds and from wounds which have suppurated and healed by granulation tissue are firmer, prominent and are attached to the deeper tissue. Stab and puncture wounds leave irregular, circular, triangular or oblong scars, Scars from superficial burns are thin and pliant, or if severe, are irregularly thickened by patches. Scars from firearm projectiles are usually rounded and slightly smaller than the original hole. Scars should always be examined in daylight to note the number of scars and the shape, size, situation and direction of each, to note the colour of each scar. It is difficult to tell the exact age of a scar. The variations in the time of healing of wounds in animals are so great that it is not possible to fix any time limit within which these reparative changes are produced.

CAUSES OF DEATH

In natural or accidental death, there are three primary modes of death, namely, coma, syncope or asphyxia since life is maintained by the interdependent action of the brain, the heart and the lungs, the arrest of the function of one of them is quickly succeeded by the arrest of the function of the others and life ceases. Death may occur due to the combined effects of coma and asphyxia.

COMA: Coma means loss of consciousness. Loss of consciousness may be partial or complete; it may be transitory, lasting for a few minutes, or may continue for some days or until death takes place.

Etiology

- Coma may be the result of traumatic injury to the brain. Direct trauma to the head is an uncommon cause of brain injury in animals. Sometimes traumatic injury to the brain is caused by an accidental collision, fall from height, animal interaction or a weapon.
- Coma may be caused by cerebral haemorrhage, thrombosis, embolism, tumours, abscess and other inflammatory conditions of the brain. Spontaneous celebral haemorrhage has been observed in cows at parturition.
- The most important cause of sudden unconsciousness in animals is poisons having specific action on the brain, e.g, bromides, carbon monoxide, zinc phosphide, nicotine, barbiturates and other anaesthetics and sedatives, atropine, hyoscine and hyoscyamine, alcohols, phenols and turpentine.
- Coma occurs subsequent to depression and lethargy in uraemia and heat stroke.

Post Mortem Appearance

1. Injuries to the skull bones.
2. The brain and its membranes are congested.

3. Blood in the cranial cavity. Blood clots may be found within membranes or in the brain.
4. The right side of the heart is usually full and the left empty
5. Tumour or cyst or abscess m the cranial cavity

ASPHYXIA: The term asphyxia, as generally employed, refers to an interference with the oxygen interchange in the lungs. The term asphyxia is also used in the broader sense of anoxia and designates the state of tissue asphyxiation produced when the oxygen and carbon dioxide interchange between the blood in the capillaries sand the tissue cells in all parts of the body is prevented.

Etiology

Fatal asphyxia may result from either natural disease pro cesses or from traumatic causes. Mechanical obstruction in the respiratory tract in animals may occur in enzootic nasal granuloma, oedema of the larynx, acute cellulitis of the throat, peri pharyngeal cellulitis with oedema, laryngeal obstruction with solid food material, chronic laryngitis, laryngeal spasm, tumour and abscesses. Asphyxia may be produced by the paralysis of the respiratory nerves, muscles or the respiratory centre from injury of disease or from the action of certain poisons. Asphyxia may result from causes operating from lungs or pulmonary circulation, Strangulation is the closure of the air passages as a result of external pressure on the neck which prevents the ingress or egress of air during respiration can cause Asphyxia, Inhalation of irrespirable gases, such as carbon monoxide, hydrogen sulphide, sulphur dioxide, nitrous oxide may cause fatal asphyxia.

Post mortem appearance

- Protruded tongue.
- Frothy blood stained fluid at the nostrils.
- Congested conjunctiva.
- Slightly frothy mucus in larynx and trachea and the mucous membrane of the trachea is congested.
- The lungs are engorged and oedematous. On section a copious, frothy, dark coloured, blood-stained exudates will be seen.
- Petechial haemorrhages on pleura, pericardium, myocardium, endocardium and substance of the brain.
- Some of the marginal portions of the lungs may perhaps show emphysematous changes.

- The cavities of the right side of the heart are engorged with dark coloured, imperfectly clotted blood.
- The cavities on the left side of the heart are comparatively empty.
- Marked venous congestion of the abdominal viscera.
- Congested brain and excess of serous fluid is found in the lateral ventricles.
- Cranial sinuses are usually filled with dark-coloured blood.
- The blood, generally, is dark in colour and is mostly fluid in the large wins.
- Microscopically, the lung tissue shows marked dilatation of both the capillaries and veins

SHOCK: The term shock is used to describe a state of collapse caused by an acute and progressive failure of the peripheral circulation. Shock is stagnant hypoxia.

These are the following types of shock

1. **Haemorrhagic Shock**: Haemorrhage is one of the most common causes of shock in animals. A normal healthy animal can tolerate a 20 per cent loss of blood volume, without developing signs of circulatory failure. Haemorrhagic shock may be hypovolemic or normovolemic. Hypovolemic shock occurs prior to the time of reinfusion and normovolemic shock following reinfusion.
2. **Traumatic Shock:** Traumatic shock is the depressed state of the vital functions that results from severe traumatic injury. There are two kinds of traumatic shock:

   i) **Immediate or primary shock:** Immediate or primary shock is caused by the overwhelming of the vital centres in the medulla by the nerve impulses originating in the injured area and conveyed to the central nervous system. Death occurs in a few minutes from vasomotor collapse in primary shock

   ii) **Delayed or secondary shock**, which does not occur immediately after the trauma but develops a few hours later. Traumatic shock is caused by loss of plasma into the injured area and it is hypovplemic.
3. **Septic Shock:** A fatal infection by pyogenic organisms may follow an injury if the animal survives the immediate complication of shock and haemorrhage. An injury of the abdomen and a perforation of the gastrointestinal tract by a weapon may introduce pathogenic bacteria into the peritoneal cavity, causing fatal acute suppurative peritonitis. A blunt force injury of the abdomen may rupture the intestines and be followed by the same complication.

4. **Thermal Shock:** Thermal shock occurs when the animal is subjected to extreme degrees of heat or cold. Shock developing after thermal injury is characterized by progressive hypovolemia, haemconcentration and circulatory failure.
5. **Anaphylactic Shock:** Anaphylactic shock is an immunologic phenomenon, depending upon a reaction between sensitized body cells and specific antigens.

Post mortem appearance

- Signs of severe injuries like fractures, crushing of the tissues, extensive lacerations and avulsions.
- Generalized visceral Congestion.
- Oedema of the lungs.
- Dark red fluid blood.
- Petechial haemorrhages in the serous membranes and parenchymatous organs.

SIGNS OF DEATH: An assessment of the various changes in the body after death enables us to arrive at an approximate idea as to the length of time that has elapsed since death. It is impossible to fix the exact moment of death. The chief signs of death are as follows:

- Cessation of respiration and circulation.
- Cooling of the body.
- Primary flaccidity.
- Rigor mortis.
- Secondary flaccidity.
- Putrefaction.
- Adipocere.
- Mummification.

VETERO-LEGAL ISSUES RELATED TO THE WILD ANIMAL CONSERVATIONS

- RESCUE of wild animals.
- Control of Rogue-Wild Animals.
- Euthanasia
- Entry of dog / sheep / goat / cattle into the wildlife areas.

- Seasonal migration of cattle and other livestock through the wildlife regions.
- Entry into wildlife sanctuary.
- Entry into national park.
- Entry into reserve forest.
- Entry in banned periods.
- Vehicle entry into the wildlife areas.
- Sound pollution (loud speakers) in wildlife regions.
- Overall pollution in wildlife regions.
- Transport inside the wildlife regions (rail / road etc.).
- Photography near wild animals.
- Trapping of any wild animal species.
- POACHING / HUNTING of wild animals.
- Poisoning of any wild animal faunaling.
- Damaging of any natural resources.
- Stealing of forest resources like wooden logs / trees / herbal plants.
- Smuggling of wild fauna (or) products of wild animals.
- Mining within the forest regions.
- Starting of industries within the prescribed distance from borders of the protected wildlife regions.
- Consumption of meat from wild animals.
- Owning of any wildlife trophies / products.
- Sale or Commercial usage of any wild animals/wild animal products.
- Theft of wild animals.
- Encroachment of forest lands.
- Confinement of wild fauna.
- Tourism inside the wildlife regions.
- Trespassing of wildlife areas.
- Straying in night without permission.
- Staying in unauthorized place.
- Carrying out of any research progrogrammes without due permission from the forest department.

Reasons for the framing and implementation of the "Wildlife Protection Act 1972"

Wildlife is a part of 'forests' and this was a state subject until the Parliament passed this law in 1972. Reasons for a nationwide law in the domain of environment particularly wildlife includes the following:

- India is a treasure-trove of varied flora and fauna. Many species were seeing a rapid decline in numbers.
- For instance, it was mentioned by Edward Pritchard Gee (A naturalist), that at the turn of the 20th century, India was home to close to 40000 tigers. But, a census in 1972 showed this number drastically reduced to about 1827.
- A drastic decrease in the flora and fauna can cause ecological imbalance, which affects many aspects of climate and the ecosystem.
- The most recent Act passed during the British era in this regard was the Wild Birds and Animals Protection, 1935. This needed to be upgraded as the punishments awarded to poachers and traders of wildlife products were disproportionate to the huge financial benefits that accrue to them.
- There were only five national parks in India prior to the enactment of this Act.

Wildlife Protection Act was subsequently amended in the year 1991 and 2002

- According to this act, "Wildlife" is defined as any animal, bee, butterflies, crustaceae, fish and moths and aquatic or land vegetation".
- Thus it is to be understood that Wildlife is the term that embraces all life forms that are wild or care themselves.

Wildlife Crime Control Bureau (WCCB)

- Wildlife Crime Control Bureau under the Director, Wildlife Preservation has been established with association by five Regional Offices viz, Delhi, Mumbai, Kolkata, Chennai and Jabalpur and 3 Sub regional offices at Amritsar, Guwahati, and Kochi, along with units called as BORDER UNITS which are located at Moreh, Nathula, Motihari, Gorakhpur and Ramanathapuram.
- This wildlife division generally deals with the policy and law-matters and knowledge management for facilitating processes and analysis for evolution of policy and law for conservation of biodiversity and Protected Area network. This wildlife division of the Ministry of Environment and Forests

in India specifically provides the technical and financial support to the State Governments for wildlife conservation under the Centrally Sponsored Scheme Integrated Development of Wildlife Habitats and also through Central Sector Scheme – Strengthening of Wildlife Division and Consultancies for Special Tasks, and through Grants in Aid to the Central Zoo Authority and Wildlife Institute of India, Dehradun.

- The Wild Life Crime Control Bureau has been created under Section 38Y of the Wild Life (Protection) Act, 1972. The mandate has been specified under Section 38(z) which includes collection, collation of intelligence and its dissemination, establishment of a centralized Wild Life crime databank, coordination of the actions of various enforcement authorities towards the implementation of the provisions of the Act, implementation of the international Conventions, capacity building for scientific and professional investigation, assistance to authorities in other countries for a coordinated universal action towards control of Wild Life crime and to advise the government on various policy and legal requirements.

35

Haematological and Biochemical Values in Captive Wild Animals

Clinical examination of animals regardless of domestic or wild ones is of utmost significance during the assessment of health status in animals. Prior to collecting samples, it is important to determine the capabilities and submission criteria of the laboratory receiving the samples. One has to determine the type of test to be conducted whether haematological or biochemical one and the practical feasibility of the tests to be carried out in the concerned clinical diagnostic laboratory attached with the captive wild animal places, like the zoo, zoological park, zoological garden, aviary centre, crocodilian centres, rescue centres etc. It is important that blood sample collection from wild animals (whether *in-situ* or *ex-situ)* should be least stressful due to the fact that stress will affect the outcome of the test-results including the baseline-haematological values. The delayed sending of the clinical samples to the associated laboratories often may have impact on the test-results. The samples need to be properly labelled with details on case number, date of collection, type of sample etc.

Significance of haematological examination basically is associated with assessment of health status overall and conditions caused by anaemia, chronic infections, bacterial as well as viral infections shall will tell upon the status of the concerned wild animal species from which blood has been collected. For example, increased PCV indicates haemoconcentration as well as dehydration. Leukopenia is common in viral infections and leucocytosis along with neutrophilia is common in case of bacterial infections and leukopenia in viral infections. Increased ESR may often be noticed in chronic infections like tuberculosis. Examination of blood smears are useful generally to rule out the haemo-protozoan infections, microfilaria etc., in addition to the differential count of WBCs. Similarly, biochemical examinations like BUN and Creatinine along with urinary parameters like protein, sediments, casts etc. are helpful towards assessment of renal functions. However, one has to be aware that increased Creatinine may also be encountered in conditions like musculo-skeletal disorders also. Similarly, the biochemical tests like total protein, ALT, AST, GGT, Total cholesterol, Total bilirubin, Direct and Indirect bilirubin levels are useful for assessment of liver function.

Cytology samples need to be detailed on site of collection in particular and haematological samples need to be mentioned on type of preservative used and dried or preferably dried and alcohol-fixed blood smears need to be sent in a properly protected package, duly labelled. Some samples need to be refrigerated like serum, urine etc. and for the distant places either a special messenger or dry ice shall be used for sending of clinical samples and formalin (10%) shall be used for storage of faecal samples. To preserve *Giardia intestinalis*DNA in faeces, 2.5% potassium dichromate solution shall be used to store faeces for one month. The chemical preservation of urine has been found to be an effective alternative to refrigeration and thymol is an excellent preservative for urine towards estimation of glucose and sediments Sodium fluoride shall be used in blood to be used for glucose-estimation for at-least three days but D-Mannose is found to be superior to sodium fluoride.

Haematological and biochemical values of captive wild animals are given below:

Spotted deer

Haematology	
PCV (%)	34.0±0.6
Hb (g/dl)	9.60±0.97
RBC (m/Cmm)	13.0±0.8
WBC (x10^3/Cmm)	4.4±0.3
Among the different leukocytes, neutrophils predominated (52.0±1.7) over the lymphocytes (44.0±1.3)	

Biochemical Parameters	
BUN (mg/dl)	10.1+0.8
AST IU/lt)	66 +5
ALT (IU/lt)	40+3
Total protein (g/dl)	8.2+ 0.15
Albumin (g/dl)	4.70 + 0.33
Glucose (mg/dl)	62+7

Wild dog

Haematology	
PCV (%)	46.88±1.31
Hb (g/dl)	16.69±0.26
RBC (m/Cmm)	7.49±0.05
WBC (x10^3/Cmm)	7.91±4.79
Neutrophils	72.63±2.81x10^3/Cmm
Lymphocytes	25.25±2.76 x10^3/Cmm
Monocytes	0.75±0.31 x10^3/Cmm
Eosinophils	1.38±0.41 x10^3/Cmm

Biochemical Parameters	
BUN (mg/dl)	20.56+0.74
Creatinine (mg/dl)	1.44+0.04
AST IU/lt)	18.97+ 0.89
ALT (IU/lt)	19.76 + 0.79
Total protein (g/dl)	6.09 + 0.30
Albumin (g/dl)	2.38 +0.22
Globulin (g/dl)	3.71+0.33
Total bilirubin (mg/dl)	0.15 + 0.07
Direct bilirubin (mg/dl)	0.39 + 0.08
Indirect bilirubin (mg/dl)	0.24 + 0.05
Glucose (mg/dl)	53.63+1.28
Cholesterol (mg/dl)	154.67+8.37
Calcium (mg/dl)	9.1+0.64
Phosphorus (mg/dl)	5.86+0.48

Elephant

Haematology	
PCV (%)	40.19±0.64
Hb (g/dl)	11.56±0.38
RBC (m/Cmm)	3.19±0.16
WBC (x10^3/Cmm)	9.19±0.23
Neutrophils	3800.63±198.51
Lymphocytes	4866.25±153.53
Monocytes	183.13±20.47
Eosinophils	-

Biochemical Parameters	
BUN (mg/dl)	9.63±0.75
Creatinine (mg/dl)	1-2
AST IU/lt)	20.40±0.20
ALT (IU/lt)	7.52±0.65
Total protein (g/dl)	7.46±0.15
Albumin (g/dl)	2.27±0.08
Globulin (g/dl)	5.19±0.19
Total bilirubin (mg/dl)	0.74±0.05
Direct bilirubin (mg/dl)	0.08±0.06
Indirect bilirubin (mg/dl)	0.66±0.04
Glucose (mg/dl)	67.56+2.07
Cholesterol (mg/dl)	64.58+7.12
Calcium (mg/dl)	9-12
Phosphorus (mg/dl)	4-6

Sloth bear

Haematology	
PCV (%)	52 ± 1.03
Hb (g/dl)	16.92 ± 0.63
RBC (m/Cmm)	6.56 ± 0.19
WBC (x10^3/Cmm)	11.72 ± 0.32
Neutrophils	8.24±0.19x10^3/Cmm
Lymphocytes	2.85±0.1 x10^3/Cmm
Monocytes	0.36±0.06 x10^3/Cmm
Eosinophils	0.2±0.44 x10^3/Cmm

Biochemical Parameters	
BUN(mg/dl)	19.08±0.55
Creatinine(mg/dl)	1.24 ± 0.9
AST IU/lt)	137.74 ± 3.11
ALT (IU/lt)	103.56 ± 1.90
Total protein (g/dl)	6.98±0.3
Albumin (g/dl)	3.89±0.19
Globulin (g/dl)	3.09±0.15
Total bilirubin (mg/dl)	0.15±0.04
Direct bilirubin (mg/dl)	-
Indirect bilirubin (mg/dl)	-
Glucose (mg/dl)	98.82+1.96
Cholesterol (mg/dl)	268.63+5.22
Calcium (mg/dl)	9.47+0.29
Phosphorus (mg/dl)	5.11+0.15

Tiger

Haematology	
PCV (%)	36-45
Hb (g/dl)	7.8-13.8
RBC (m/Cmm)	4.66-9.15
ESR (hrs)	14-26
Icterus index	2-5 U/l
WBC (x10^3/Cmm)	6.20-11.05
Neutrophils (%)	57-75
Lymphocytes (%)	18-35
Monocytes (%)	2-6
Eosinophils (%)	2-6
Basophils (%)	0-4

Biochemical Parameters	
BUN (mg/dl)	6.5-48.2
Creatinine (mg/dl)	1.6-4.6
AST IU/lt)	14.4-84.0
ALT (IU/lt)	21.2-109.0
Total protein (g/dl)	3.7-8.7
Albumin (g/dl)	2.1-4.6
Total bilirubin (mg/dl)	0.4-3.2

Panther

Haematology	
PCV (%)	46.88 ± 1.31
Hb (g/dl)	12.98 ± 0.85
RBC (m/Cmm)	7.06 ± 0.56
ESR (mm/hr)	42.22 ± 3.67
WBC (/Cmm)	13,100 ± 975
Neutrophils (%)	69.89 ± 4.04
Lymphocytes (%)	25.56 ± 1.81
Monocytes (%)	1.44 ± 0.88
Eosinophils (%)	5.56 ± 1.51

Biochemical Parameters	
ALT (IU/lt)	46.8 + 26.8
Total protein (g/dl)	7.0 + 1.4
Bun (mg/dl)	27.6 ± 11.4
Cocatinine (mg/dl)	1.6 ± 0.7
AST (Iu/lt)	41.3 ± 19.2
Total cholesterol (mg/dl)	115 - 254
Glucose (mg/dl)	58.6 ± 26.9
Triglyceride (mg/dl)	29.5 ± 12.5
Calcium (mg/dl)	9.9 ± 3.2
Prosphorus (mg/dl)	5.5 ± 1.8

Crocodile

Haematology	
PCV (%)	22.75 ± 1.16
Hb (g/dl)	7.21 ± 0.39
RBC (m/Cmm)	0.85 ± 0.07
WBC (x10^3/Cmm)	10.14 ± 0.48
Neutrophils	4.92 ± 0.34x10^3/Cmm(heterophils)
Lymphocytes	2.45 ± 0.1 x10^3/Cmm
Monocytes	0.02 ± 0.0 x10^3/Cmm
Eosinophils	0.04 ± 0.2 x10^3/Cmm

Biochemical Parameters	
BUN (mg/dl)	6.62±0.23
Creatinine (mg/dl)	0.42 ± 0.02
AST (IU/lt)	45.41 ± 1.46
ALT (IU/lt)	51.13 ± 1.70
Total protein (g/dl)	5.75±0.09
Albumin (g/dl)	2.35±0.04
Globulin (g/dl)	3.4±0.08
Total bilirubin (mg/dl)	0.46±0.01
Direct bilirubin (mg/dl)	-
Indirect bilirubin (mg/dl)	-
Glucose (mg/dl)	66.25+5.04
Cholesterol (mg/dl)	222.27+15.21
Calcium (mg/dl)	10.55+0.55
Phosphorus (mg/dl)	4.18+0.11

36

Collections of Samples During Necropsy

SAMPLING IN IMPORTANT BACTERIAL DISEASES

Actinobacillosis (*Actinobacillus lignieresi*)

- Hard tongue due to fibrous tissue proliferation (termed as wooden tongue) is a characteristic feature.
- Swab and smear from abscess and tissue samples including tongue and lymphnodes.

Actinomycosis (*Actinomyces bovis*)

- Cut surface is white, glistening, abscess with yellowish pus having sulfur granules at mandible and maxilla regions and is characteristic
- Swabs from discharging pus from the cut surface of maxilla and mandible regions.

Anthrax

- Absence of rigor mortism, splenomegaly and oozing of unclotted blood from body- orifices are characteristic features.
- Examine the air dried blood smear from oozing and unclotted blood sample of natural orifices or by puncturing the peripheral area (Ear) and smear from oedema fluid.
- Don't open up carcass (due to the risk of spore dissemination), until examination of blood smear is negative for anthrax. If accidentally opened up, collect formalinised and freshly refrigerated tissue like spleen in particular and parts of all internal organs and fluids (csf, blood, ocular and other body fluids).
- Swab from blood for culture.

Brucellosis

- Placenta or intact foetal stomach under refrigerated condition.
- Foetal stomach contents under refrigerated condition.

- Milk, serum, vaginal mucus etc. shall be submitted under refrigerated condition.

Contagious bovine pleuropneumonia (CBPP) (*mycoplasma mycoides var. Capri*)

- Fibrinopurulent exudate in lungs and pleura is a characteristic feature.
- Nasal swabs under refrigerated condition.

Listeriosis

- Half the brain under refrigerated condition for bacterial isolation.
- Half the brain fixed in 10% formal saline for histology.
- Foetal stomach contents and CSF under refrigerated condition.

Blackleg

- Excise a cube of affected muscle and place it under refrigerated condition.
- Smears and swabs from fluid of lesions.

Leptospirosis

- Tissue samples esp. liver and kidneysunder refrigerated condition.

Pasteurellosis (Haemorrhagic septicaemie/HS)

- Petechiae on pericardium and swelling in neck regions extended to the brisket between forelegs and congestion of conjunctivae and other mucosal membranes are significant features.
- Heart blood smears and swabs under refrigerated condition.
- Nasal swabs under refrigerated condition.

Necrobacillosis (*Spherophorus necrophorus*)

- Necrotic plaques in larynx, pharynx and trachea, necrotic foci in spleen, liver, ulceration in rumen oral region in addition to foot rot/pododermatitis are characteristic features.
- Swabs from foot lesions, and nasal regions along with affected tissue samples under refrigerated condition.

Tuberculosis

- Tubercles in lungs, liver and emaciated body conditions are the characteristic features.

- Tissues from the tubercular lesions under refrigerated condition.
- Impression smears from cut surface of the affected lung regions.

Mycoplasmosis

- Special transport medium is a must and often it may consist basically the brain-heart infusion broth, yeast extract, the antifungal agent–nystatin and an antibiotic such as ampicillin. The sample to medium ration is to be 1:10.

Johne's disease (*Mycobacterium Paratuberculosis*)

- Corrugated folds in mucosa of intestines, evidence of chronic diarrhea including emaciation and tubercules in mesenteric lymph nodes and small and large intestines.
- Rectal mucosa-pinch under refrigerated condition.

SAMPLING IN IMPORTANT VIRAL DISEASES

Sampling for diagnosis of viral agents

- Use sterile mode of collection like usage of sterile needle, containers etc. and tissues shall be kept in 50% glycerol saline and special transport media also shall be used.

  NOTE: Viral and mycoplasma transport media should be stored frozen at -20 degree C. and when required, the bottles are to be removed, thawed slowly and then to be used within 12 hrs. Once thawed, the media should not be refrozen.

Rabies

- Dissected brain tissue must include a complete cross section of the brain stem and either cerebellum or hippocampus and is to be sent under frozen conditions.

Pseudo-rabies / Aujeszky's disease (Herpes virus)

- Tissue samples esp. lung, liver and adrenal cortex under refrigerated condition

Bovine malignant catarrh (Herpes virus)

- Erosions on oral mucosa and large intestine leading to zebra strippings in addition to necrosis of epithelium and enlargement of liver and kidneys with mottling are notable features in this disease.
- Tissues from organs esp. liver and kidneys and nasal discharge.

Neonatal calf diarrhea (Rota virus)

- Yellowish watery diarrhea is a characteristic feature and length of intestinal villi is reduced.
- Feces, intestinal contents and tissue samples esp. intestinal epithelium under refrigerated condition.

Bovine viral diarrhea-Mucosal disease (Pesti virus)

- Zebra markings of small and large intestine are characteristic features, in addition to the ulcers in oesophagus and abomasum.
- Intestinal contents and tissue samples esp. intestinal tissues.

Contagious bovine ecthyma / or Parapox virus

- Papular, vesicular and pustular lesions on lips, oral mucosa, udder, feet, with necrosis and sloughing of affected areas.
- Skin lesions are to be sampled.

Bovine popular stomatitis (Parapox virus)

- Erythema, papule on lips, muzzle, nostrils, tongue, oral mucosa, oesophagus, rumen, reticulum and abomasum are characteristic features.
- Skin lesions are to be sampled.

Bovine ulcerative mammilitis (Herpes virus)

- Erythema, oedema, vesicles and ulcers covered with scab on teats.
- Scabs, vesicles and tissues are to be sampled.

Cow Pox (Orthopox virus)

- Papule, vesicle, pustule and cab on hairless parts of body like teats and udder.
- Scab samples are to be sent for examination.

SAMPLING IN IMPORTANT PARASITIC DISEASES

Babesiosis

- Swollen spleen and anaemic and emaciated carcass are characteristic.
- Carcass is anaemic or sometimes yellowish.
- Kidneys are congested and enlarged and haemorrhages are in heart, stomach and intestines.

- Collect impression smears from spleen and lymph nodes.
- Brain crush-smear.

Theileriosis

- Often kidneys are pale in color.
- Abomasum is with ulcers and haemorrhages.
- Collect smears from spleen and lymph nodes.

Anaplasmosis

- Emaciated carcass.
- Dark brownish urine (not red) in the bladder.
- Spleen and lymph nodes are enlarged.
- Collect smear from spleen and lymph nodes.

Trypanosomosis

- Emaciated carcass with pale mucosa.
- Enlargement of spleen, liver and lymph nodes and blood is watery in nature.
- Collect smear from liver, spleen and lymph node.
- Smear from CSF also shall be examined.

  NOTE: Trypanosomes could not be diagnosed in smears, if postmortem is delayed for a few hours.

Trichomonosis

- Affected tissue samples are to be placed in Trichomonas media (oxoid) to enhance the chances of isolation.

SAMPLING IN POISONINGS

Caution during collection of samples for diagnosis of poisoning:

- Act based on letter from Police department.
- Use chemically clean plastic containers and should make photographic evidences.
- Collect appropriate samples depending on poison suspected and properly label it and have duplicate samples and store the duplicate samples.
- Get acknowledgement letter from police officials for dispatch of samples in proper manner to forensic laboratory.

Cyanide Poisoning

- Stomach or rumen contents and parts of liver and muscle under refrigerated condition.
- Use 1% mercuric chloride as preservative with tissue samples.

Copper

- Liver tissue

Nitrate-Nitrite

- Stomach contents and 10 ml clotted blood sample **under** refrigerated condition.

Mercury

- Fresh liver and kidney tissues under refrigerated condition.
- Stomach and intestinal contents under refrigerated condition.

Ammonia

- Rumen contents under frozen condition.

Phosphorus

- Liver and stomach contents along with 30 ml oxalated blood under refrigerated condition.

Sodium Chloride

- Liver and whole brain under refrigerated condition.

Chlorinated Hydrocarbons

- Cerebrum in glass containers under refrigerated condition.

Organophosphorus

- Nervous tissues (brain), muscle or liver for estimation of choline esterase in freshly dead animals.
- One ml of heparinized blood.

Oxalates

- Kidney fixed in formalin.

Strychnine

- Liver, kidneys and stomach contents under refrigerated condition.

Arsenic

- Liver, kidney, vomitus and stomach contents under refrigerated condition.
- Urine samples under refrigerated condition.
- Hair samples (for diagnosis of chronic arsenic poisoning).

Fluoride

- Affected bone and urine samples under refrigerated condition.

Lead

- Liver and kidney (20 gm of tissue is required and all the containers must be lead free eg. plastic.
- Rumen contents and intestinal contents under refrigerated condition.

Phenols

- Rumen contents in air tight containers.

Selenium

- Liver and hair cloppings

Sulphates

- Brain fixed in formalin

Dicoumoral

- Liver

Zinc Phosphide

- Liver and gastric contents under frozen conditions.

CAUTIONS DURING SAMPLING OF BIOLOGICAL SAMPLES

Caution during collection of urine samples from bladder

- Use always sterile needle and syringe and use sterile bottle or tube with cap and transfer it under refrigerated condition.
- Don't store urine samples at room temperature for more than a few hours esp. if urine-culture is to be undertaken.

Caution during collection of fecal and worm samples

- Place the moist faecal samples from GI tract into tube with cap and placc it under refrigerated condition.
- If delay is expected for examination, use 10% formalin with the faecal sample to prevent the embryonation.
- If adult worms are encountered, use 5% formal-saline as preservative for them.

Caution during collection of swabs

- Always use sterile swabs to collect materials and place it in transport media like Stuart's (or) Amies' media, if bacterial examination is warranted and use PBS, if examination for virus is warranted.

Caution during collection of serous cavity-fluids

- No preservative is to be added to the serous cavity-fluids.
- If the inflammatory lesion is suspected and the protein content of the fluid is likely to be high, it is wise to place the samples into EDTA to prevent coagulation.
- Always transport the serous fluid collected in a sterile container under refrigerated condition.

The following materials are needed for documenting a necropsy:

- Field note book
- Measuring cylinder
- Measuring tape
- Spring balance
- Camera / Videocamera

Necropsy personnel should protect themselves against contracting infectious diseases from wild animals:

The protective clothing includes-

- Rubber / polythene apron
- Latex gloves
- Gum boots
- Face shield / masks / Eye goggles

The minimal equipments needed for conducting necropsy include the followings:

- Small and large scissors
- Small and large knives
- Knife sharpening reel
- Bone cutters and saw
- Chisel and hammer
- Small and large forceps

The basic specimen sampling kit should include the followings:

- Microscopic slides, with container for storing slides
- Microscopic glass cover slips
- Tissue paper roll / Cotton.
- Filter paper
- Marker pen & fluorescent-stickers.
- Histopathological tissue containers- 500 ml capacity (leak proof ones).

The kit for microbiological sampling includes the followings:

- Sterile cotton swabs.
- Spirit lamp and match box.
- Spatula
- Bardparker handle and blades.
- Sterile syringes and needles- 2, 5, 10, 20 ml
- Sterile containers, leak proof – 2, 50, 100 ml
- String, sealing tape / Parafilm.
- Phosphate-buffered saline solution (PBS for diagnosis of viral pathogens).

Storage materials for biological samples:

- 10% buffered formalin for histo-pathology
- 100% acetone for cytology
- Normal saline / 70% ethyl alcohol for parasites
- Sterile transport media for bacteria & virus
- Ice box

Pre-requisites for post-mortem

- Collect Details of Animal Particulars

  (Name, Zoological Name, Sex, Species, Age)
- Enquire Time,Date And Place of Death
- Obtain Clinical History- Signs & Therapy
- Conduct Necropsy Under Good
- White Light
- Knowledge on Taxonomy

ORDER	:	Primates
SUB-ORDER	:	Anthrapoidea
SUPERFAMILY	:	Hominoidea
FAMILY	:	Pongidae
GROUP	:	Greater apes
ZOOLOGICAL NAME	:	*Pan troglodytes*

External examination of the carcase

- Check the identity of the carcass
- Assess the condition of carcass
- Check for wounds, injuries, fractures
- Examine for external parasites
- Examine the natural orifices for any discharge
- Examine the visible mucosa
- Examine for fractures/dislocations

Smear preparation

- Collect thin peripheral blood smears before opening the carcass for internal examination
- Collect smears from discharges
- Collection of peripheral blood for smear preparation

Examination of individual organs:

- Examine the surface of organs.
- Incise the parenchymatous organs in multiple locations and examine the cut surface.

- Examine the contents of organs with lumen.
- Examine the mucosa for lesions.
- Examine the digestive tract at the end.

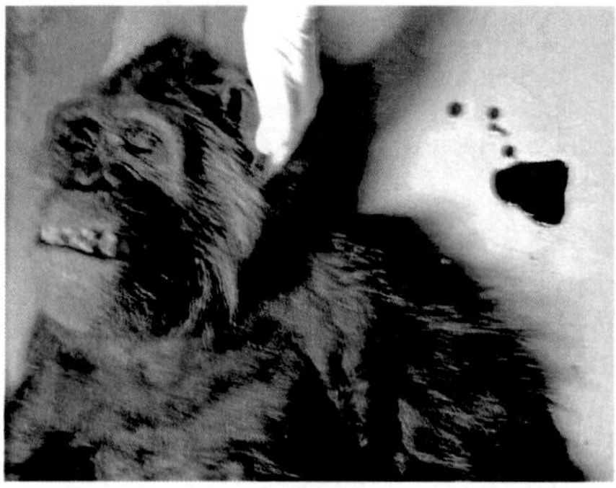

Fig. 1. (Carcase of Chimpanzee)

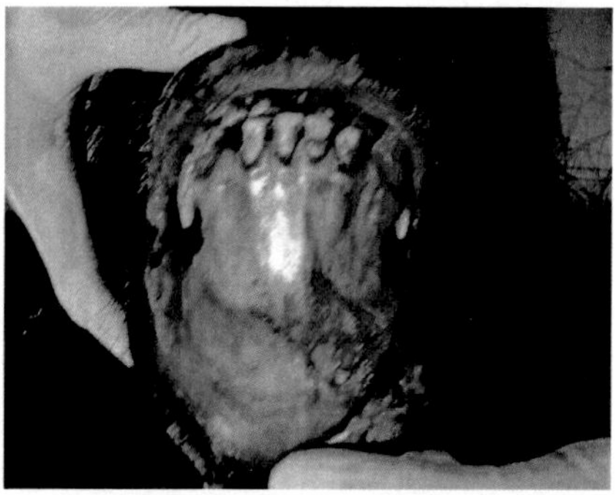

Fig. 2. (Ulceration in buccal cavity)

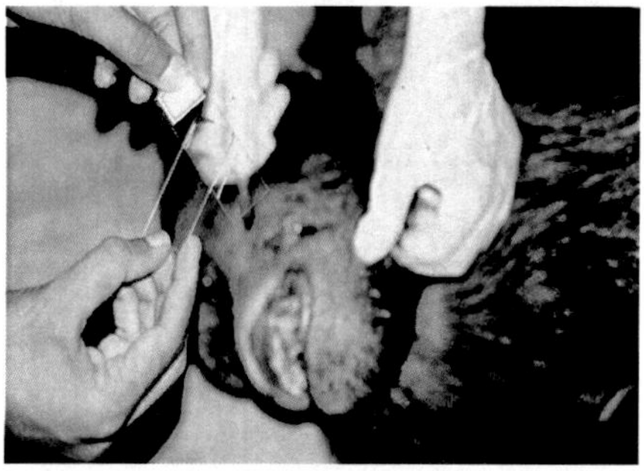

Fig. 3. (Blood smear-collection to rule out anthrax)

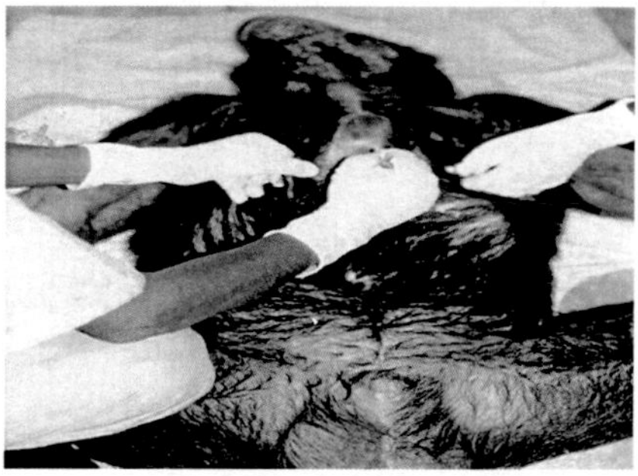

Fig. 4. (Longitudinal incision at thorax)

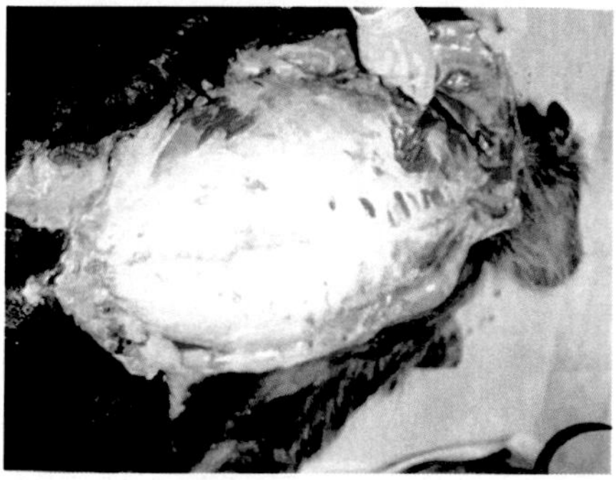

Fig. 5. (Separation of skin in ventral region)

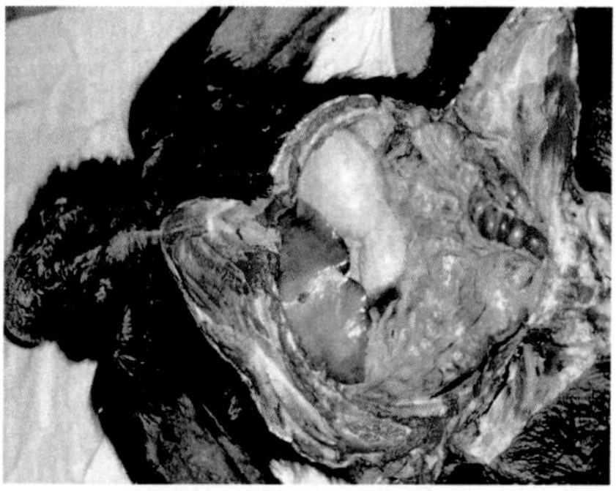

Fig. 6. (Exposure of viscera in ventral abdomen)

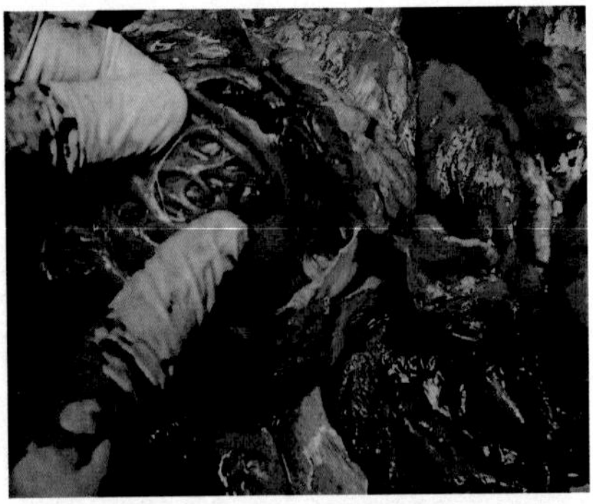

Fig. 7. (Examination of cardiac chambers)

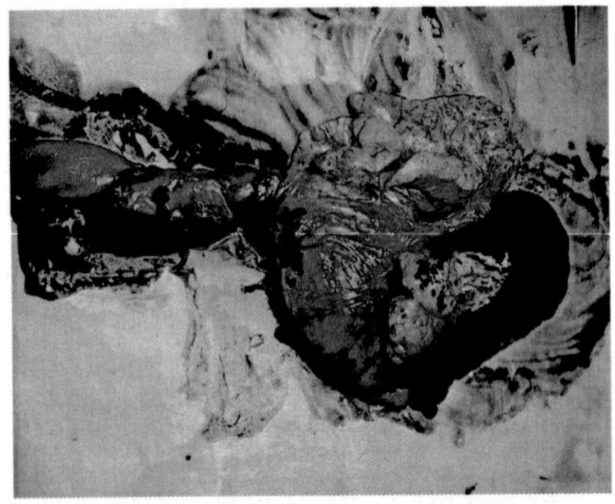

Fig. 8. (Haemorrhagic Lung: unilateral)

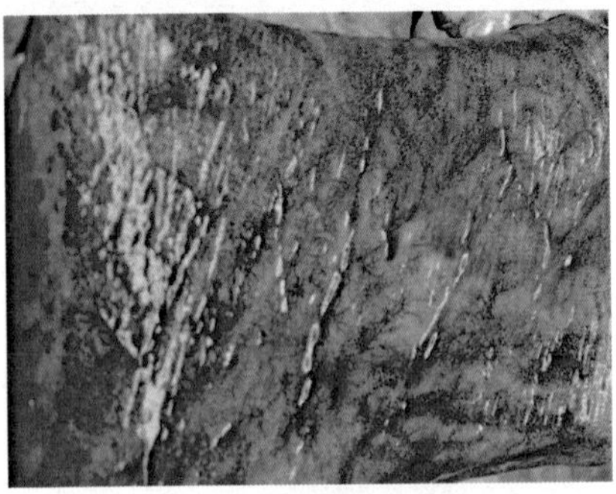

Fig. 9. (Pyloric region revealing haemorrhagic lesions)

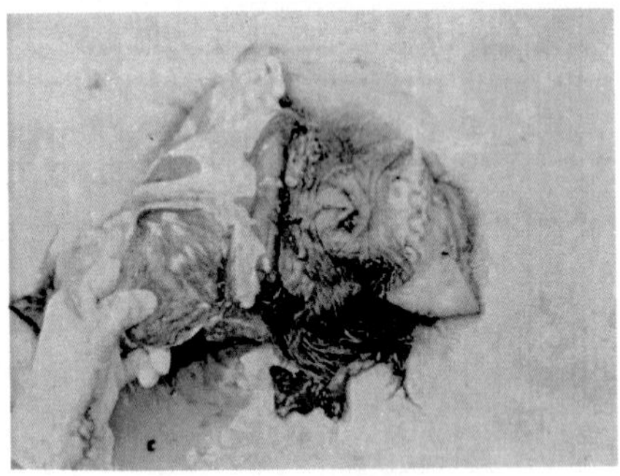

Fig. 10. Exposure of brain-region

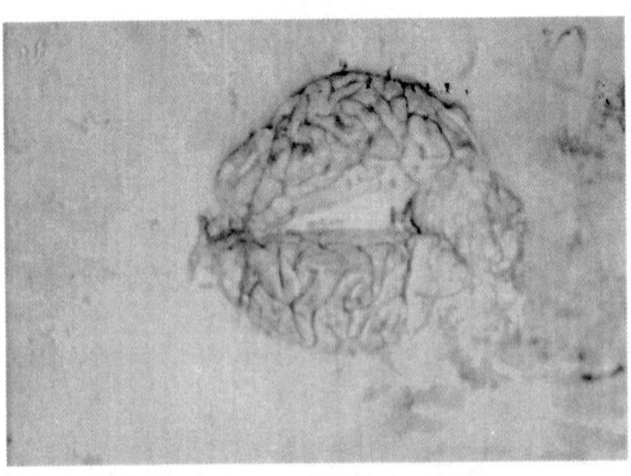

Fig. 11. Examination of brain

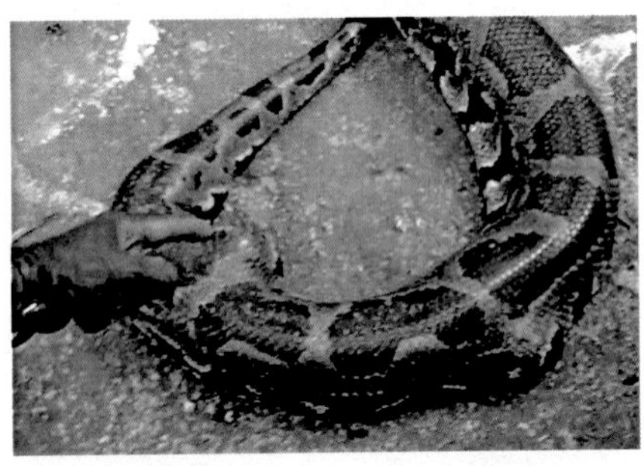

Fig. 12. Examination of skin-lumps in python

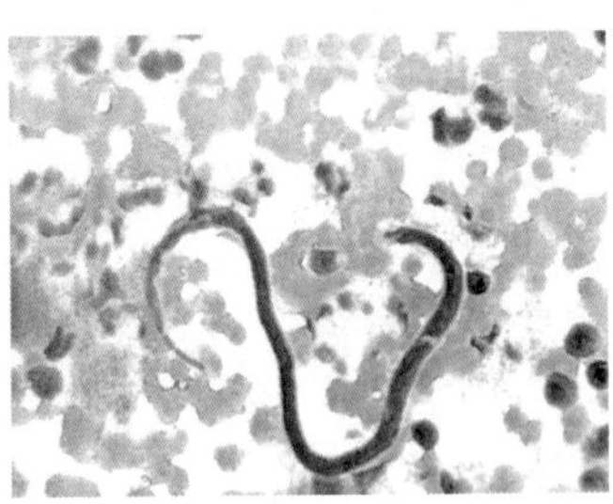

Fig. 13. (Microfilaria in blood smear of elephant calf)

Colour Plates

Chapter 9: Bacterial Diseases in Wild Animals

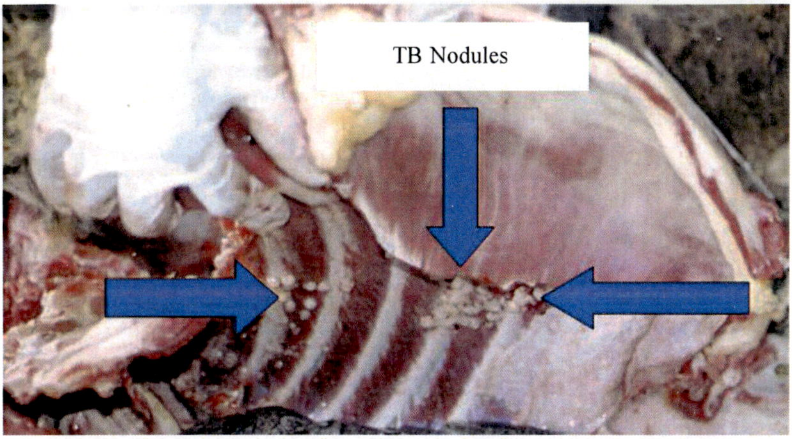

Fig. 1. (TB nodules on organs)

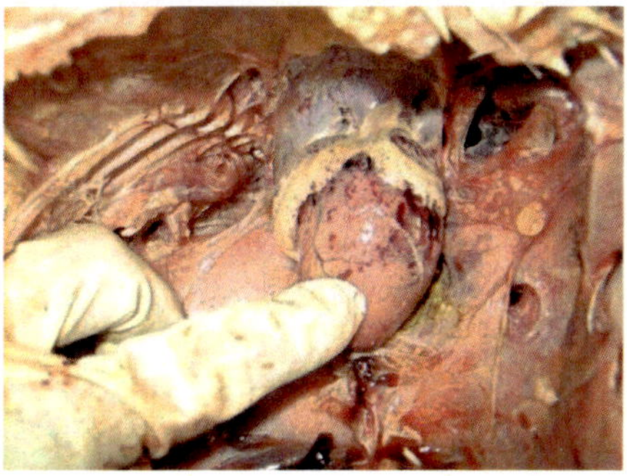

Fig. 2. (Haemorrhagic spots on heart)

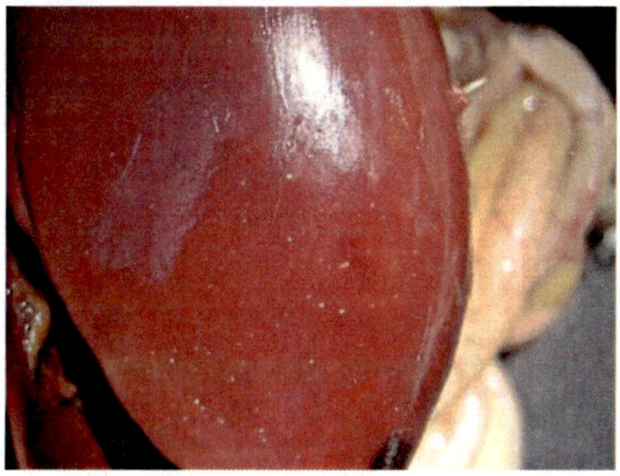

Fig. 3. (Necrotic foci on liver)

Chapter 10: Viral Disease in Wild Animals

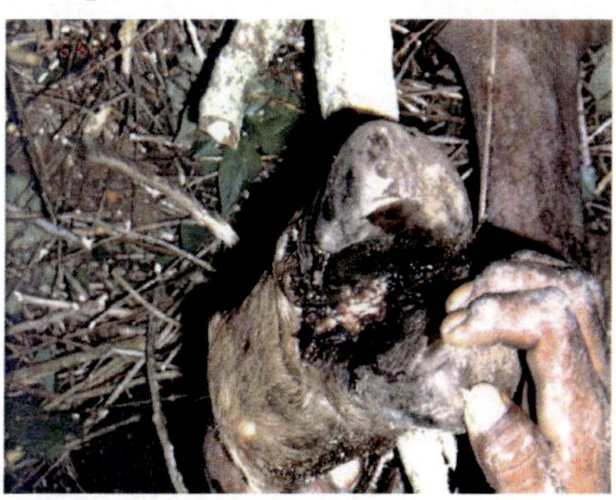

Fig. 5. Ulcer in inter-hoof area

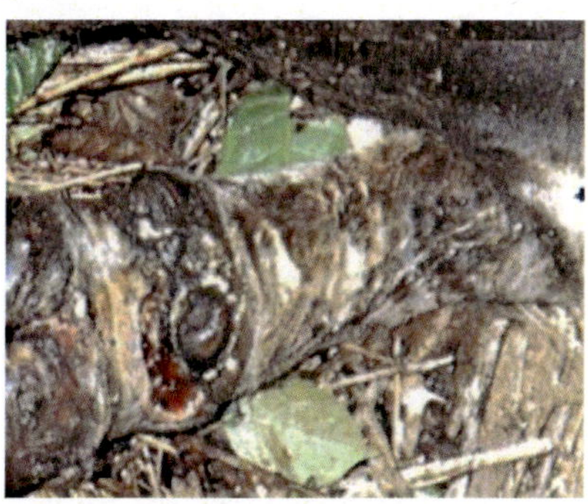

Fig. 6. Ulcer at skin near hoof

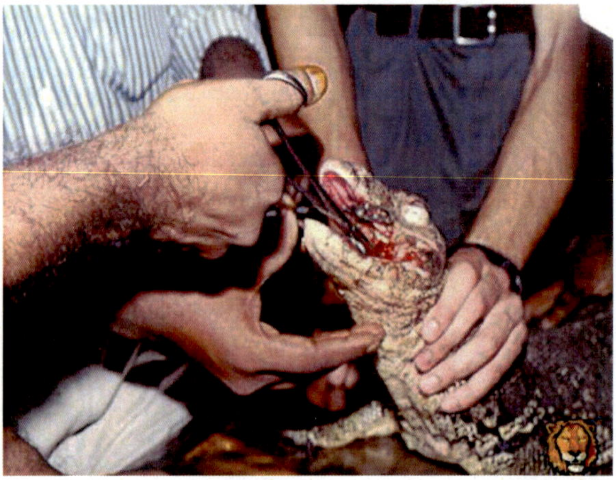

Fig. 7. Extraction of tumour like growth from oral region of reptile

Chapter 11: Parasitic Diseases in Wild Animals

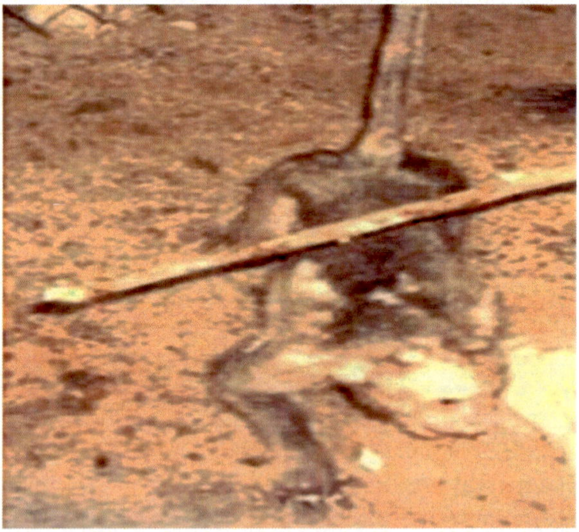

Fig. 1. Patchy distribution of hairless patches in Bonnet macaque

Chapter 12: Field Based Identificationof Evidences on Different Parasitic Fauna in Captive Wild Animals

Ancylostoma sp. egg (oval, thin-shell, segmented yolk containing usually 8 cells)

Spirocerca sp. egg (thick shelled and gelatin shape with fully developed larvae inside).

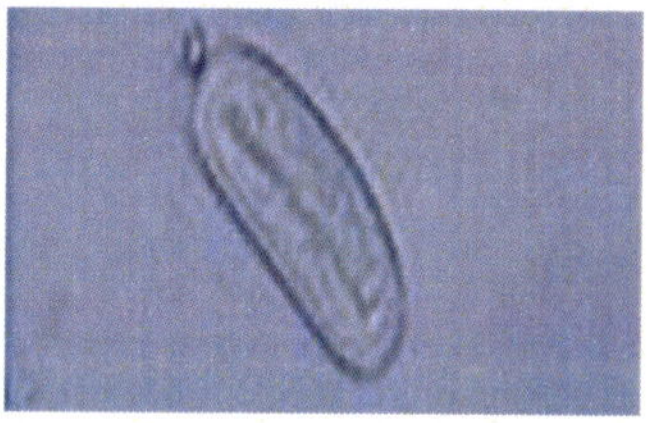

Paragonimus sp.egg (yellowish brow with operculum & shell thickened at opposite pole).

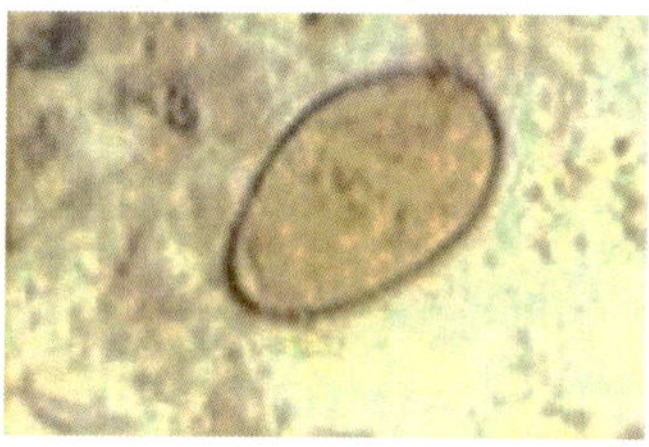

Dipylidium sp. egg (thick plain shell with hexacanth embryo).

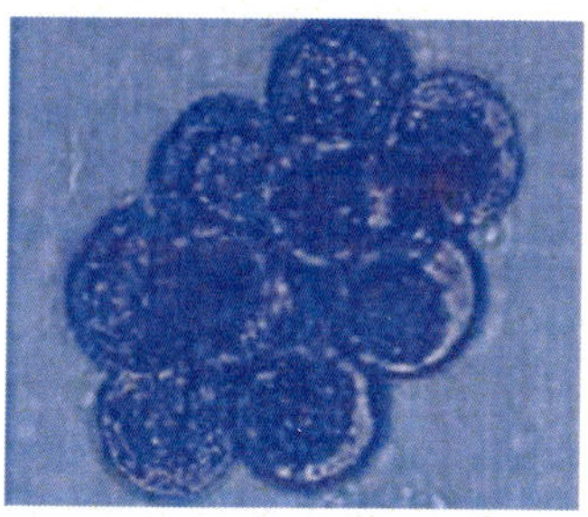

Spirometra sp. egg (yellowish brown, both ends are pointed, presence of operculum and contains yolk cells).

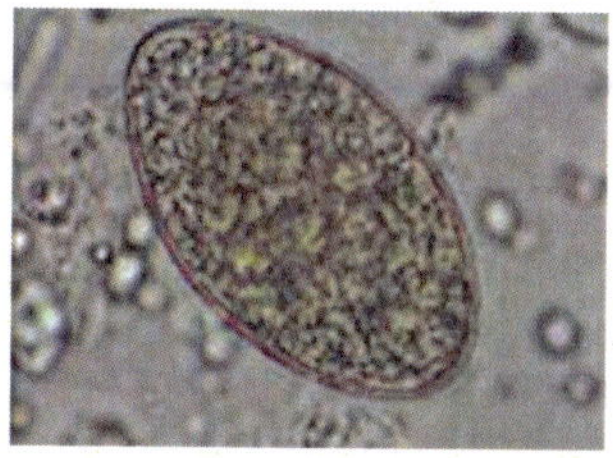

Echnococcus sp. egg (typical taenid egg, circular, thick shelled with radial striations, yellow tinted and hexacanth embryo).

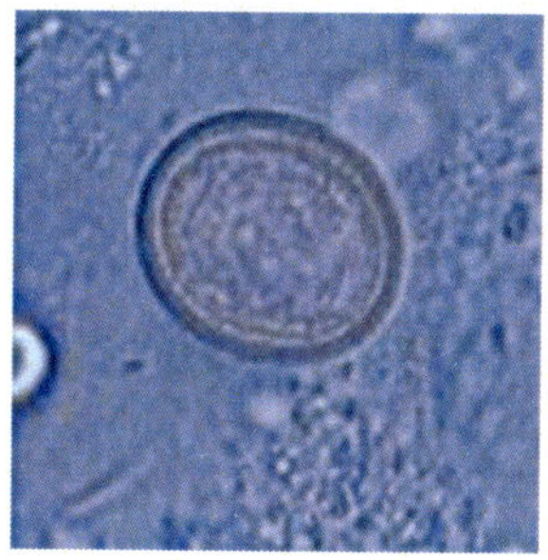

Diphyllobothrium sp. egg (oval shape, yellowish brown, rounded ends, operculum & contains yolk cells).

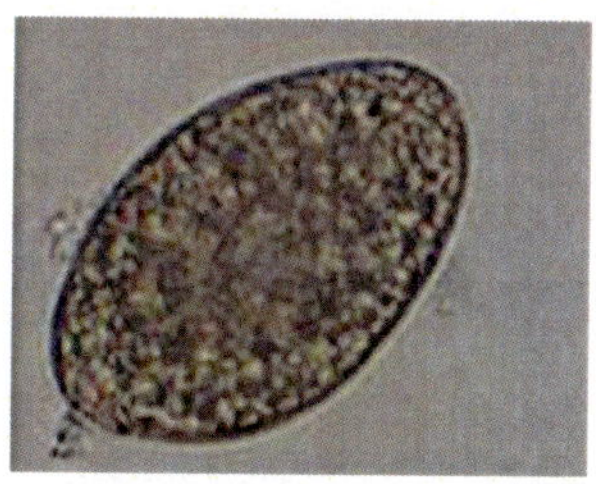

Toxocara canis egg (thick and finely pitted shell with compact yolk inside and egg of *Toxocara cati*is also similar to this).

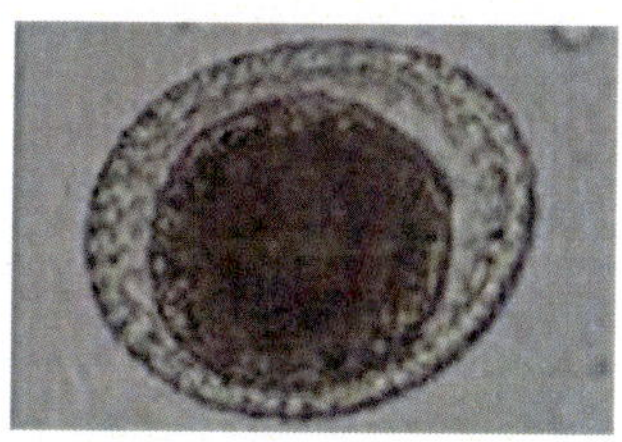

Toxocara leonina egg (mildly oval with thick & smooth shell).

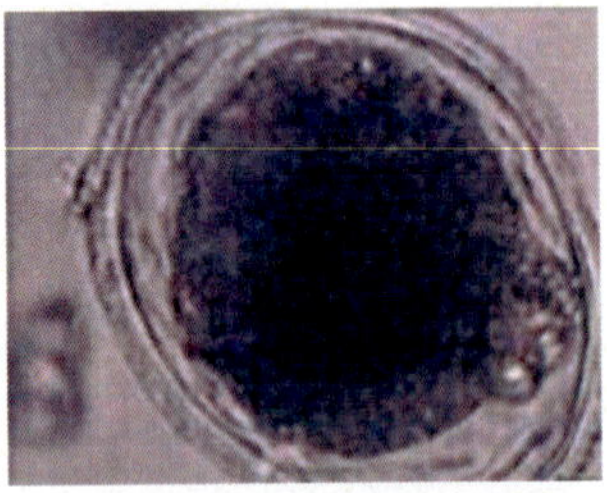

Microfilaria of (***Dirofilaria*** sp.) in blood smear(elongate with a straight tail and tapered head).

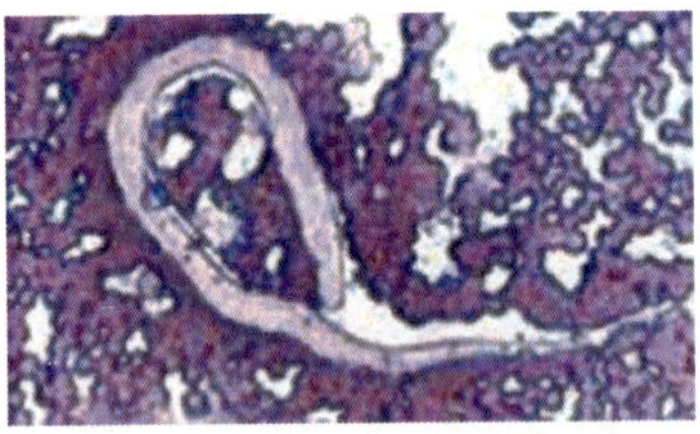

Physaloptera sp.

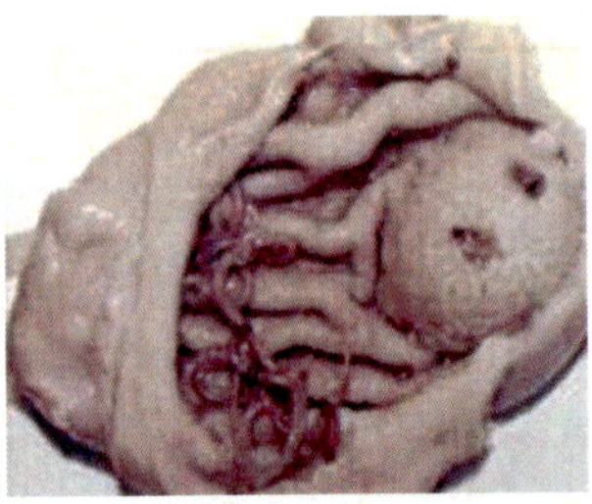

Trichuris sp. egg (brownish, transparent plug at either pole, with unsegmented embryo inside)

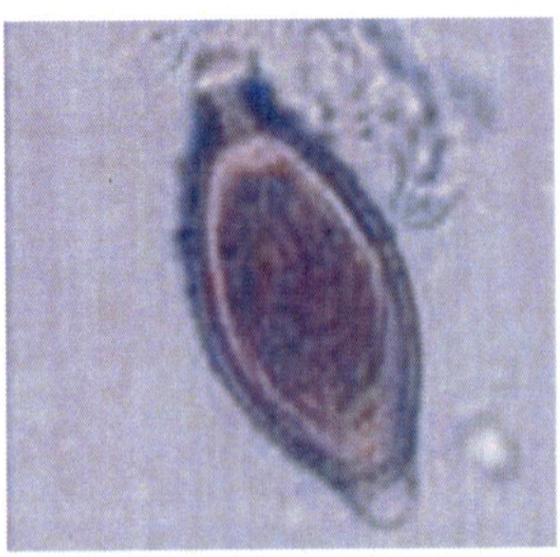

Babesia canis *in blood smear* (Merozoite inside RBC with pyriform bodies lying at an angle to one another but the merozoite of B. gibsoni in the RBC is annular or oval or signet ring form).

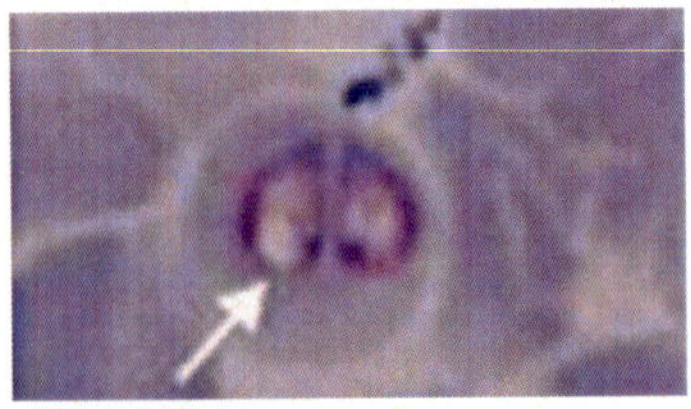

Trypanosoma evansi in blood smear (Free flagella and well developed undulating membrane).

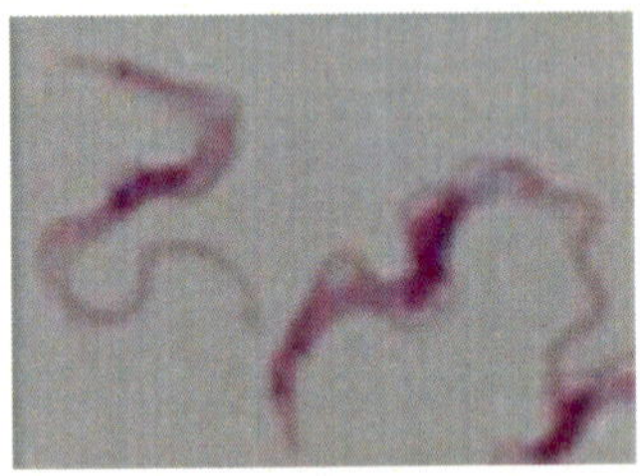

Hepatozoon canis in blood smear(garments commonly occur in leukocytes, gelatin globule shape, dark reddish purple nucleus with horse-shoe shaped chromatin usually at one end).

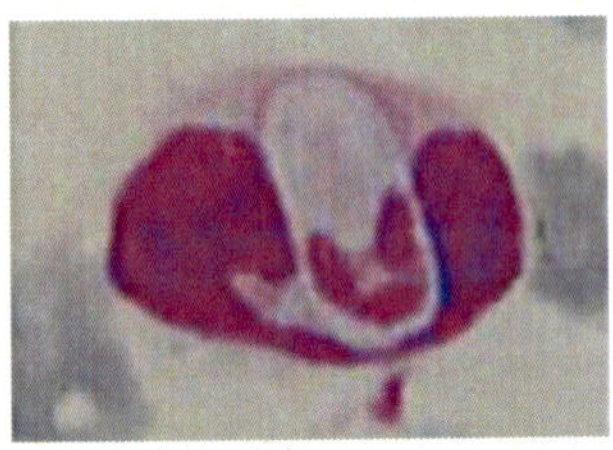

Ehrlichia canis in blood smear (single or compact colonies of inclusion bodies ie. morulae, as intracytoplasmic forms in the circulating WBCs).

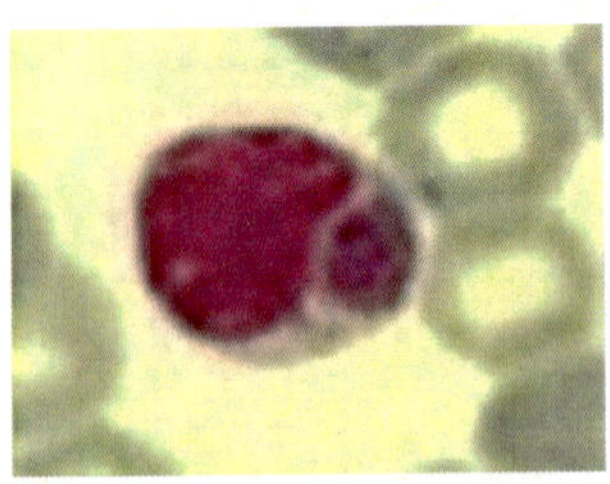

Isospora felis (ovoid and sporulated oocyst with 2 sporocyst and each sporocyst with 4 sporozoites).

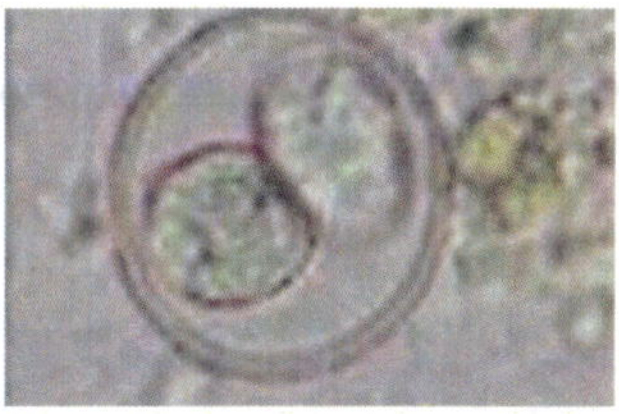

Toxoplasma gondii (spherical and sporulated oocyst with 2 sporocysts and each sporocyst with 4 sporozoites).

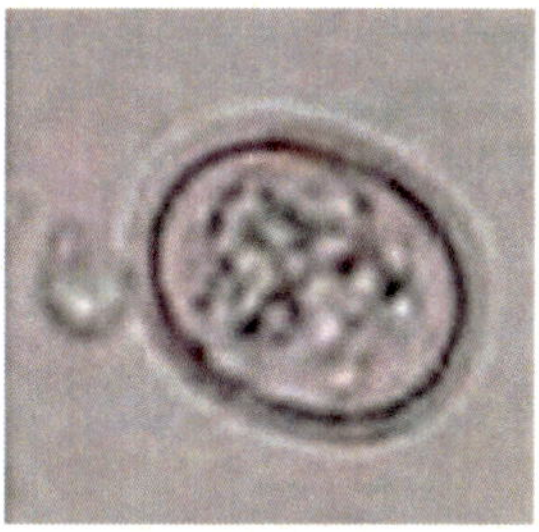

Fasciola gigantica egg (large, oval and yellowish with indistinct operculum and contains yolk cells and germ cells).

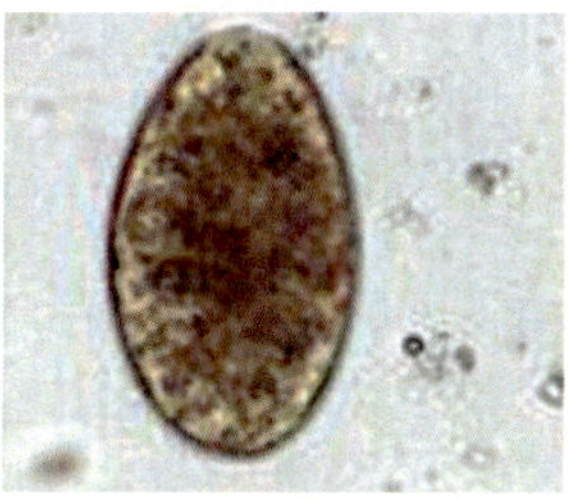

Amphistome egg (clear and pearly in appearance ie. non-tinted and distinct operculum and contains yolk cells and germ cells).

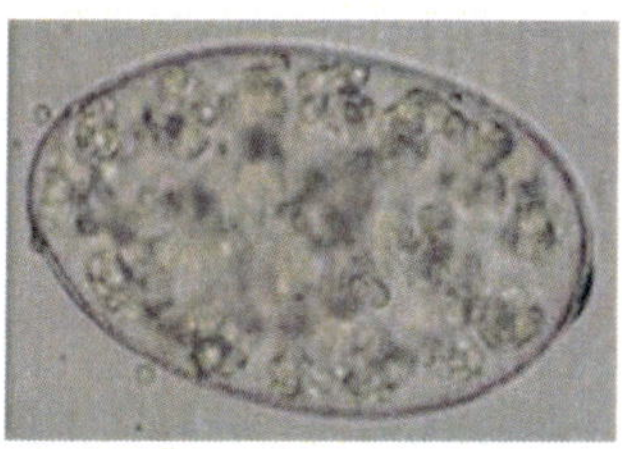

Amphistomes in wall of rumen.

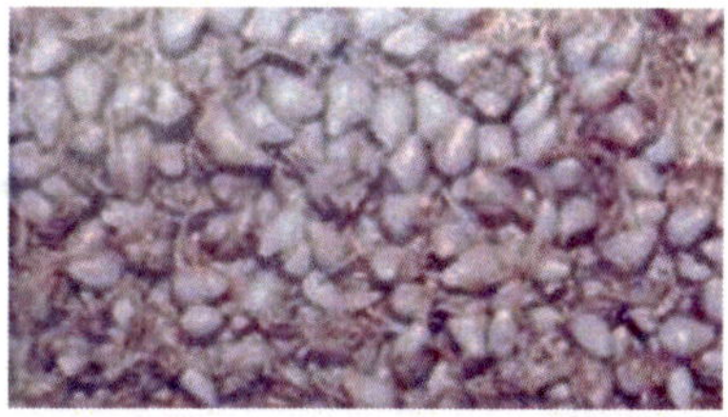

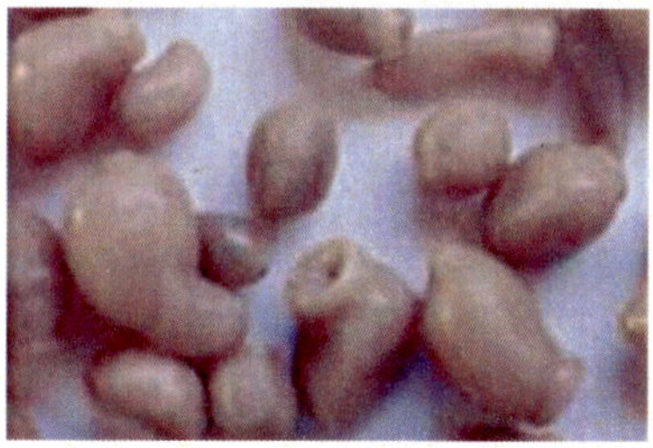

Moniezia spp. (Triangular or squarish shape with well developed pyriform apparatus and contains hexacanth embryo).

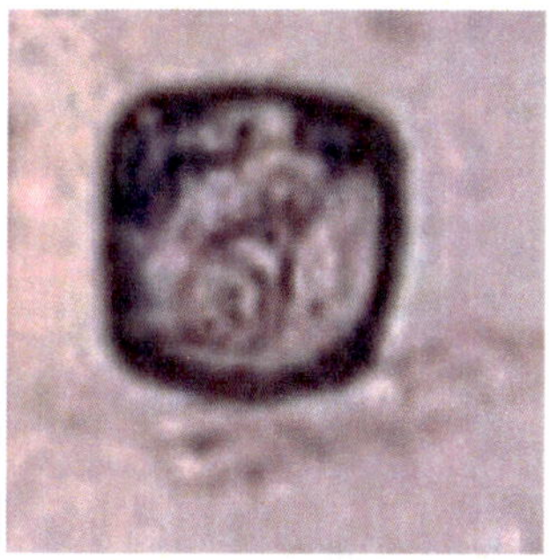

Anoplocephala sp. worm (in small intestine of elephant / rhinoceros).

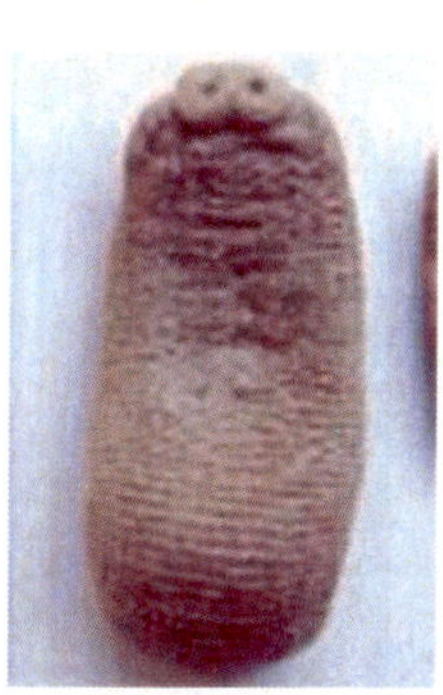

Hydatid cyst (liver)

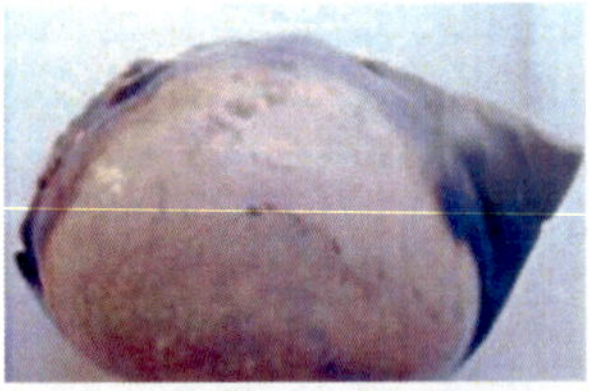

Protoscolices from the hydatid cyst- fluid

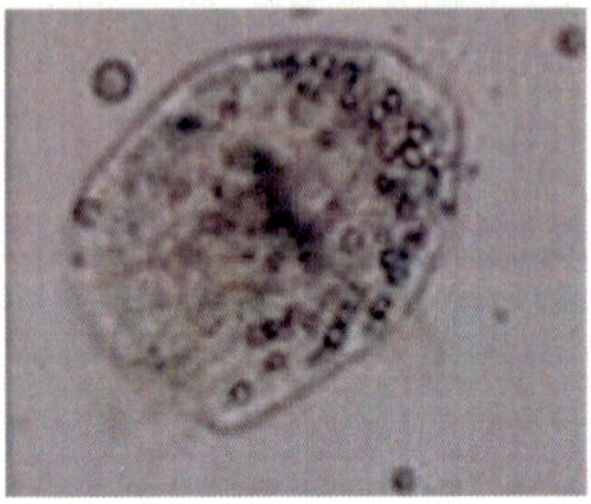

Cyst in Cysticercosis due to ***Cysticercus tenuicollis***

This is associated with the tape worm-*Taenia hydatigena* and the cyst is fluid filled and is about 5 cm in diameter, attached to various organs on the peritoneal surface.

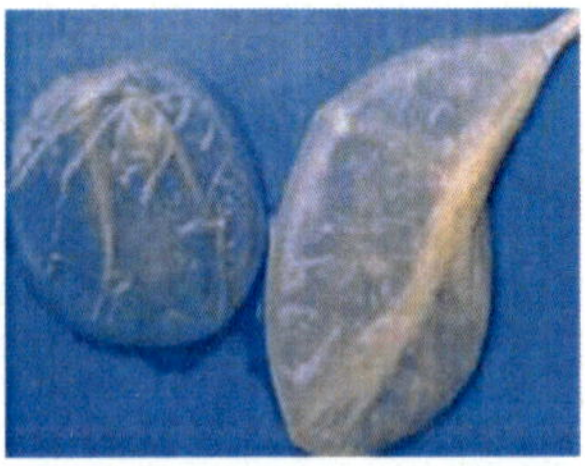

***Ascaris suum* egg** (ovoid, thick shelled with prominent projections and brownish yellow and the unsegmented yolk seen as a compact mass).

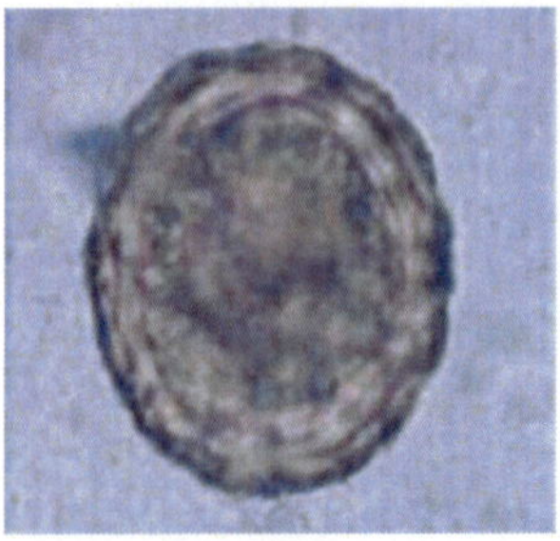

Toxocara vitulorum egg (subglobular, finely pitted albuminous layer and thick shelled with compact yolk).

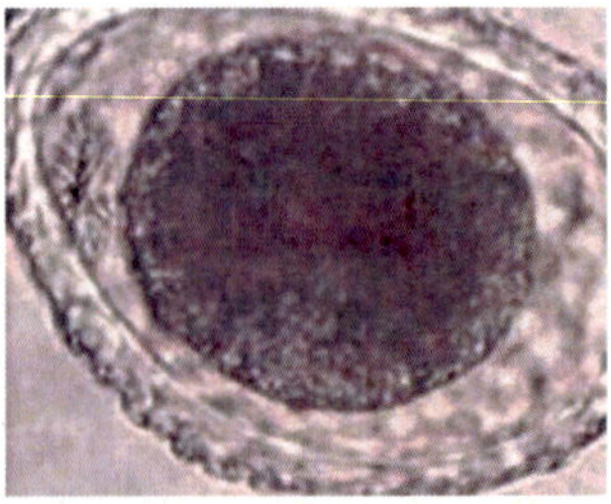

Strongyle egg (eg. *Haemonchus* sp. and *Bunostomum* sp.): oval, thin shelled and segmented yolk inside).

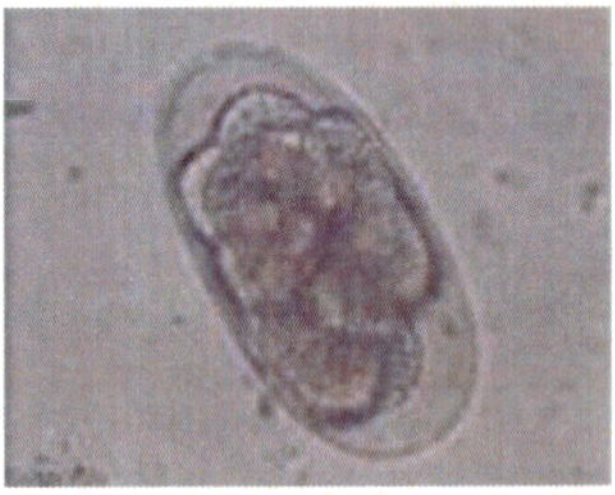

Strongyloides spp. egg (thick shell with both ends blunt and well developed embryo inside the egg).

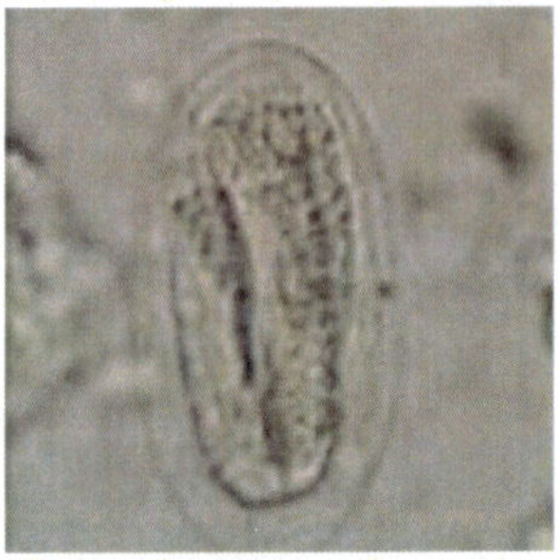

Trichuris sp. egg (brownish, barrel shaped, transparent plug at either pole and contains unsegmented embryo).

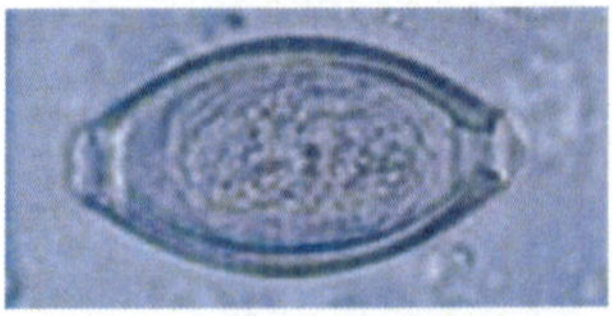

Oxyuris equi egg (creamy colored masses of eggs, flattened one side and presence of plug at one pole; egg in enterobiosis ie. pinworm infection, caused by *enterobius vermicularis* is also similar to egg of *Oxyuris equi*).

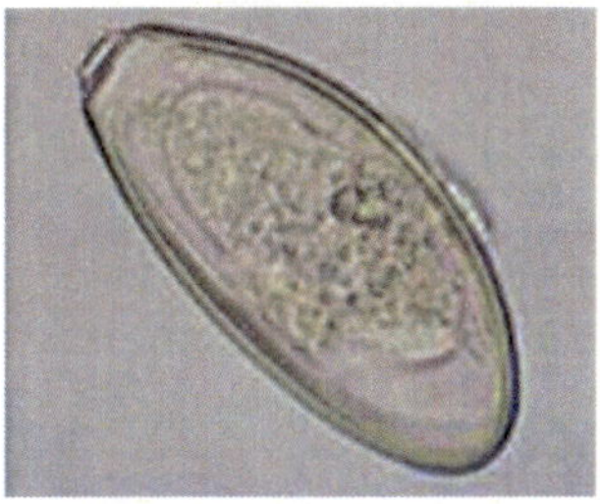

Theileria spp. (merozoites of multiple shapes ie. round, oval, comma or shaped, within the RBCs and schizonts called as Kochs blue bodies as irregularly oval or rounded matrix with numerous chromatin particles in the cytoplasm of the lymphocytes).

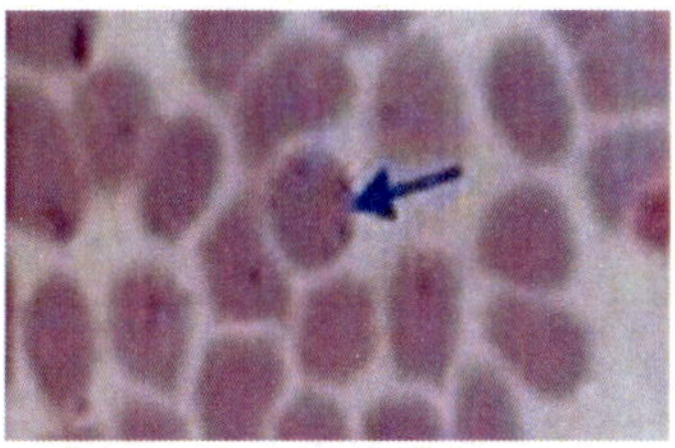

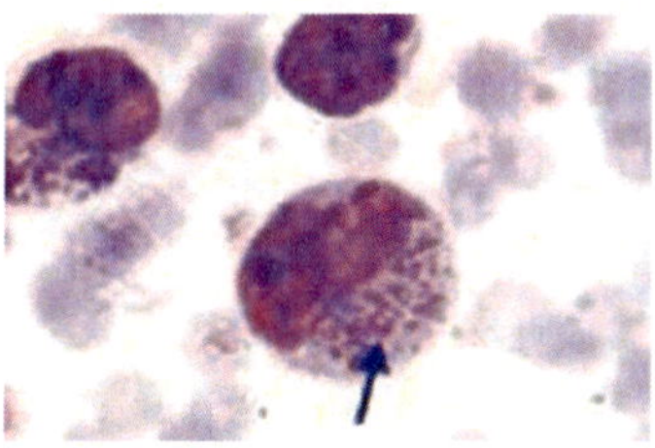

Anaplasma marginale (small spherical red to dark red bodies in the margin of RBCs).

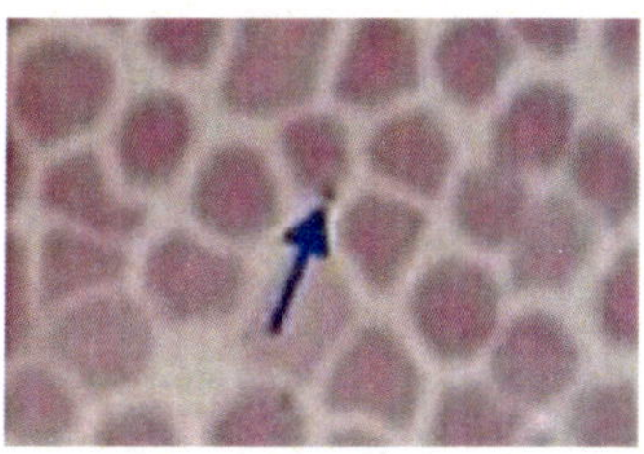

Cysts of ***Entamoeba histolytica*** (round shape with 4 distinct nuclei and chromatoid bodies).

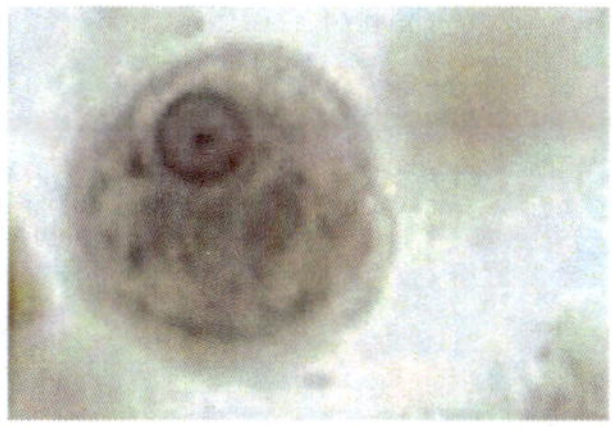

Cysts of ***Giardia lamblia*** (ellipsoidal, bilarterally symmetrical resembling a pear that is cut in half longitudinally) and anterior end is broad and round, while the posterior end is drawn out and presence of two or four nuclei).

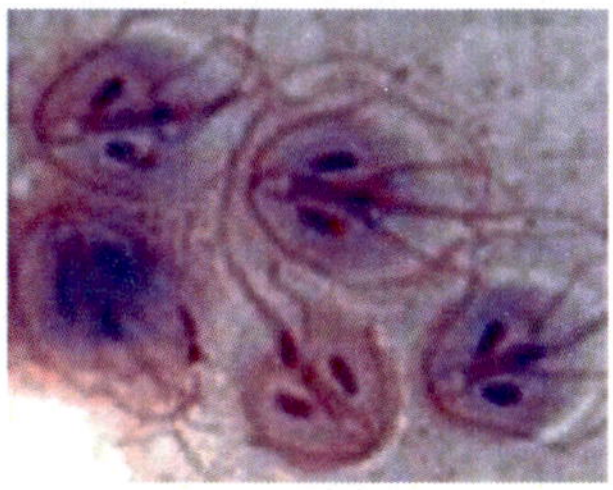

Coccidial oocyst (presence of sporocysts containing sporozoites within the oocyst).

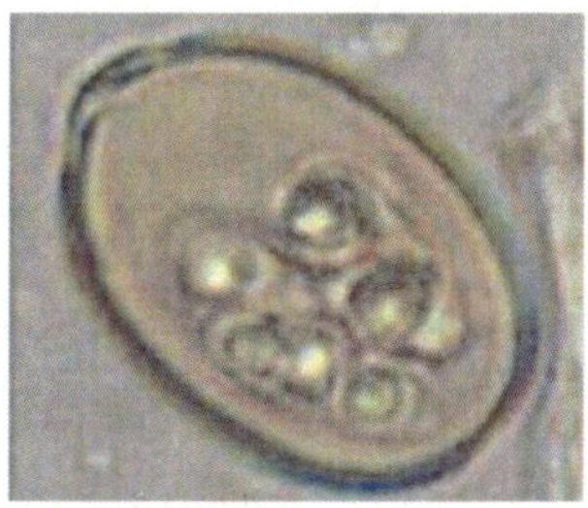

Cyst of ***Balantidium coli*** (ovoid or spherical and is faintly yellowish or greenish with presence of macronucleus and the cyst wall has 2 membranes).

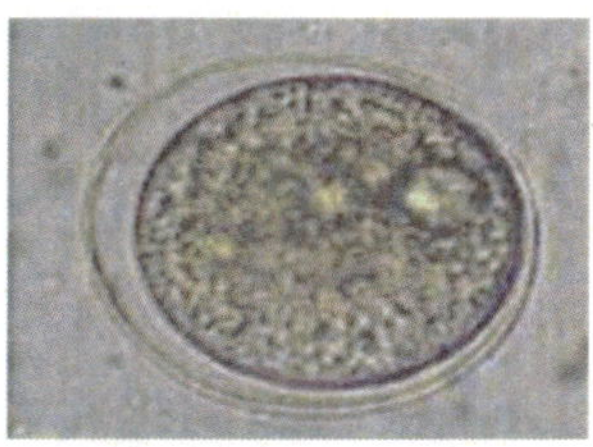

Cobboldia cobboldi maggot (in stomach of elephant).

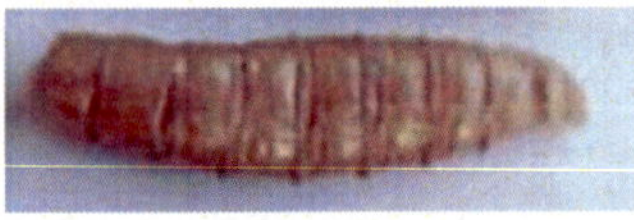

Ctenocephalides felis (flea)

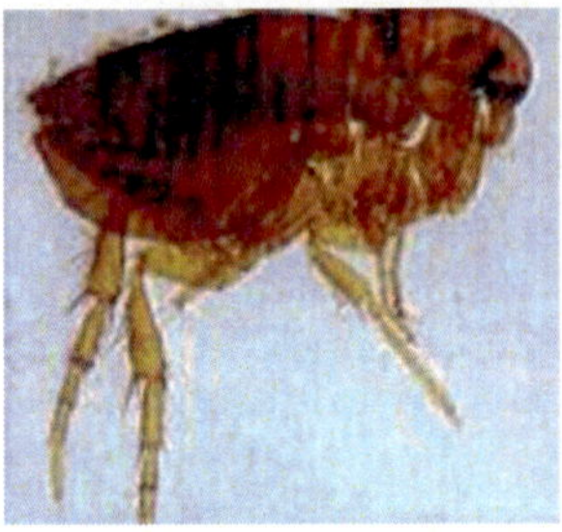

Rhipicephalus sanguineus (tick)

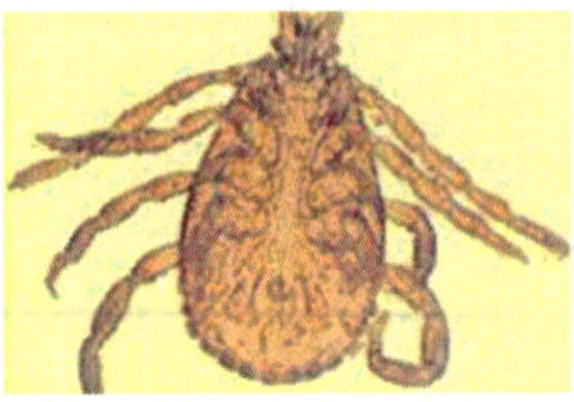

Nits (egg of lice)

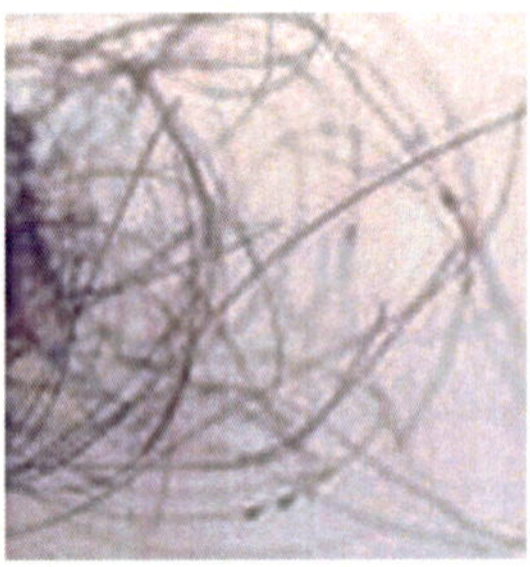

Demodex sp. (burrowing mite)

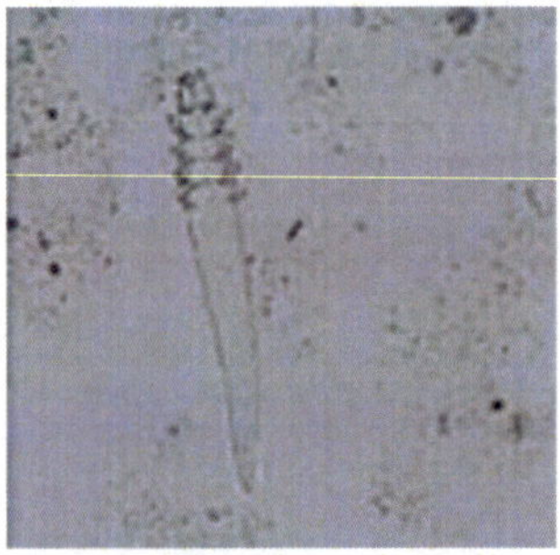

Sarcoptes sp. (mite)

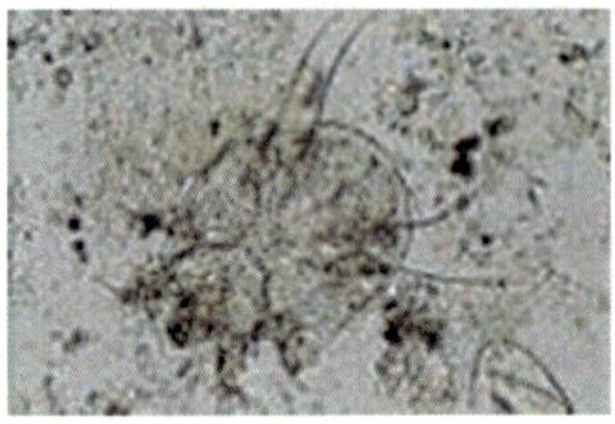

Chapter 20: Reptilian Features

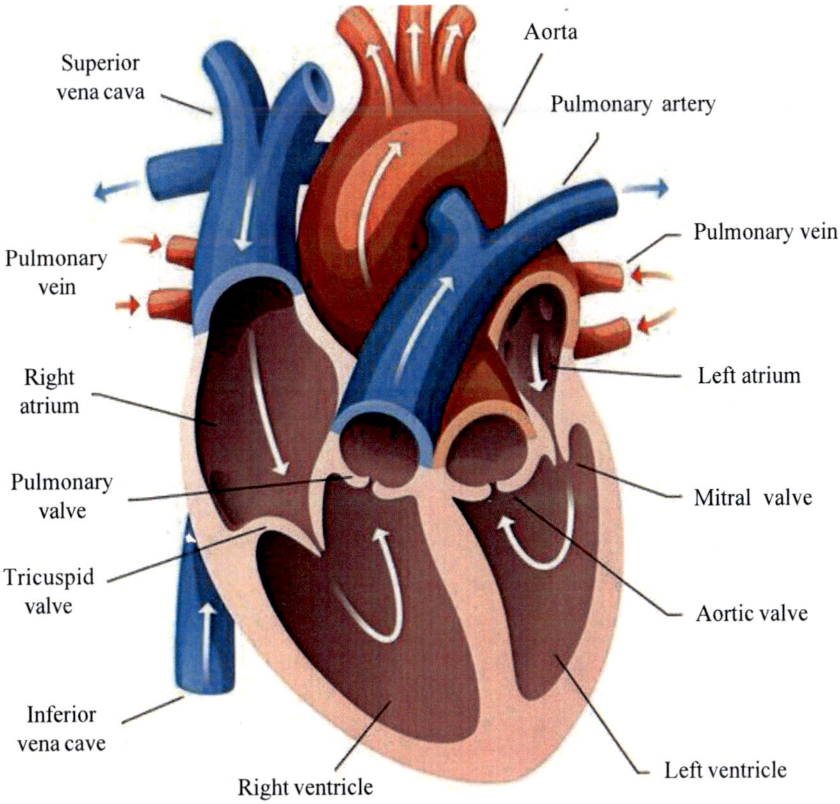

Fig. 1. Normal mammalian heart

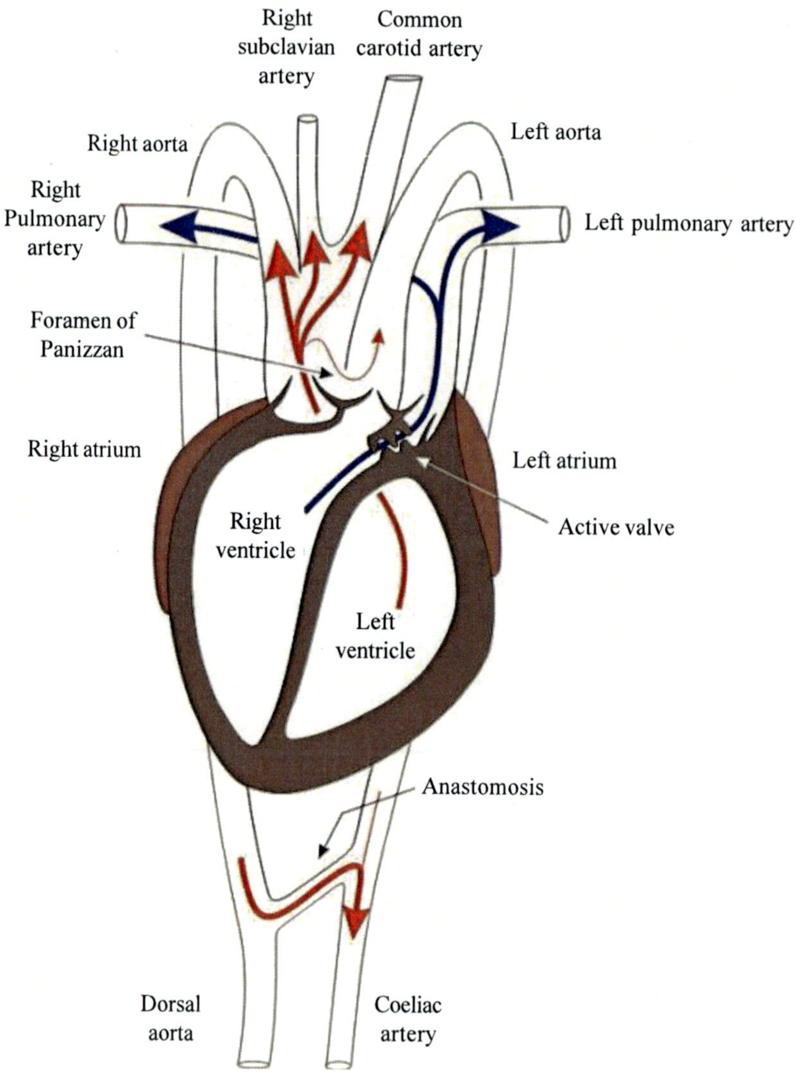

Fig. 2. Blood circulation in crocodile

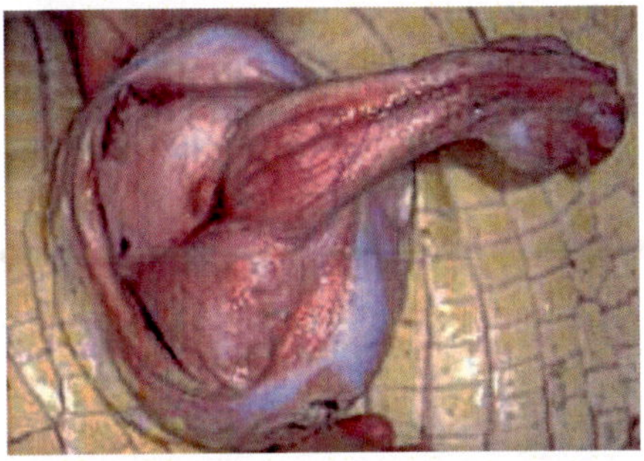

Fig. 3. Rigid penis ie. os penis of crocodile

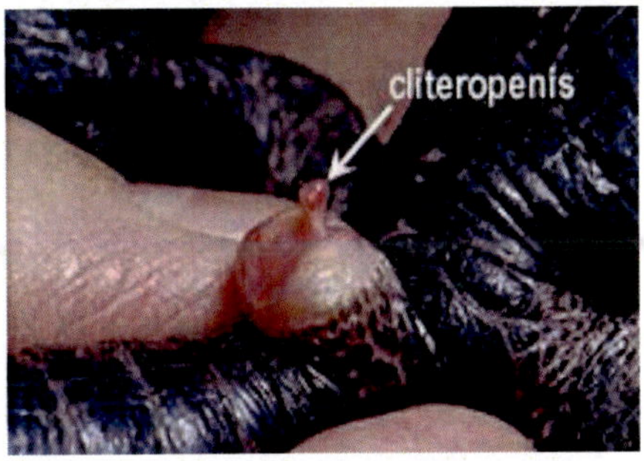

Fig. 4. Cliteropenis of crocodile

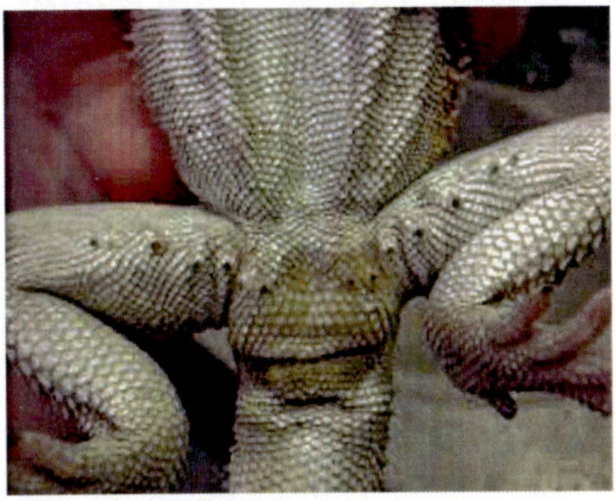

Fig. 5. Femoral pores in lizard

Chapter 21: Clinical Examination of Aves

The Respiratory System

The Respiratory System

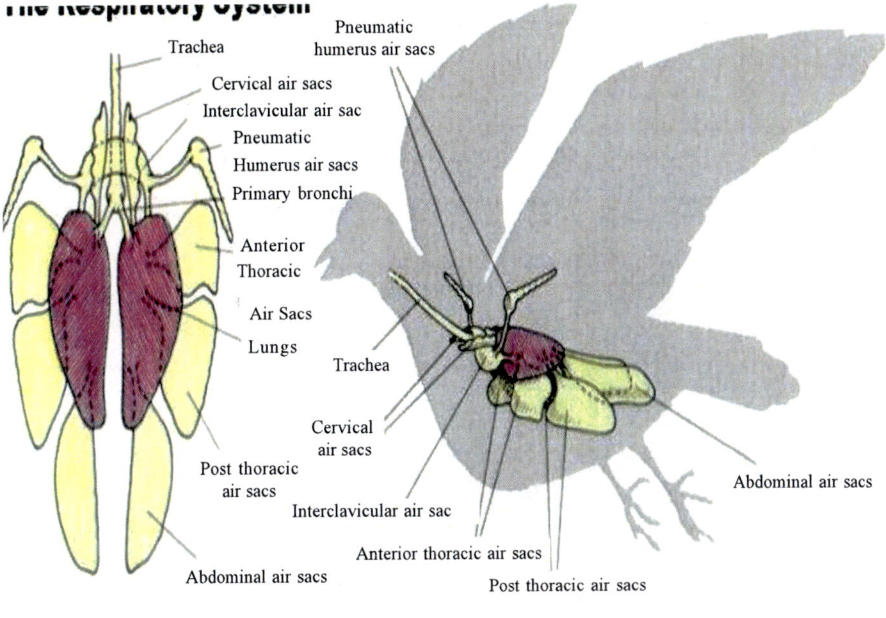

Fig. 1. Air sacs in aves-a speciality

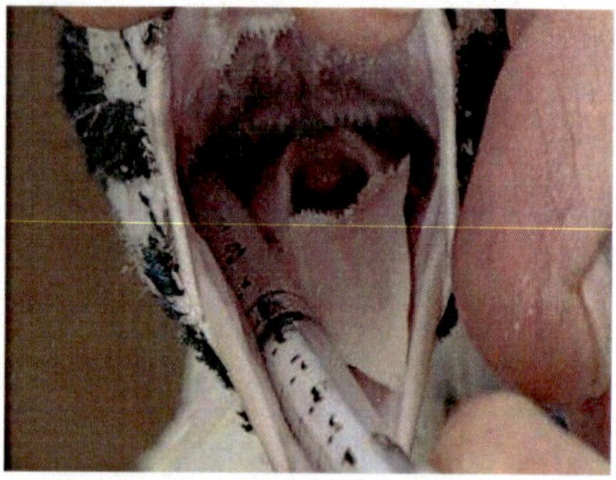

Fig. 5. Oral delivery of drugs in birds

Chapter 33: Blood Collectionin Different Species of Wild Animals

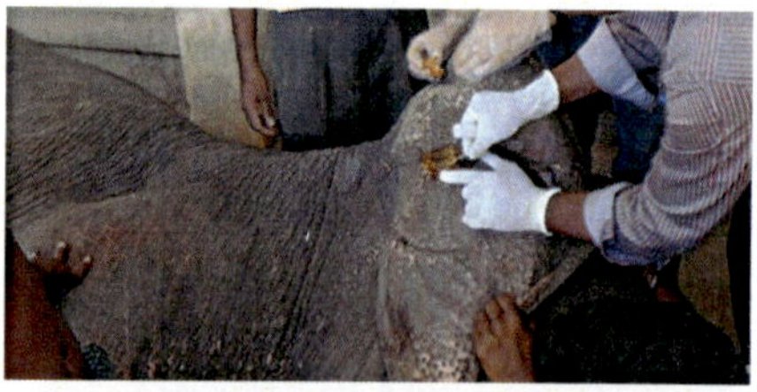

Fig. 5. Loacation of external-ear vein in elephant

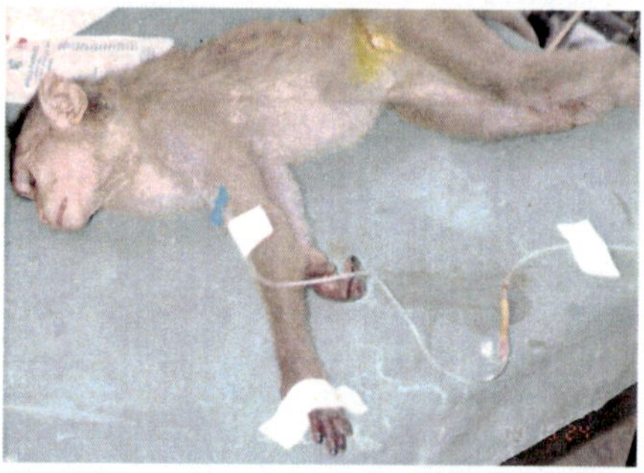

Fig. 8. Loacation of cephalic vein in Bonnet macaque

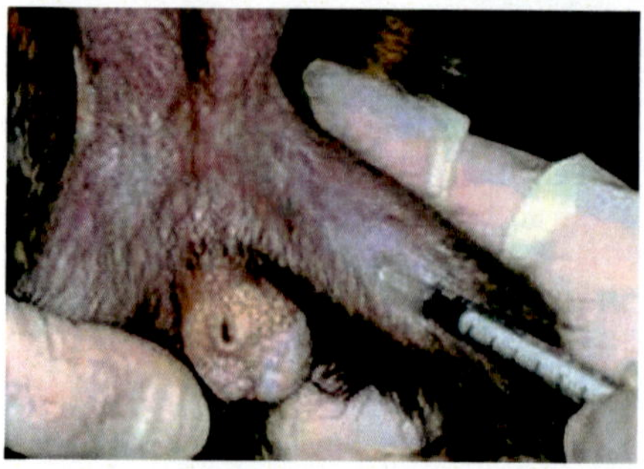

Fig. 9. Loacation of femoral vein in NH primate

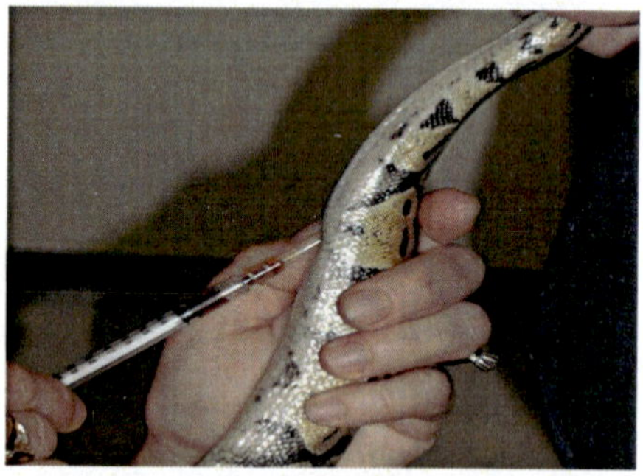

Fig. 10. Loacation of tail-vein: posteriror area to cloaca in snake

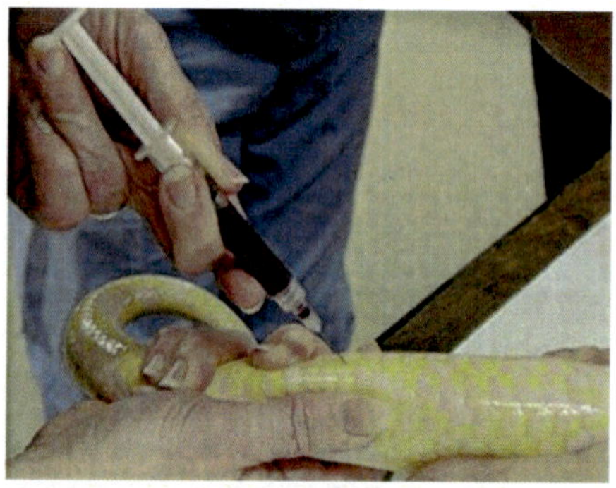

Fig. 11. Loacation of tail-vein for collection of blood

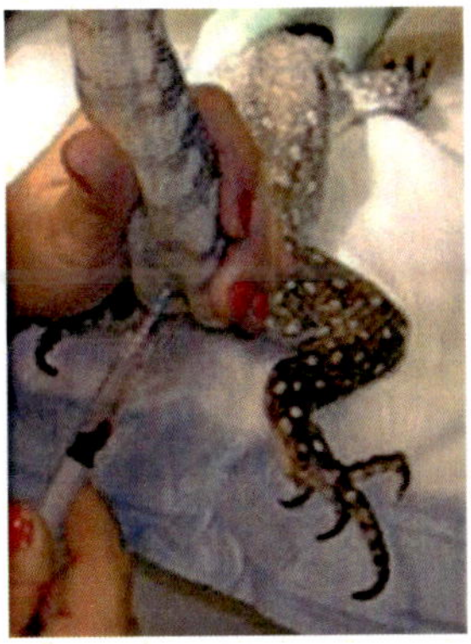

Fig. 12. Loacation of tail-vein in lizard

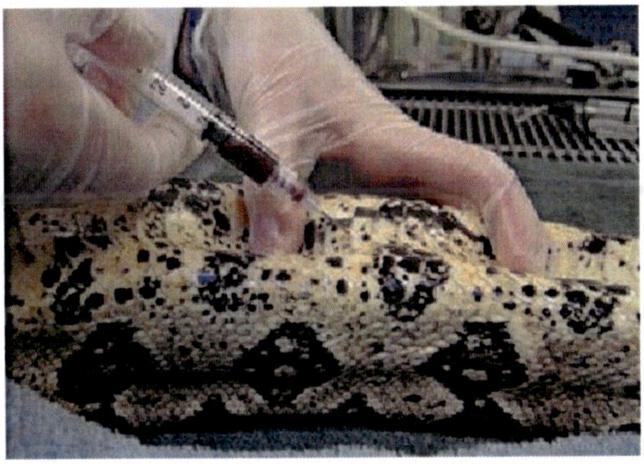

Fig. 13. Intra-cardial blood collection from snake

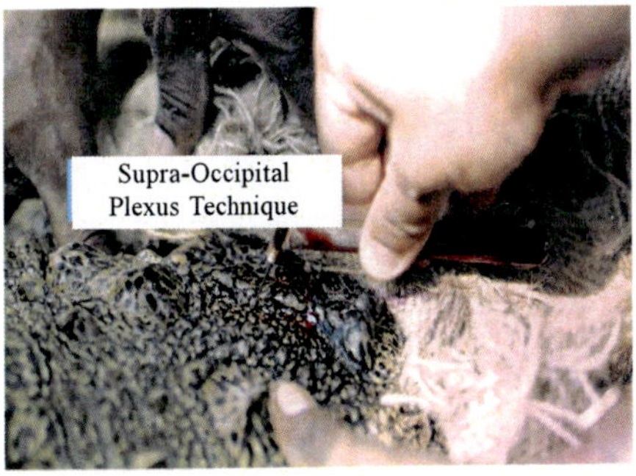

Fig. 14. Blood collection in crocodile using supra-occipital sinus technique

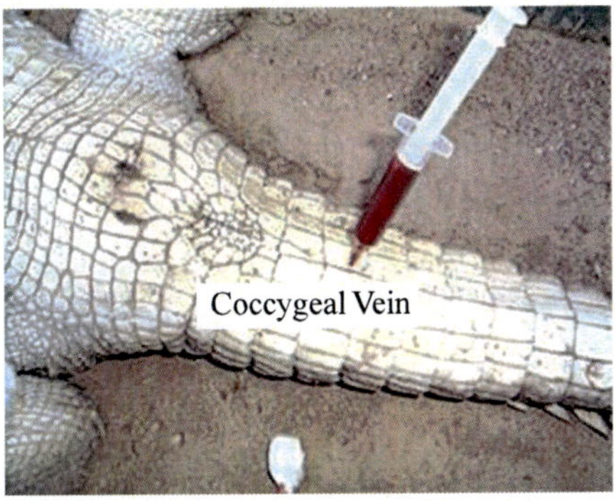

Fig. 15. Site of ventral-coccygeal vein in crocodile

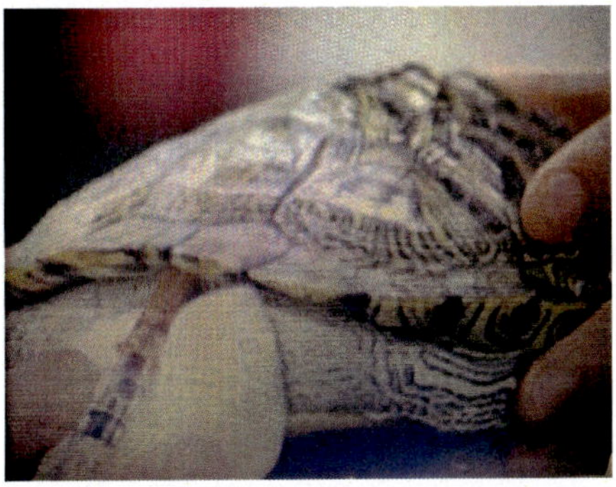

Fig. 16. Sub-vertebral sinus based blood-collection from chelonian

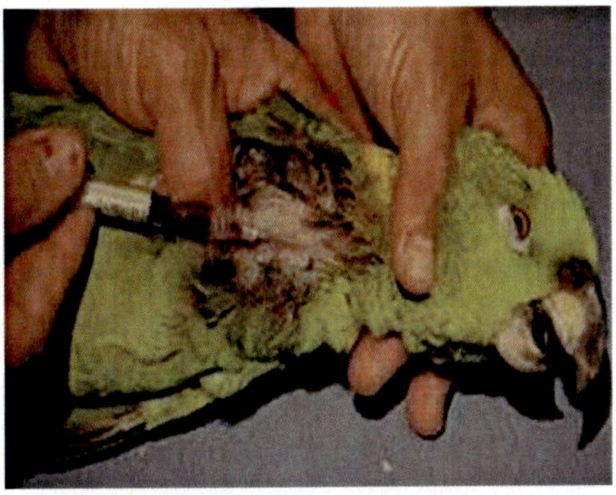

Fig. 17. Jugular vein based blood-collection

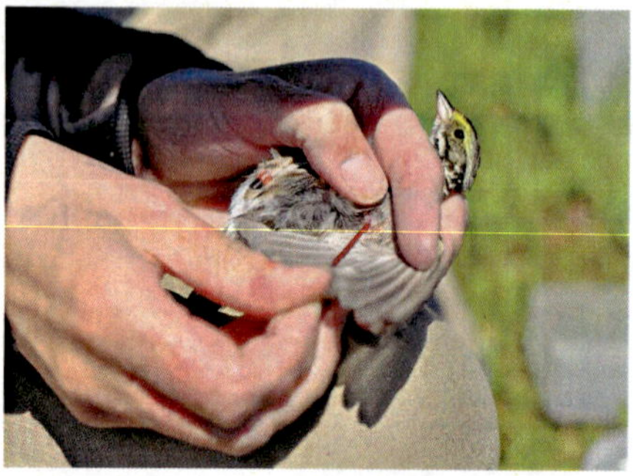

Fig. 18. Wing vein & capillary tube based blood-collectioin

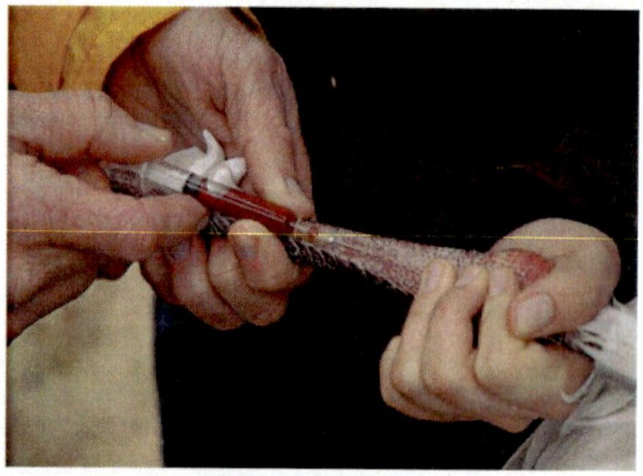

Fig. 19. Blood collection from blood vessel in leg

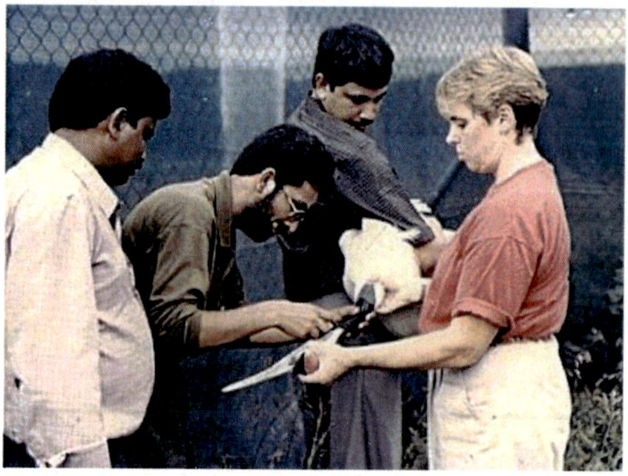

Fig. 20. Blood collection using jugular vein in long-necked bird

Chapter 36: Collections of Samples During Necropsy

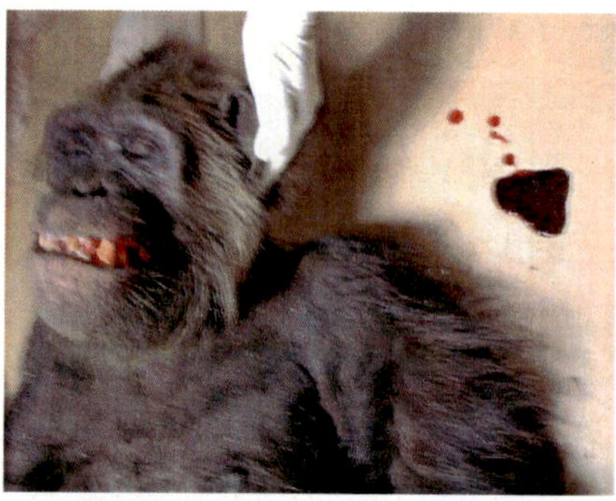

Fig. 1. (Carcase of Chimpanzee)

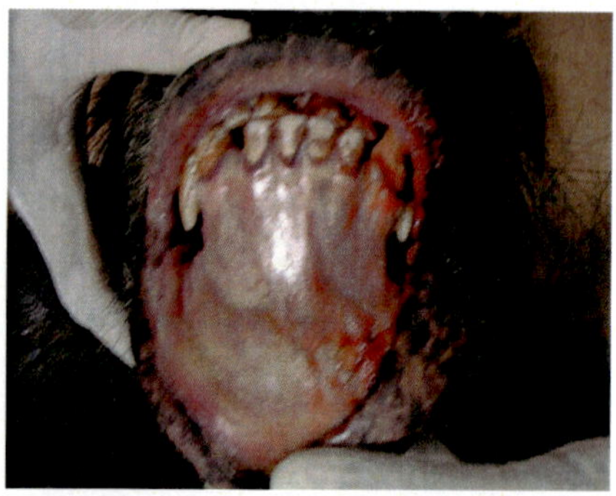

Fig. 2. (Ulceration in buccal cavity)

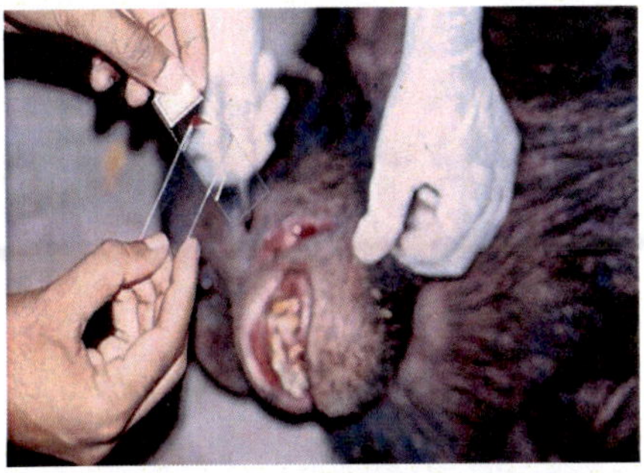

Fig. 3. (Blood smear-collection to rule out anthrax)

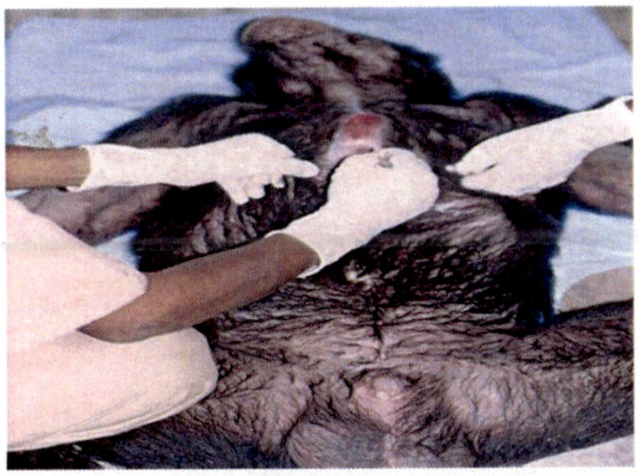

Fig. 4. (Longitudinal incision at thorax)

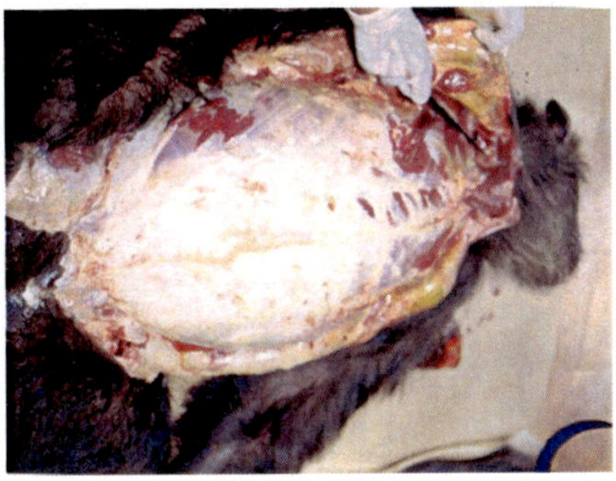

Fig. 5. (Separation of skin in ventral region)

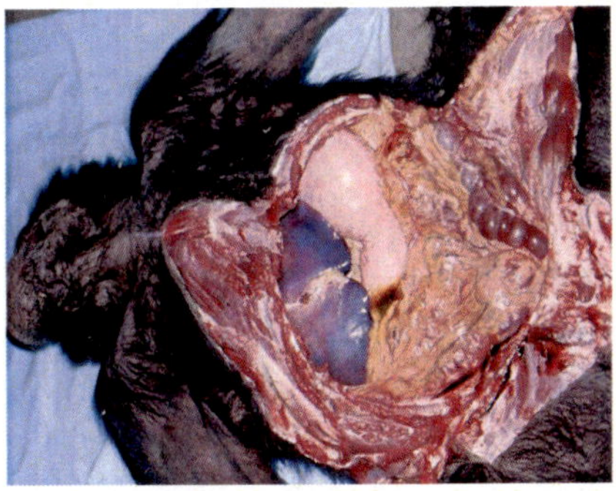

Fig. 6. (Exposure of viscera in ventral abdomen)

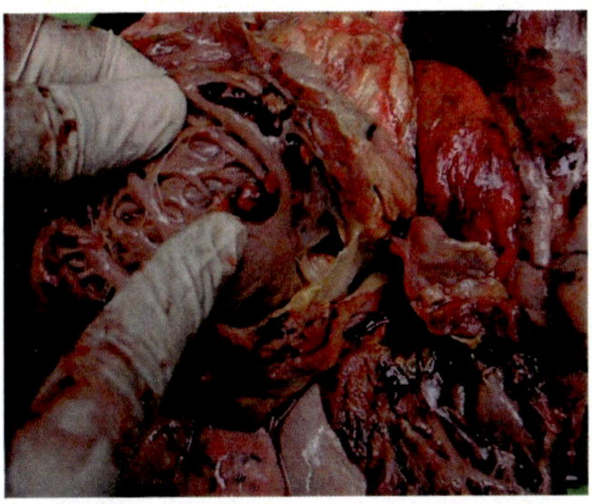

Fig. 7. (Examination of cardiac chambers)

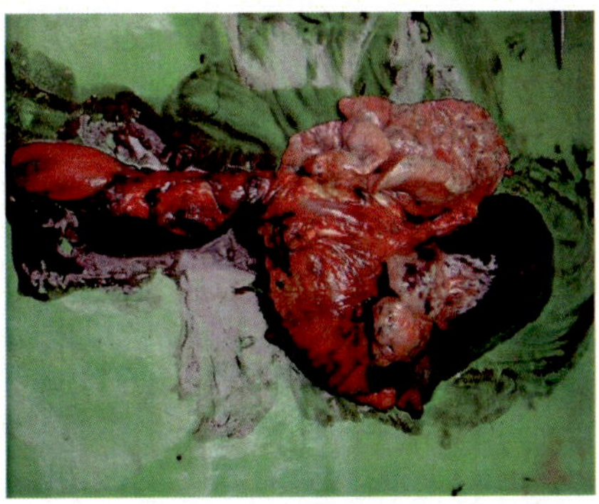

Fig. 8. (Haemorrhagic Lung: unilateral)

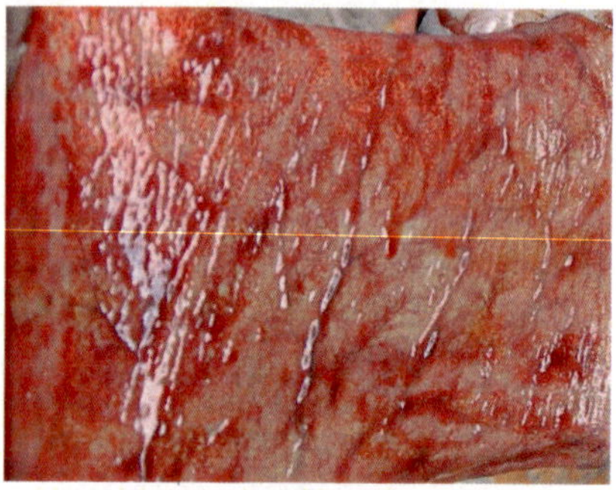

Fig. 9. (Pyloric region revealing haemorrhagic lesions)

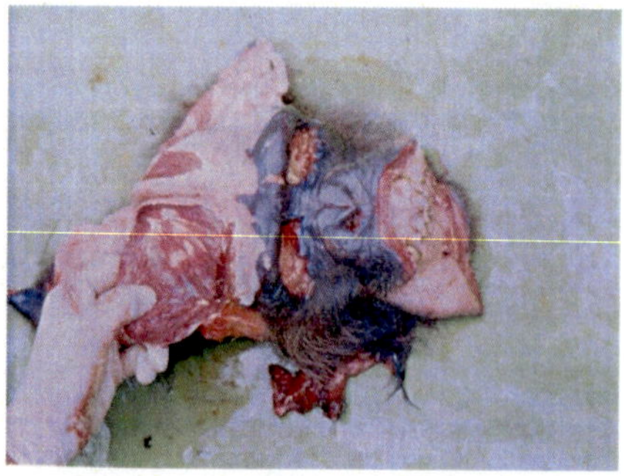

Fig. 10. Exposure of brain-region

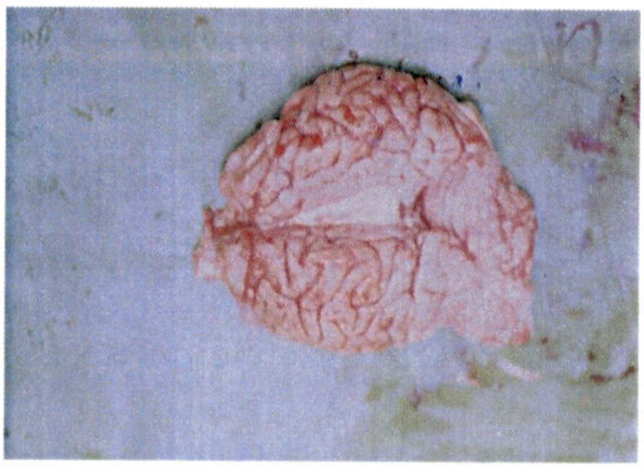

Fig. 11. Examination of brain

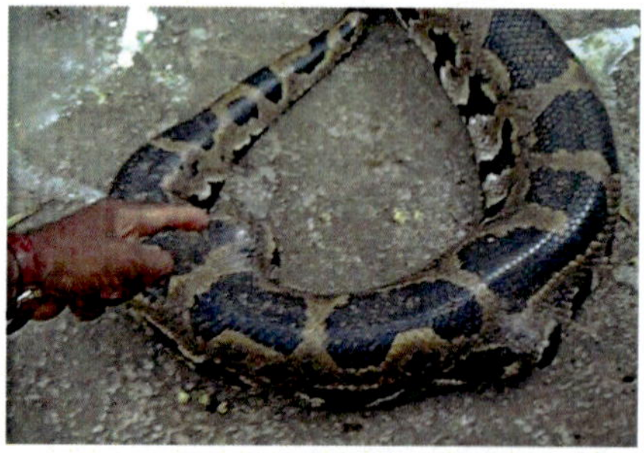

Fig. 12. Examination of skin-lumps in python

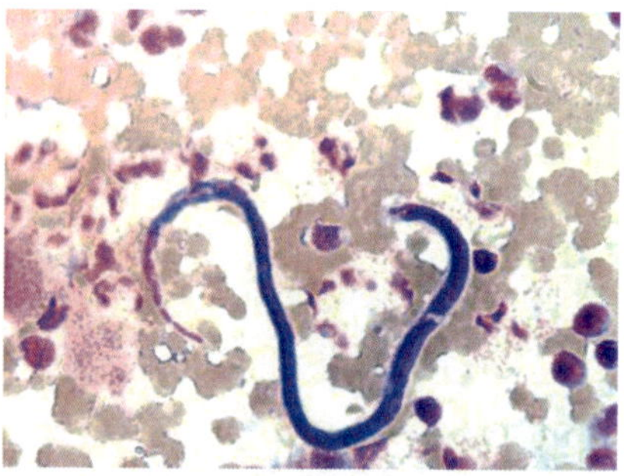

Fig. 13. (Microfilaria in blood smear of elephant calf)

References

1. Arora, B.M. (2003). Indian Wildlife Diseases and Disorders.Association of Indian Zoo and Wildlife veterinarians, India.
2. Chauhen, R.S. (2003). Veterinary Laboratory Diagnosis. International Book
3. Constable, P.D., K.W.Hinchcliff, S.H. Done and W.Grunberg. Veterinary Medicine. (2017). 11th ed. Vol.One. Elsevier, Missouri.
4. Constable, P.D., K.W. Hinchcliff, S.H. Done and W. Grunberg. Veterinary Medicine. (2017). 11th ed. Vol.Two. Elsevier, Missouri.
5. Cork, S.C. and Halliwell, H.W. (2002). The Veterinary Laboratory and Field Manual. University Press, Nottingham Distributing Co., Lucknow.
6. Doxey, D.L. (1983). Clinical pathology and Diagnostic Procedures. Bailliere Tindall, London.
7. Fowler, M.E. (1986). Zoo and Wild Animal medicine, 2nd edn. W.B. Saunders Company, HongKong.
8. Hosetti, B.B. (2008). Wildlife Management.3rd edn. Daya Publishing Company, New Delhi.
9. Internet resources and discussions with forest department veterinarians and wildlife experts and informations from Dpt.of Wildlife Science, TANUVAS, Arignar Anna Zoological Park, Tamil Nadu and other state forest departments, Wildlife Institute of India and Central Zoo Authority of India.
10. Miller, R.E., N. Lamberski and P.Calle (2019). Fowler's Zoo and Wild Animal Medicine.Current Therapy.Vol.9, ELSEVIER, Missouri.
11. O.I.E. Manual of Standards for Diagnostic tests and Vaccines for lists A and B diseases of Mammals, Birds and Bees (1992). 2nd edn. Office International Des Epizooties, France.
12. Radostits, O.M., Gay, C.C., Hinchcliff, K.W. and Constable, P.D. Veterinary Medicine: A Textbook of the Diseases of Cattle, Horses, Sheep, Pigs and Goats. 10th edn. Elsevier Saunders, U.K.
13. Sabapara, R.H., R.G. Jani and C.N. Bhuva (2008). Haematological reference intervals for Indian Leopards (*Panthera pardus*). Veterianary World. 1(6): 173-174.
14. Sahoo, A. and B.M.Arora (2002). Haematological and blood biochemical Profile of spotted deer (*Axis axis*) reared in semi-captive environment. Indian J.Anim. Sci.72(9): 762-765.

15. Shrivastav, A.B. and K.P.Singh. Tigers Blood: Haematological and Biochemical studies (2012). CHAPTER METRICS OVERVIEW.DOI: 10.5772/50360

16. Soulsby, E.J.L. (1982). Helminths, arthropods and protozoa of domesticated animals. The ELBS and Bailliere Tindall, UK

17. Sukumar, R. (1989). Ecology of the Asian elephant in South India. 1. Movement and habitat utilization patterns. *Journal of Tropical Ecology*, 5: 1-18.

18. Wallach, J.D., and W.J. Boever (1983). Diseases of Exotic Animals-Medical and Surgical Management. W.B. sounders company, Tokyo.

19. Internet resources, Discussions with all staff of the forest department-staff esp. the veterinarians, AAZP, MoEF & CC, GOI and Dean and Department of Wildlife Science, Madras Veterinary College, Chennai and Tamil Nadu Veterinary and Animal Sciences University and Central Zoo Authority of India.

Index

B

C

D

E

I

O

T

U

V

W